Studies in the Psychosocial

Studies in the Psychosocial seeks to investigate the ways in which psychic and social processes demand to be understood as always implicated in each other, as mutually constitutive, co-produced, or abstracted levels of a single dialectical process. As such it can be understood as an interdisciplinary field in search of transdisciplinary objects of knowledge. Studies in the Psychosocial is also distinguished by its emphasis on affect, the irrational and unconscious processes, often, but not necessarily, understood psychoanalytically. Studies in the Psychosocial aims to foster the development of this field by publishing high quality and innovative monographs and edited collections. The series welcomes submissions from a range of theoretical perspectives and disciplinary orientations, including sociology, social and critical psychology, political science, postcolonial studies, feminist studies, queer studies, management and organization studies, cultural and media studies and psychoanalysis. However, in keeping with the inter- or transdisciplinary character of psychosocial analysis, books in the series will generally pass beyond their points of origin to generate concepts, understandings and forms of investigation that are distinctively psychosocial in character.

Series Peer Review Policy:

Proposals for books in this series are single-blind peer reviewed by experts in the field as well as by the Series Editors. All manuscripts will be reviewed and approved by the Series Editors before they are accepted for publication.

More information about this series at
http://www.palgrave.com/gp/series/14464

Belinda Mandelbaum · Stephen Frosh ·
Rafael Alves Lima
Editors

Brazilian Psychosocial Histories of Psychoanalysis

palgrave
macmillan

Editors
Belinda Mandelbaum
Department of Social and Work Psychology
University of São Paulo
São Paulo, Brazil

Rafael Alves Lima
Laboratory of Social Theory
Philosophy and Psychoanalysis
University of São Paulo
São Paulo
Brazil

Stephen Frosh
Department of Psychosocial Studies
Birkbeck, University of London
London, UK

ISSN 2662-2629 ISSN 2662-2637 (electronic)
Studies in the Psychosocial
ISBN 978-3-030-78508-6 ISBN 978-3-030-78509-3 (eBook)
https://doi.org/10.1007/978-3-030-78509-3

Cover illustration: A Psicanálise/Severino Borges (1998). Woodcut print (xilogravura). Used with permission.

This Palgrave Macmillan imprint is published by the registered company Springer Nature Switzerland AG
The registered company address is: Gewerbestrasse 11, 6330 Cham, Switzerland

Acknowledgements

This book arose out of a symposium on the history of psychoanalysis in Latin America held at the University of São Paulo in September 2019. The symposium itself was part of a research project run by Belinda Mandelbaum and Stephen Frosh with financial support from The São Paulo Research Foundation (Fundação de Amparo à Pesquisa do Estado de São Paulo, FAPESP).

The editors would like to thank Cathy Gardner for her work on the text and the following translators of Portuguese versions of the chapters into English:

Gabriel Castro de Siqueira Jr.
Renata Luder
Evan Morson-Glabik
Mariana Nacif Pinto Coelho Mendes
Francine Natasha Alves de Oliveira
Naomi J. Sutcliffe de Moraes
Renata Takatu

Chapter 12 of this book was originally published in Portuguese in *Revista USP* (126), 85-98, 2020 as *O 'bandeirante destemido' Durval Marcondes, a Psicanálise e a modernização conservadora no Brasil*. The authors are grateful to the editors for permission to publish it in English.

Contents

Notes on Contributors

Lucas Charafeddine Bulamah is a psychoanalyst with a Ph.D. in Clinical Psychology from the University of São Paulo. He is a member of the Brazilian Sándor Ferenczi Research Group (GBPSP) and the Laboratory of Research and Interventions in Psychoanalysis (psiA). His publications include *História de Uma Regra Não Escrita* (Zagodoni, 2020) and the forthcoming *O self anônimo* (Zagodoni, 2021).

Francisco Capoulade is a psychoanalyst with a Ph.D. in Psychology from the Federal University of São Carlos and in Psychopathologie et Psychanalyse from l'Université Sorbonne Paris Cité (Paris-Diderot). He made the documentary *Histories of psychoanalysis: readers of Freud* (2016). He is currently director of the Institute for Research and Studies in Psychoanalysis in Public Spaces (IPEP). He was president of the Campinense Psychoanalysis Association from 2018 to 2020.

Thiago Bloss de Araújo is a social psychologist, college professor and Ph.D. student at the Federal University of São Paulo. He is the author of *The Birth of Social Psychology in Brazil: a Critique of Raul Briquet* (2021).

Raquel Saad de Avila Morales has a Bachelor of Psychology from the Pontifical University of São Paulo (PUC-SP/2020) and in Performing Arts from the University of São Paulo (USP/2012). She is currently a doctoral student in the Social Psychology Program at the University of São Paulo and participates in the following study groups: "History of Psychoanalysis in Latin America" (Psychology Institute/USP), "History, Memory and Public Health" (Public Health Faculty/USP) and "Salus—Study Group on the History of Medical and Health Practices" (Medicine Faculty/USP).

Rafael Dias de Castro holds a doctoral degree in History of Sciences and Health from Casa de Oswaldo Cruz (COC/Fiocruz- Rio de Janeiro). Currently, he is Assistant Professor in the Department of History and Graduate Program at the State University of Montes Claros (Unimontes—Minas Gerais).

Carmen Lucia M. Valladares de Oliveira is a sociologist and psychoanalyst, Professor of Psychoanalysis at the COGEAE-PUC/SP in São Paulo. She is the author of several scientific articles and the book *Histoire de la Psychanalyse au Brésil: São Paulo (1920-1969)*, published in 2005 by L'Harmattan of Paris, and translated into Portuguese and published by Escuta in 2006.

Fernando A. Figueira do Nascimento is a social psychologist and public health worker and a doctoral student in social psychology at the University of São Paulo. He is a member of the Brazilian Association of Social Psychology—ABRAPSO—Regional São Paulo.

Christian Ingo Lenz Dunker is a psychoanalyst, Full Professor of Psychoanalysis and Psychopathology at the Institute of Psychology of the University of São Paulo. He is an Analyst Member of the School of Forums of the Lacanian Field, twice awarded the Jabuti Prize, and he coordinates the Laboratory of Social Theory, Philosophy and Psychoanalysis of USP. He is the author of more than 100 scientific articles and 10 books, including "*Paixão da Ignorância*" (Contracorrente, 2020), "*O Palhaço e o Psicanalista*" (Planeta, 2018), *Transformações da Intimidade* (Ubu, 2017), "*Mal-Estar, Sofrimento e Sintoma*" (Boitempo, 2015) and "*The Constitution of the Psychoanalytic Clinic*" (Routledge, 2012).

Cristiana Facchinetti, is a Brazilian psychoanalyst, Professor at the Graduate Program in the History of Sciences and Health at Casa de Oswaldo Cruz (Fiocruz—Brazil). She is a researcher on the cultural history of psychoanalysis and psychiatry (DEPES/COC/Fiocruz), and her research follows two intersecting lines: reconstructing the circulation and appropriation of psychoanalysis in Brazil from the beginning of the twentieth century onwards, and reconstructing the Brazilian modernisation process and its transcultural scientific relations, especially those related to *psy* knowledge.

Stephen Frosh is a Professor in the Department of Psychosocial Studies at Birkbeck, University of London. He is an Academic Associate of the British Psychoanalytical Society and a former Vice Dean of the Tavistock Clinic, London. His many books on psychoanalysis and psychosocial studies include *The Politics of Psychoanalysis*, *Psychoanalysis Outside the Clinic*, *Hate and the Jewish Science*, *Hauntings* and *Those Who Come After*.

Daniel Kupermann is a psychoanalyst and a Professor at the Institute of Psychology, University of São Paulo. He is currently the president of the Sándor Ferenczi Brazilian Research Group and a member of the board of the International Sándor Ferenczi Network. He has authored articles published in French, English, Spanish, Italian and Portuguese, and books published in Brazil and in France.

Rafael Alves Lima is a psychoanalyst with a Ph.D. from the Department of Clinical Psychology at the University of São Paulo. He is a member of the Laboratory of Social Theory, Philosophy and Psychoanalysis (LATESFIP-USP), the Clinical Network of Jacques Lacan Laboratory (IP-USP) and the collective Margens Clínicas, which offers psychoanalytic assistance to victims of State violence. He is a visiting researcher at the Centro de Investigación Clínica en Psicología, Facultad de Psicología, Universidad de la República (Udelar), Uruguay. He is co-founder of the Institute for Research and Studies in Psychoanalysis in Public Spaces and author of articles and book chapters in the area of the history of psychoanalysis, with a focus on Brazil.

Belinda Mandelbaum is a psychoanalyst and Associate Professor at the Department of Social Psychology of the University of São Paulo, where she coordinates the Laboratory of Family, Gender Relations and Sexuality Studies. Her teaching and research deal with the interface between psychoanalysis and psychosocial studies, methods of qualitative research, families in vulnerable psychosocial conditions, families in Brazilian literature and the history of psychoanalysis in Brazil. Her publications include *Psicanálise da família* (Artesã, 3rd. ed., 2019), *Trabalhos com famílias em Psicologia Social* (Casa do Psicólogo, 2014), *Desemprego: uma abordagem psicossocial* (Blucher, 2017) and *Família, contemporaneidade e conservadorismo* (ed., Benjamin Editorial, 2017).

J. Guillermo Milán-Ramos is Associate Professor at the Institute of Clinical Psychology of the Faculty of Psychology, University of the Republic, Uruguay. He is coordinator of the research group *Formación de la Clínica Psicoanalítica en el Uruguay* (FCPU), which is currently developing research on the emergence of the psychotherapeutic field in Uruguay and the region, in collaboration with the Laboratory of Social Theory, Philosophy and Psychoanalysis (LATESFIP) from the University of São Paulo. He is author of the books *Hombres de palabra*(Lapzus, Montevideo, 2005), *Passar pelo escrito: uma introdução ao trabalho teórico de Jacques Lacan*(Mercado de Letras, Campinas, SP, Brazil, 2007) and *Análise Psicanalítica de Discursos: Perspectivas Lacaniana* (Estação das Letras e Cores, São Paulo, Brazil; together with Ch. Dunker and C. Paulon). He has published numerous articles in scientific journals and book chapters on language and psychoanalysis.

Fuad Kyrillos Neto has a Ph.D. in Psychology (Social Psychology) from the Pontifical Catholic University of São Paulo (PUC-SP). His post-doctorate studies were at the Department of Clinical Psychology at the Institute of Psychology of the University of São Paulo (USP) and the Faculty of Philosophy and Theology (FAJE). He is former coordinator of the Graduate Program in Psychology at the Federal University of São João del-Rei (2018-2020). He is Associate Professor, Department of Psychology, Federal University of São João Del Rei (UFSJ). He is the editor of books and author of several articles on psychoanalysis, psychiatric reform, and the institutions and history of psychoanalysis.

Mariano Ben Plotkin is currently principal researcher at the CONICET (National Council of Scientific and Technological Research) in Argentina and Professor of History at the Universidad Nacional Tres de Febrero. He obtained his Ph.D. in history at the University of California, Berkeley. He has taught at Harvard University, Colby College, Boston University, and has been visiting professor at Université Paris VII; Jonian University (Corfú, Greece); Universidad del Rosario (Bogotá), and held the Sarmiento Chair at the Universidad de Salamanca. He has published extensively on the history of psychoanalysis in Latin America, and in 2010 was awarded a Guggenheim Fellowship.

Aline Librelotto Rubin is a clinical psychologist who holds a Master's Degree in Psychoanalytic Studies from Birkbeck, University of London, and a Ph.D. in Social Psychology from the Universidade de São Paulo (USP). Her research concerns the history of psychoanalysis in Brazil, particularly in the context of the civil-military dictatorship (1964–1985).

Rodrigo Afonso Nogueira Santos is a psychologist and psychoanalyst with an MA in Psychology from the Federal University of São João del-Rei (UFSJ). He is a doctoral student in Psychology at the University of São Paulo (USP) and a substitute professor at UFSJ.

Part I

Introduction and Prelude

1

Introduction

Belinda Mandelbaum, Stephen Frosh, and Rafael Alves Lima

Psychoanalysis, History, Brazil

Despite the growth of a postcolonial perspective on psychoanalysis (e.g. Khanna, 2004), there has been only a slow emergence of understanding about psychoanalysis that properly locates its international dimension. Derrida (1991), in his account of 'geopsychoanalysis,' famously

B. Mandelbaum
Department of Social and Work Psychology, University of São Paulo, São Paulo, Brazil
e-mail: belmande@usp.br

S. Frosh (✉)
Department of Psychosocial Studies, Birkbeck, University of London, London, UK
e-mail: s.frosh@bbk.ac.uk

R. A. Lima
Laboratory of Social Theory, Philosophy and Psychoanalysis, University of São Paulo, São Paulo, Brazil

B. Mandelbaum et al. (eds.), *Brazilian Psychosocial Histories of Psychoanalysis*, Studies in the Psychosocial,
https://doi.org/10.1007/978-3-030-78509-3_1

commented scathingly on the International Psychoanalytic Association's (IPA) division between its societies in Europe, America and the 'Rest of the World.' The 'rest of the world' thesis may give the impression that there is limited work in English on the history and identity of the psychoanalytic movement beyond Europe and America, overlooking the reality of what is actually available, and this is especially striking in the case of Latin America, which has a reasonable claim to be currently one of the most vibrant psychoanalytic cultures in the world.

It is certainly true that, until recently, the growth and importance of Latin American psychoanalysis was neglected by English-language historians of the discipline. For example, Zaretsky (2004) offers only a few passing comments, despite his book being subtitled 'a social and cultural history of psychoanalysis.' According to Plotkin (2012), studies of the transmission, diffusion and production of psychoanalysis in the so-called peripheral areas within which Latin America fits date back to no earlier than the 1980s. In regard to this 'peripheral' group, Plotkin stresses the fact that Argentina at his time of writing had six IPA-affiliate societies; in Brazil there were eleven, whereas in France the number dropped to two. This would not only point to the questionability of terms like 'periphery,' but also to the wealth of information one might be missing both about the history of the psychoanalytic movement as a whole and the specificity of a psychoanalytical culture that has been developed in turbulent dialogue with its social and historical contexts.

In fact, books like those of Ruben Gallo (2010) or Nancy Caro Hollander (1997, 2010) attest to the complexity of the social and political factors that determine the place of psychoanalysis in the culture of some Latin American countries, as well as the local political reasons that sometimes made of Freudianism a suspicious practice, or even a subversive intellectual resource. In line with the 'official history' linked to the IPA, Pieczanski and Pieczanski (2014) provide a compilation of the Latin American 'pioneers' of psychoanalysis, and there are also excellent outlines in the 'historical dictionary' organised by Alain de Mijolla (2005). Bruno Bosteels (2012) offers us a kind of intellectual history of the presence of the thoughts of Marx and Freud in Latin American art and literature, whilst Daniel Gaztambide (2019) has written a 'people's history' of the encounter between psychoanalysis, the psychology of liberation and Paulo Freire's intellectual militancy in the field of education within a political agenda of social justice. Recognising the importance of creating conditions for the publication of Latin American material that would enable the psychoanalysts of the region to participate in a broader psychoanalytic debate, since 1996 the IPA has invited distinguished Latin American psychoanalysts to edit collections of essays on different aspects of Latin American work (e.g. Lewkowicz & Flechner, 2005). Some historical accounts are now available; for example, a special issue of the journal *Psychoanalysis and History* (2012) included an important paper written by Russo (2012a) about Brazil that recounts in detail the early history of psychoanalysis there, attending to the social and political context of the time. A separate paper by Russo (2012b) dealing with the history of Brazilian psychoanalysis during the dictatorship of the 1960s to 1980s was included in Damousi and Plotkin's (2012) edited collection subtitled, *Histories of Psychoanalysis under conditions of restricted political freedom*. Other psychoanalysts have traced some of the institutional histories and begun to formulate what is specific about the way psychoanalytic ideas and practices have developed in the region (e.g. in English: Azevedo et al., 2005; Plotkin, 2001). Therefore, it is not necessarily that the scholarship does not exist; rather, that the dispersal of historiographical perspectives of research dedicated to 'the rest of the world' may be responsible for the impression that the work is limited. This poses three challenges: systematisation of the work already produced; evaluation of this material; and, obviously, the incentive to promote more research on this subject.

In the Brazilian case, the national literature on the history of psychoanalysis in the country is quite rich (e.g. Coimbra, 1995; Dunker, 2015; Facchinetti, 2001; Facchinetti & Ponte, 2003; Oliveira, 2003). Yet there is still only a limited amount of Brazilian psychoanalysis available in English translations. In particular, there is a paucity of psychosocial reflection that might show how politics, culture and society contributed to the history of ideas in Brazilian psychoanalysis, and also the converse, how psychoanalysis impacted on Brazilian culture and society—a fascinating field of studies that has been better explored in the case of Argentina and Chile (Plotkin, 2001; Veto, 2013). Nevertheless, Brazil is an important case study for the history of psychoanalysis: not only is this history long and rich in its professional and cultural dimensions, but there was an especially important period of conflict for psychoanalysis during the civil-military dictatorship (1964–1985), which can be seen as dramatising some of the issues concerning the erasure of memory in psychoanalysis, especially in connection with political difficulties.

The first evidence of the arrival of psychoanalysis in Brazil is as old as psychoanalysis itself. There are controversies about the inaugural Brazilian psychoanalytic act—as ever, it is difficult to establish the initial origin of an area of knowledge, which, like all historical events, always take place in a field of forces in dispute. 'The legend says' that the psychiatrist Juliano Moreira, considered the founder of modern psychiatry in Brazil, quoted Freud in his classes at the Bahia Medical School in 1899, but the best *documented* evidence places this origin in 1914, when Juliano Moreira presented the new psychoanalytic theses to the Brazilian Society of Psychiatry, Neurology and Legal Medicine, in Rio de Janeiro. In the same year, the first PhD thesis on psychoanalysis was defended at the university, by Genserico Aragão de Souza Pinto. After that, psychoanalysis began to circulate in Brazil in a more systematic way. Whatever the correct date, the historical data shows that in the early days of Freudian work in Europe psychoanalytic ideas were introduced in 'distant' Brazil, within the psychiatry that was practiced there. Psychoanalysis offered a new, profound and systematic understanding of the causes of 'mental illnesses' based on Freudian theory as it developed between the end of the nineteenth century and the beginning of the twentieth century, which promised to renew local psychiatric science and its treatments. In dialogue with knowledge from other human and social sciences, psychoanalysis also participated in the construction of a new psychological, social and cultural understanding of the human being. Crucially, this new theory of the psyche arrived in Brazil at the turn of the twentieth century as part of a context of modernisation, industrialisation and urbanisation that impacted on the local economy, society and culture. In Brazil, both aristocratic and new bourgeois elites sought to build a modern country, and psychoanalysis came to contribute not only with new conceptions of mental suffering, but, more broadly, all these processes of national transformation demanded a new identity for Brazilians, for whom the new science of the mind promised to have something to say.

In the years following, psychoanalysis, both as a theory about the origin and functioning of the mind and as a transformative practice, had a profound impact on local society. For the elites, it was offered as a new therapy for the treatment of so-called neuroses, as an alternative to organic and asylum psychiatric practices. In relation to the poorest populations, it offered concepts that promised to civilise and educate them, in an evolutionary process that would free the country from ways of functioning considered 'primitive,' originating from Brazil's mix of races, towards participation in the set of developed nations. Brazilians learned throughout the twentieth century that they belonged to a developing country, a term that changed, in the first decades of the twenty-first century, to that of 'emerging power.' Whether 'in development' or 'emerging,' Brazilians continue to wait for the fulfilment of this promise, whilst having to deal, effectively, with successive ruins of national projects. Brazil was forced to abolish slavery in 1888, with the English fleet and its cannon preventing the slave trade from Africa, and without any measure of social support or compensation from the State to ex-slaves; it was proclaimed as a republic in 1889, inaugurating a series of military governments; it went through two periods of dictatorial regime, the first between the 1930s and 1950s, the second between the 1960s and 1980s; in the second half of the 1980s, it entered into a process of openness and democratisation through a pact of general and unrestricted amnesty under which those who fought for democracy and their opponents were left equally unpunished; and it is currently returning, since general elections in 2018, to an authoritarian, fascist-inspired government.

Psychosocial Histories

Within these broad background historical processes, the chapters on the history of psychoanalysis in Brazil gathered together in this book start from a common question: how did the psychoanalysis that arrived in the country integrate, develop and flourish in a society whose history, although shaken by modernising transformations, manifests a permanently unequal, authoritarian and violent character? How did psychoanalysis, which, according to Roudinesco (1995), depends on democracy to be practiced and unfolded, survive in Brazil alongside authoritarianism, censorship and repression? Whence the question, in our view needing to be answered by Brazilian psychoanalysts, about which of the many possible 'types' of psychoanalysis took hold in Brazilian lands, and how this came about. How have psychoanalytic theories and practices been adapted to coexist, often uncritically and silently,[1] in relation to the reality in which they have taken root and grown up? Through a variety of lenses, focusing on different aspects of its history in Brazil, we see how psychoanalysis presented itself as progressive and transformative, maintaining this self-image whilst at the same time developing institutional structures that reproduce the authoritarian hierarchies crystallised in the wider society. For instance, throughout the twentieth century, psychoanalysis offered itself as a high-cost therapy for local elites, inviting them to seek the causes of their malaise within their psychic interiors. As a conception about the human being that has deeply penetrated culture, we can see psychoanalysis transmuted into complex forms that pass through arts, media, ideology and common sense, contributing to processes of rupture and transformation, at times registering resistance by some psychoanalysts to social oppression, but also acting in the service of preservation of the social status quo.

The chapters of this book seek to shed light on these relations of conservative accommodation, but also of transformation, between psychoanalysis and Brazilian society, with their historical specificities. The work presented here is located in a field of knowledge that has aroused, since the 1980s, a lively interest amongst academic research

[1] There is a form of coexistence that remains intriguing for Brazilian historians of psychoanalysis, which is that between psychoanalysts who remained silent and those who expressed themselves critically even in the most acute moments of political repression in the country, inside and outside the IPA. Although silence was the major position of official psychoanalysis, coexistence did not always indicate connivance, resignation, complicity or intellectual and political harmony between the agents. It is yet to be fully described and explained in the history of psychoanalysis in Brazil how this imagery of tacit cordiality would create a certain lack of differentiation that overshadowed the psychoanalysts' resistance to these repressive regimes.

groups in several countries in which psychoanalysis has taken root and grown. This has especially been concerned with the relationship between psychoanalysis and repressive political systems in different countries (e.g. Damousi & Plotkin, 2012; Frosh, 2005). Our common interest is focused not only on the impact of psychoanalysis on conservative societies, but on *which* psychoanalysis is produced in these contexts. Research on this carried out by the editors and their associates (e.g. Mandelbaum et al., 2019; Rubin et al., 2016) is one of the sources of this volume; it instantiates a collaboration between Brazilian and UK researchers that combines the type of psychosocial studies characteristic of UK work with the psychoanalytic and historical orientation of Brazilian critical social psychology. The volume itself arises from a symposium on the history of psychoanalysis in Latin America held at the University of São Paulo in September 2019. This symposium focused mainly on Brazil and offered papers on the methodology of historical research on psychoanalysis; the specific history of Brazilian psychoanalysis; and the contribution of Brazilian researchers to wider histories of psychoanalysis. These papers defined a specific orientation of Brazilian work that is neglected in the wider anglophone literature—a Southern Cone perspective that is psychoanalytically saturated, yet politically radical and that is marked especially by the legacies of colonialism and by the history of dictatorship and of resistance. This particular stance gives the work represented in this volume a strong psychosocial grounding, as it draws both on 'internal' histories and psychoanalytic perceptions, and an alert understanding of the situated sociality of the Brazilian psychoanalytic and academic movement.

Although this book has a mainly historical focus, almost all authors are psychoanalysts and psychosocial researchers. The book gathers a set of psychoanalytic psychosocial histories, that is, histories in which the psychic and social dimensions that constitute the psychoanalytic field itself, its institutions and authors—dynamised in the relations they establish with the broader social environment—are central to our attention. The journey into the complex and contradictory social history of Brazil was a challenge that each author faced seriously, drawing on the work of the best Brazilian historians of the contemporary period, but the fact that many of the authors are themselves psychoanalysts brings advantages to the investigation of psychosocial histories of psychoanalysis. This is because, first of all, the research presented here is, to a large extent, due to the motivations (or inconveniences) arising from their experiences as psychoanalysts in Brazil, within the ideologies and practices of their training and member institutions. This context means being psychoanalysts of their own history, or rather, of histories that involve each one in interactions with others and with their objects of study and intervention, in their personal, professional and institutional trajectories. It means making the psychoanalysis they know and practice *reflexive*, necessarily attentive to the narratives that have been built throughout the history of psychoanalysis in Brazil, around a multiplicity of themes: what are the theories prevalent in each context? What are the objects of study? Who are the patients? With what conceptions and techniques do they approach them? With what objectives? How do they dialogue with the wider social and cultural context? Psychoanalysis, as can be seen throughout the chapters, is present in the method of researching history and in the way of understanding it. In analysing their material, the authors make use of psychoanalytic conceptions of trauma and its relations with personal and collective history, impediments to knowing, thinking and speaking, repetitions, the mechanisms of repression and denial, secrets, pacts, the limits and possibilities of memory and its erasure, and reparation. If the work presented here takes place at the confluence of history and Brazilian psychoanalysis, now presented to English-speaking readers, we hope that it will contribute to a critical international and intercultural dialogue on the possible conditions for the creation, debate and development of the psychoanalytic field in different contexts—conditions that, for psychoanalysis, can only come from the possibility of contact, recognition and criticism of its own history.

Chapter Outlines

Brazilian Psychosocial Histories of Psychoanalysis is organised into three main sections, the first consisting of this Introduction and a 'prelude' from Mariano Plotkin, one of the foremost historians of Latin American psychoanalysis. In this prelude (Chapter 2), Plotkin sets a broader Latin American context for our focus on Brazil, suggesting that psychoanalysis gained a strong foothold there in part because of its relatively comprehensive theoretical apparatus that could be applied not only to explain and treat many 'mental disorders' as well as to analyse social issues, but also because it could be used as a 'battering ram' against positivism at a moment in which Comte's and Spencer's theories were in crisis. Plotkin also offers some reflections about a possible research agenda on the emergence of local 'psychoanalytic cultures' that take into consideration some Latin American cultural specificities.

Part II of the book explores methodological issues that arise in relation to developing a historiography of psychoanalysis in Brazil, paying particular attention to the way its social and political conditions are reflected in the problematics of research practice. In Chapter 3, Lucia Valladares de Oliveira asks a number of questions that reflect on some difficulties in the writing of this history. How can we write about characters or heirs that are still alive? How might we deal with memory and memory loss in an analytical community? How might we handle a deficient history with insufficient files? How can we preserve relevant files and other sources, including the places where the files are stored and research sources that are able to restore previous generations' experiences? This chapter argues that the university, as a site that promotes diversity, might be crucial for maintaining and recovering these sources and the history they contain.

In Chapter 4, *Wounds of Dictatorship in Brazilian Psychoanalysis: Traumatic Revivals in Research on the History of Psychoanalysis*, Belinda Mandelbaum draws on her experience as a psychoanalyst and researcher in the field of Brazilian psychoanalytic history to reflect on the impact of powerful research events and findings on the subjectivity of the researcher. She argues that the threads that weave the personal history of Brazilian researchers into the history of the country and psychoanalysis are important determinants of the direction of the research process, from the motivation to carry it out, to the choice of sources, the reading of the findings and their publication. Mandelbaum gives special attention to the way in which experiences lived in childhood and adolescence during the period of the civil-military dictatorship (1964–1985) are re-presented in the research field in various ways: difficulty in accessing information, reading documents and viewing photos in police records that refer to lived memories, censorship of papers by interviewed subjects and editorial committees. The Ferenczian notion of trauma in two temporalities helps her to reflect on the personal and social impact of the impediments to acknowledging, working through and sharing the recent history of the country, particularly, in the case of this research, of the ways in which Brazilian psychoanalysis went through and participated in the 'years of lead' of the dictatorship.

In Chapter 5, writing as a researcher based outside Brazil, Stephen Frosh takes up an argument made by the British historian of science John Forrester for the value of an approach to knowledge based on case histories, with the psychoanalytic case being its exemplary instance. Forrester's arresting account of the value of the individual case is applied in this chapter to the study of psychoanalysis itself. Do specific 'cases' of psychoanalytic institutional functions, such as those in Brazil, reveal general attributes of psychoanalysis? And to what extent can reports of such 'cases' be trusted when there are often problems about confidentiality and ethical concerns that block publication or wide discussion of their findings? One problem with psychoanalytic case reports is that they are often fictitious in their published form; Frosh asks whether this is also the situation with institutional cases and if so, what can be rescued from them when trying to trace a reliable history of psychoanalysis. The experience of researching the history of Brazilian psychoanalysis during the dictatorship provides the backdrop to these questions.

Chapter 6 is an account by Christian Dunker and J. Guillermo Milán-Ramos of transformations in the history of psychoanalysis in Brazil from the perspective of clinical cases. Writing from a Lacanian perspective about what they term the function of psychoanalytic 'casuistry' within the psychiatric, anthropological and literary discourse, they suggest that it becomes possible to better understand the path of assimilation and autonomy of psychoanalysis in Brazil. In particular, they distinguish four moments in this history, proposing first that the period of the pioneers (1914–1949) was marked by a hybrid discourse and allegorical connection between psychoanalysis, psychiatry and anthropology. The period of institutionalisation (1950–1984) was characterised by normative descriptivism, with recourse to illustration and a concern with legitimacy in conceptual use. The period of re-democratisation of the country (1984–2000) presented clinical cases with a greater content of authorial function and the search for more singular stylistics. In the contemporary period (after 2000), with the rise in importance of Lacanianism, there is a kind of inversion of the previous traits: a search for unique cases, sovereignty of concepts in their hybrid relationship with other concepts, criticism of the aspirations of normativity and consensus.

Finally, Rafael Alves Lima presents in Chapter 7 an account of how the archival policies of the psychoanalytic field are organised according to the category of secrecy. Drawing on a range of theoretical resources that reflect the resonance of secrecy in the psychoanalytic field, from Freud and Ferenczi to Lacan, Lima establishes a horizon of debates on private (psychoanalytical institutions) and public (state) archival policies in order to understand the direct repercussions that the maintenance or suspension of the secret archive have on the labour of the historian. The chapter concludes by discussing the implications of the fascination with the secret archive in the historiography of psychoanalysis, highlighting those that dedicate themselves to periods of democratic suspension (as in the case of research on the civil-military dictatorship in Brazil), with the objective of raising issues that the historian of psychoanalysis should not ignore.

Part III of the book consists of chapters devoted to specific historical issues surrounding the development of psychoanalysis in Brazil, several of them in relation to its early emergence but others to the 1960's to 1980's dictatorship and to more recent events. Some of these chapters examine particular individuals who were influential in the development of psychoanalysis in the country, and who are either insufficiently well known, or ripe for reconsideration. The section begins with Cristiana Facchinetti and Rafael Castro, who discuss in Chapter 8 a strand of colonial and racist thought underpinning elements of early Brazilian psychoanalysis. They describe some intellectual and academic traditions in Brazil that paved the way for the appropriation and circulation of psychoanalysis in local psychiatry. The locus of their analysis is the Hospital Nacional de Alienados (HNA), the first psychiatric institution in the country. The time frame begins in 1914, the year of the Faculty of Medicine of Rio de Janeiro's first thesis on psychoanalysis for inpatients under treatment, and covers the developments that occurred there until 1944, when the HNA closed. The chapter demonstrates the engagement of psychoanalytic theory with matters of race and degeneration, with treatments of 'pathologies' referring to sex and gender, as well as with therapeutic practices that started to take into account the notion of the unconscious as a concept that arose from articulations between psychoanalysis and the country's modernist vanguard.

Raquel Saad de Avila Morales continues this section with her chapter (Chapter 9) on Francisco Franco da Rocha, who was one of the main people responsible for the establishment of psychiatry in São Paulo and who also promoted psychoanalysis there. In 1927, da Rocha helped found the first psychoanalytic society in Latin America, of which he was also president. Morales argues that in the early days of the Republic both psychiatry and psychoanalysis, in order to be recognised as scientific areas and to become institutionalised in Brazil, contributed to the process of Brazilian conservative modernisation.

Chapter 10, by Thiago Bloss, describes some theoretical and political contributions of psychoanalysis to the process of introducing social psychology in Brazil, which can be understood as the result of an important historical movement present in the 1930s at the national and international level. Specifically, on national soil, social psychology was pioneered by the physician Raul Carlos Briquet, who in 1935 published the first Brazilian book in this discipline and was part of the intellectual elites who spearheaded a conservative modernisation project in the country. As the chapter reveals, psychoanalysis had a strong presence in this process of constitution of social psychology, which was characterised by profound contradictions and attempts at ideological conciliation guided by authoritarianism at both the theoretical and political level.

The next three chapters continue with the theme of how the foundations of psychoanalysis fed the conditions of conciliation with conservative social trends, despite the existence of countervailing progressive tendencies. In Chapter 11, Fernando Figueira examines the case of Arthur Ramos, who from the 1920s to 1940s was part of a group of Brazilian intellectuals dedicated to reflect on the direction, identity and modernisation of the country, especially on health issues and education. From his reading of Freud's *Totem and Taboo* and *The Interpretation of Dreams*, Ramos devoted himself to analysing the phylogenetic origin of primitive fantasies and to understanding the similarities between the mental dynamism of children, 'primitive' peoples and schizophrenics. In his consideration of the content of psychosis, he argued that it would be possible to perceive the relationship between an ancestral unconscious, depositary of the phylogenetic legacy, an ethnic soul and an interpsychic unconscious, which would rest on the complex influences of the social environment on the individual. Ramos also elaborated the notion of social maladjustment, a fundamental object for Mental Hygiene that would become an Applied Social Psychology and would expand psychiatric practices beyond the asylum walls to reach 'normal' individuals and, with a view to health promotion and prevention of mental illness, elect children as privileged subjects.

The next contribution (Chapter 12) has Belinda Mandelbaum and Stephen Frosh explore the academic and professional trajectory of the psychiatrist, psychoanalyst, poet and university professor Durval Marcondes, which runs through the period of the 1920s to the 1980s. Marcondes pioneered the implementation of psychoanalysis in São Paulo, both in his private practice and in the School Mental Health Service, of which he was director, and in the creation of the first specialisation course in Clinical Psychology at the University of São Paulo. The chapter shows, however, that his trajectory in all these fields was marked by conservatism regarding (1) psychoanalysis itself, when looking to institute in Brazil the hegemonic model recommended by the International Psychoanalytic Association and put its theories and uncritical techniques in the service of society; (2) the prevailing social customs, publishing psychoanalytic knowledge about childhood, womanhood and family serving the reproduction of the traditional status quo; (3) explicitly reactionary attitudes as Professor of Clinical Psychology at the University of São Paulo. In all these ways, his modes of import and incorporation of psychoanalysis in the middle decades of the twentieth century reproduce patterns that scholars of Brazilian culture named 'conservative modernisation,' a broad process of rapid cultural changes that left untouched social, economic and political traditions in the country.

Finally, in this sequence, Chapter 13, by Rodrigo Afonso Nogueira Santos, discusses the figure of Karl Weissmann, an Austrian who became very well known in Brazil as a psychoanalyst willing to comment on social, political and cultural phenomena. Using Weissmann's book *Masochism and Communism: Contribution to a political pathology* as a focus of discussion, Santos analyses the relations of Weissmann with psychoanalysis, attending particularly to his development of the argument that makes a pathologisation of communism possible. It becomes apparent that, by claiming himself as a bearer of a psychoanalytic truth, and by positioning himself as an 'infectologist' facing a plague, Weismann used psychoanalysis as a political tool in an ambitious way. What can be observed is a proposal for using psychoanalysis as a device for clinical and pedagogical work aimed at curing communists of their supposed illness, in the context of the Cold War.

In Chapter 14, Aline Rubin offers an analysis of psychoanalytic discourse about adolescence during the Brazilian dictatorship. She argues that in psychoanalytic publications of the time, which only rarely made reference to the dictatorship and its apparatus of violence, the phenomena of adolescence and its deviances occupied a privileged position. This was coupled with a concern with conflict between different generations, the theme of the *IV Brazilian Congress of Psychoanalysis* in 1973. In this way, this chapter analyses the psychoanalytic discourse about adolescence and, more specifically, about student rebellion and the counter-culture movements. In addition, it seeks to offer an overview of the different conceptions and approaches to these themes within the psychoanalytic movement more widely in Brazil. Lastly, it explores whether this kind of investigation can help change the relation with the past, re-signifying it and working through traumatic situations such as repressive political times.

Chapter 15, by Lucas Charafeddine Bulamah with Daniel Kupermann, investigates the silent practice of proscribing male homosexual candidates in the training offered by the International Psychoanalytical Association (IPA) in São Paulo. Supported by the Civil Rights initiatives, gay visibility movements arose in western countries in the 1970s and hit institutionalised psychoanalysis with the charge of prejudice during selection and training of candidates, inviting proscribed gay candidates and silent trained analysts to speak up. The development of the psychoanalytical theory of homosexuality, which after Freud's death progressively turned homosexuality into a disease, along with the model of institutionalisation of psychoanalysis, are counted as major factors in excluding homosexuals from the contingent of psychoanalysts trained by IPA societies and institutes. This situation has slowly changed, but the authors claim that the 'enunciators of the homophobic silence of the institutionalized psychoanalytic movement in São Paulo seem to slowly wither, in a silence not unlike the one that allowed the unwritten rule to act for such a long time.'

Our two final chapters are concerned with the Lacanian movement in Brazil, which has been strikingly influential over the past thirty years. Francisco Capoulade (Chapter 16) presents an investigation into the arrival of Lacan's ideas in Brazil in the 1970s, specifically with the group that would form the Centre for Freudian Studies (CFS). From the discovery of two previously unknown documents—one referring to the postgraduate course in clinical psychology at the Pontifical Catholic University of Campinas, and the other referring to the report of the initial national meetings of the CFS—it can be said that as early as the first half of the 1970s Lacan's teaching was being propagated in the university environment, as well as influencing psychotherapists from various parts of Brazil who either had contact with Lacan himself or with his ideas through his disciples. These pioneers of Lacan's ideas had at least two traits in common, namely, they were ex-religious Catholics and had not done any psychoanalytical training in Brazil.

Lastly, Fuad Kyrillos Neto and Rodrigo Afonso Nogueira Santos examine the Brazilian Lacanian movement through the book *The Black Legend of Jacques Lacan: Élisabeth Roudinesco and her historical method*, by Nathalie Jaudel. As a member of the École de la Cause Freudienne and of the World Association of Psychoanalysis, Jaudel critiqued Elisabeth Roudinesco's famous biography of Lacan. To Jaudel, this book presents methodological problems, since the work is marked by an alleged negative transference in relation to Lacan. The authors draw out from this debate two irreconcilable positions that present distinct ways of writing the history of Lacan, resulting also in methodological effects on how to think a history of psychoanalysis. Starting from that, they map and discuss the basis of both positions, aiming to extract their methodological foundations and consequences for the history of psychoanalysis.

A Note on the Text

Most of the chapters in this book were originally written in Portuguese. After their translation to English, there was an editorial effort to reduce the unevenness between the chapters, but we are aware that something of the 'aura' of texts in translation still remains. Our hope is that the anglophone reader will be compensated by hearing voices that would otherwise remain unknown. And maybe part of the experience of getting in contact with Brazilian culture comes through reading texts which are not in their original language.

References

Azevedo, A. M., Vannucchi, A. M., & Sandler, E. H. (2005). Yes, we have bananas! *International Journal of Psycho-Analysis, 86*, 993–1009.

Bosteels, B. (2012). *Marx and Freud in Latin America: Politics, psychoanalysis and religion in times of terror*. Verso.

Coimbra, C. (1995). *Guardiães da ordem. Uma viagem pelas práticas psi no Brasil do 'Milagre'*. Oficina do Autor.

Damousi, J., & Plotkin, M. (Eds.). (2012). *Histories of Psychoanalysis under conditions of Restricted Political Freedom*. Oxford University Press.

de Mijolla, A. (2005). *International dictionary of psychoanalysis*. Thomson Gale.

Derrida, J. (1991). Geopsychoanalysis: "...And the rest of the World". *American Imago, 48*, 199–231.

Dunker, C. (2015). *Mal-Estar, Sofrimento e Sintoma: uma psicopatologia do Brasil entre muros*. Boitempo.

Facchinetti, C. (2001). *Deglutindo Freud: Histórias da digestão do discurso psicanalítico no Brasil. 1v. Tese (Doutorado)*. IP. Universidade Federal do Rio de Janeiro.

Facchinetti, C., & Ponte, C. (2003). De barulhos e silêncios: contribuições para a história da psicanálise no brasil. *Psychê (São Paulo. Impresso), v. AnoVII, n.11*, 59–83.
Frosh, S. (2005). *Hate and the Jewish science: Nazism, anti-semitism and psychoanalysis*. Palgrave.
Gallo, R. (2010). *Freud's Mexico*. MIT Press.
Gaztambide, D. (2019). *A people's history of psychoanalysis: From Freud to liberation psychology*. Lexington Books.
Hollander, N. (1997). *Love in a time of hate: Liberation psychology in Latin America*. Rutgers University Press.
Hollander, N. (2010). *Uprooted minds: Surviving the politics of terror in the Americas*. Routledge.
Khanna, R. (2004). *Dark continents: Psychoanalysis and colonialism*. Duke University Press.
Lewkowicz, S., & Flechner, S. (Eds.). (2005). *Truth, reality, and the psychoanalyst: Latin American contributions to psychoanalysis*. Karnac.
Mandelbaum, B., Frosh, S., Rubin, A., & Theodoro, A. R. (2019). Antropofagia e Autoritarismo na Psicanálise Brasileira. *Calibán Revista Latino-Americana De Psicanálise, 17*, 112–125.
Oliveira, C. (2003). *História da psicanálise. São Paulo 1920–1969*. Escuta/FAPESP.
Pieczanski & Pieczanski. (2014). *The pioneers of psychoanalysis in South America: An essential guide*. Routledge.
Ploktin, M. (2012). Dossier: Psychoanalysis in Latin America. *Psychoanalysis and History, 14*, 227–235.
Plotkin, M. (2001). *Freud in the pampas: The emergence and development of a psychoanalytic culture in Argentina*. Stanford University Press.
Roudinesco, E. (1995). *Genealogias*. Relume-Dumará.
Rubin, A., Mandelbaum, B., & Frosh, S. (2016). 'No memory, no desire': Psychoanalysis in Brazil during Repressive Times. *Psychoanalysis and History, 18*, 93–118.
Russo, J. (2012a). Brazilian psychiatrists and psychoanalysis at the beginning of 20th century: A question for national identity. *Psychoanalysis and History, 14*, 297–312.
Russo, J. (2012b). The social diffusion of psychoanalysis during the Brazilian Military Regime: Psychological awareness in an age of political repression. In J. Damousi & M. Plotkin (Eds.), *Psychoanalysis and politics: Histories of psychoanalysis under conditions of restricted political freedom*. Oxford University Press.

Vetö, H. (2013). *Psicoanálisis en estado de sitio.* Facso/El buen aire.
Zaretsky, E. (2004). *Secrets of the soul*. Knopf.

2

Prelude: 'Global' Psychoanalysis in Latin America: Some Reflections

Mariano Ben Plotkin

Can psychoanalysis be characterised as a global phenomenon of the twentieth century? The answer to this question partially depends on the scope we give to the word 'global.' Throughout the century, psychoanalysis has introduced a new conceptual framework to re-think such issues as sexuality, subjectivity, family and the unconscious, among others. In large portions of what is usually called the *Western World*, psychoanalysis, like Marxism, has changed the way people think about themselves and their relationships to others. I am emphasising the expression *Western World* for two reasons: first, because it is an imprecise construction: What are the limits of the 'Western World'? Is Latin America part of it? French scholar Alain Rouquié has characterised Latin America as the 'extreme West' (Rouquié, 1987). Second, because, no matter how we define 'the West,' there are 'other Worlds' (certainly much larger than the 'Western'

M. B. Plotkin (✉)
CIS-CONICET-IDES, Buenos Aires, Argentina
e-mail: mplotkin@ides.org.ar

Universidad Nacional Tres de Febrero, Buenos Aires, Argentina

B. Mandelbaum et al. (eds.), *Brazilian Psychosocial Histories of Psychoanalysis*, Studies in the Psychosocial,
https://doi.org/10.1007/978-3-030-78509-3_2

one), where the impact of psychoanalysis has been far more superficial, if it existed at all. Thus, I prefer to think of psychoanalysis as a transnational (meaning that it travels across national and cultural borders) rather than as a global phenomenon.

In this chapter, I shall focus on one specific area, what is usually called *Latin America*. Once again, I added the italics because *Latin America* is also a weak notion: it is a 'region' (another imprecise term) that is inhabited by people who belong to many different cultures and who speak a variety of languages besides Spanish and Portuguese. Just to give an example, the Mexican census of 1910 (around the time when psychoanalysis started to be known and discussed in various Latin American countries) revealed that there were over 100 languages spoken in that country alone. Today, countries like Paraguay, Bolivia and Mexico continue to be plurilingual. Therefore, when I refer to Latin America, I am talking about a culturally heterogeneous geographical entity, and particularly, given the nature of the topic to be examined here (psychoanalysis), large urban conglomerations.

Defining psychoanalysis is not any simpler than defining 'Latin America.' Psychoanalysis was born at the end of the nineteenth century in the decadent capital of a decadent European Empire, and it was invented by a Jewish medical doctor who occupied a relatively marginal position within the local scientific field. Surprisingly, within thirty years, psychoanalysis became a transnational discipline, anchored in a relatively centralised institutional system, which had branches in different countries on both sides of the Atlantic, and as far away as in India. However, as recent scholarship has shown, in each cultural space, psychoanalysis (particularly in the period before its institutionalisation) was read, interpreted, appropriated and reformulated in different ways.[1] Uffa Jensen, for instance, has recently shown the different meanings that the material object that symbolises psychoanalysis, the couch, had in Europe and in India. To put it simply, lying on a couch did not have the same meaning in London or in Calcutta (Jensen, 2019). If we consider that the history of a system of thoughts and beliefs cannot be separated from the history

[1] For an enlightening analysis of contemporary uses and interpretations of psychoanalysis in marginal areas of the US, see Gherovici and Christian (eds.) (2019).

of its multiple receptions and forms of circulation (both material and non-material), then we have to admit that the history of psychoanalysis in Latin America, or in India, for that matter, is as important to the general history of psychoanalysis as it is its development anywhere else. This, however, has been largely ignored by the current scholarship.

In this presentation, I concentrate on the development of psychoanalysis in Latin America, knowing the risks and the unavoidable simplifications that the use of such notions imply. Just to clarify my concepts: when I refer to psychoanalysis, I am considering it as a 'folk term': in other words, I am using it as the actors do, usually referring to any system of ideas that legitimises itself in its (real or imagined) Freudian origins. Therefore, I am not concerned here with discussions about the level of 'accuracy' of different appropriations and uses of psychoanalysis; I take them all at face value. The first part of this chapter discusses the early reception of psychoanalysis in a few Latin American countries (in many others, it went virtually unnoticed until much later). The second part offers a more general, methodological reflection on how to understand the place of psychoanalysis in the region.

Psychoanalysis in Latin America or Latin American Psychoanalysis

Generally speaking, histories of psychoanalysis have ignored its early reception and development in Latin American countries. A recent book that presents itself as a 'Globalgeschichte der frühen Psychoanalyse,' for instance, focuses on three cities, none of which is located in Latin America. The word 'global' is associated with the fact that one of the cities is Calcutta; the other two are Berlin and London (Jensen, 2019). Most 'general histories' of psychoanalysis only concentrate on Europe and the US (Makari, 2008; Zaretsky, 2005, among others). However, psychoanalysis became known, used and discussed in some Latin American cities—including Lima, São Paulo, Rio de Janeiro and Buenos Aires—earlier than in many European cities, let alone in India. By the time that Girindrasekhar Bose (one of the earliest psychoanalysts in India) had sent to Freud an imagined portrait (of Freud) painted by another Indian enthusiast of psychoanalysis (they had no idea how Freud really looked, because they had not had access to his actual photograph), the creator of psychoanalysis had been corresponding and exchanging photos and publications with the Peruvian psychiatrist Honorio Delgado for some years (Plotkin & Ruperthuz, 2017; Scheib, 2012). By the 1920s, there had been several doctoral dissertations defended in Rio de Janeiro (the first one is from 1914—Stubbe, 2011), Lima (1918), Mexico City (1926) and elsewhere, that not only focused exclusively on the Freudian system, but also made references to psychoanalytic treatments that had been carried out since earlier times in those cities by prestigious doctors. As early as in 1932, Brazilian doctor Julio Pires Porto Carrero wrote a history of the reception and circulation of psychoanalysis in his own country (Porto Carrero, 1934). By the 1930s, moreover, psychoanalysis and psychoanalytic terms had become common staple among some sectors of the middle classes of several major Latin American cities and it also had an impact in that imprecise area usually referred to as 'popular culture.'

In cities like Buenos Aires, Rio de Janeiro or Santiago de Chile, popular newspapers, novels and publications (and even a few radio shows) disseminated different versions of the Freudian system. However, psychoanalysis was not implanted in the same way in all countries. Thus, while there existed in Brazil a small, but very active group of popular diffusers of psychoanalysis who wrote notes in the popular press and widely read books during the 1930s, nothing like this seems to have happened in Peru, a country where, nonetheless, since the 1910s, a tiny group of prestigious psychiatrists had been discussing and practising eclectic forms of psychoanalysis. In the 1930s, the name of Freud had become so popular in some Latin American cities (particularly in Brazil) that some music-hall artists mentioned their supposed proximity to the inventor of psychoanalysis in order to promote their shows. Such was the case of a certain Maximilien Langsner, who claimed that he was one of Freud's dearest disciples and closest friends (Nosek, 1994). While Langsner announced that he was opening a psychoanalytic sanatorium in Brazil, he also offered popular shows at theatres in São Paulo, where he displayed telepathic and 'magnetic capacities,' including the ability of safely driving a car, blindfolded, on the stage. This episode provoked an agitated exchange of letters between the Paulista Durval Marcondes (one of the first psychoanalysts in Brazil recognised as such by the international psychoanalytic community and who had been corresponding with Freud) and one no less than Sigmund Freud himself, who denied knowing anyone under the name of Langsner (Nosek, 1994; Plotkin & Ruperthuz, 2017). Both Freud and Marcondes were scandalised by the episode. The apparent success of Langsner's show suggests that Freud's name was familiar to the public in São Paulo, to the extent that it could be used for promotional purposes. However, the same public still associated psychoanalysis with the kind of performances that Langsner was offering in theatres (let us remember that Freud himself did not discard possible connections between psychoanalysis and telepathy) (Freud, 1974 [1921]; 1974 [1922]). A few years later, *carioca* doctor Gastão Pereira da Silva (who had also corresponded with Freud) ran a popular radio show on psychoanalytic interpretation of dreams in Rio de Janeiro. This time, Freud did not complain.

All nuances and cultural differences notwithstanding, it is still possible to find some common characteristics in the general process of reception, circulation and dissemination of psychoanalysis in some Latin American cities. The first noteworthy characteristic of the reception of psychoanalysis in the region was its speed, compared to some European countries. In France, for instance, well-established psychiatric and psychological traditions combined with the rejection of all things German (particularly after the debacle of 1870 and, later, of World War I) and a visible distaste for cultural artefacts of Jewish origins, posed a barrier against the early diffusion of psychoanalysis within the medical profession. French literary circles, in contrast, for reasons that have been studied by Élisabeth Roudinesco, among others, were more receptive of Freudian ideas than were medical doctors (Roudinesco, 1988). Psychoanalysis—particularly in its French (and therefore non-German and non-Jewish) version, promoted by Jacques Lacan—would only become a broadly accepted theory and a therapeutic practice of choice in France after World War II. Lacan's version of psychoanalysis would later, in the 1980s, became hegemonic in Argentina and Brazil. In the US, by contrast, psychoanalysis had an early reception, popularisation and institutionalisation; however, it was adapted to already existing cultural traditions and, in the last decades, it has largely been rejected and replaced by other forms of therapy.

In most Latin American countries, there was nothing like an established psychiatric (or, for that matter, scientific) tradition that could pose a strong resistance against the entrance of new theories; therefore, many Latin American intellectual and professional elites were receptive of everything coming from Europe. This was particularly so in the southern cone of the continent. Moreover, in many Latin American countries, scientific (as well as religious) syncretism was far more common than in Europe. The early reception of psychoanalysis in Latin America was highly syncretic, as many of the members of Freud's inner circle did not fail to notice, while Freud, interested as he was in the diffusion of his discipline in far-away countries, was ready to overlook these 'deviations' from his theory (Plotkin & Ruperthuz, 2017). In his personal library, Freud kept many 'unorthodox' books on psychoanalysis written by Latin Americans, and he took more than a few of them with him when he went to his exile in London in 1938.

For Latin American doctors and intellectuals, psychoanalysis had an advantage over other psychiatric ideas that were current during the first decades of the twentieth century: for them, it offered a coherent theory. Moreover, psychoanalytic theory could be applied to explain and treat a variety of mental disorders, and also to analyse social and cultural issues, such as the malaise associated with modernity, or the fast changes of social (and particularly sexual) mores. Furthermore, even the somatic therapies that became available around the 1920s and 1930s to treat mental disorders were, generally speaking, not grounded on a firm theoretical basis, but rather on empirical (and many times dubious) results. Doctors knew that some therapeutic methods could (although did not always) alleviate certain symptoms, but they did not know exactly why.

Psychoanalysis, on the contrary, offered a theory based on the centrality of unconscious desires: whether it was true or false, empirically demonstrable or not, psychoanalysis still had a theory to offer. For instance, shock therapies were widely used during the 1930s in Latin America and elsewhere to alleviate certain forms of schizophrenia; however, nobody knew exactly how or why they worked (when they worked at all). The utilisation of shock therapies was based on the empirical evidence that there was an apparent incompatibility between epilepsy and schizophrenia. Thus, the shock therapies (whether the shock was produced by medication or electricity) were designed to provoke artificial epileptic fits. Dr Enrique Pichon Rivière, a highly respected psychoanalyst who was one of the founding members of the Argentine Psychoanalytic Association and a pioneer in the use of electroshock in Argentina, in contrast, developed a psychoanalytic theory to explain the usefulness of electroshocks: according to Pichon Rivière, they operated as a substitute for a punitive super-ego that was absent in some schizophrenics. Therefore, psychoanalysis, usually combined with other European theories, filled a void in psychiatric theory and practice in contexts that lacked a well-established scientific tradition (Plotkin, 2001). Something similar could be said about the reception of psychoanalysis within psychological circles. In Argentina, for instance (but this could be easily extended to other Latin American countries as well), the lack of a tradition associated with scientific or experimental psychology, and its early clinical orientation, generated a theoretical void that was eventually filled by psychoanalysis (Dagfal, 2009; Plotkin, 2001).

At the same time, psychoanalysis could also be used to fill another, more general, gap in the realm of ideas. Many nineteenth-century Latin American intellectuals and scientists had been very much influenced by evolutionism and positivism in its different versions (in Brazil, one can still find today a few 'positivist temples,' at least in Rio de Janeiro) that led to monistic and materialistic interpretations of reality. This was particularly so in countries like Argentina, Brazil or Mexico (Hale, 1989). During the first decades of the twentieth century, and particularly after World War I, positivism lost much of its previous prestige in favour of various idealist and intuitivist philosophic currents. To some extent, Henri Bergson (but also Benedetto Croce and Giovanni Gentile, at least until the latter became the Fascist Minister of Education) replaced Herbert Spencer as an intellectual beacon for many Latin American intellectuals. The visits of Spanish philosopher José Ortega y Gasset to Latin America from the 1910s, when he introduced and popularised elements of neo-idealistic German philosophy, were very important in generating a new climate of ideas among intellectuals. Later, as a consequence of the Spanish Civil War and the rise of fascism, prominent disciples of

Ortega y Gasset would move to Mexico. Many Latin American intellectuals (particularly in Argentina and Chile) found in psychoanalysis (or in some version of it) a weapon, legitimised by the prestige provided by its supposedly scientific nature, for their struggle against positivism. Psychoanalysis' emphasis on unconscious fantasies offered explanations for the origins of mental diseases and, more importantly, of human behaviour and human nature, in general, that contradicted the traditional materialistic and monistic explanations that had been in fashion since the nineteenth century (Plotkin & Ruperthuz, 2017).

Moreover, psychoanalysis could be easily associated with a Lamarckian version of evolutionism. Freud himself was a firm adherent of Lamarckian evolutionism (Freud, 1987; Maffi, 2012) to the despair of some of his closest disciples, including Ernest Jones who wrote in his biography of Freud: 'We begged him to omit the passage where he applied it [the Lamarckian view] to the whole field of biological evolution, since no responsible biologist regarded it as tenable any longer' (Jones, 1957, p. 313). Works like *Totem and Taboo* (Freud, 1974 [1913]) or *Moses and Monotheism* (the book Jones was referring to) (Freud, 1974 [1939]) are firmly anchored in Lamarckian evolutionary thought. Since that theory, originated in early nineteenth-century France, claimed that evolution took place as a result of adaptation to changing environmental conditions and not as a consequence of random changes and natural selection, as Darwin would propose half a century later, one of the conclusions that could be drawn from it was that the whole process of evolution could be, to some extent, manipulated by voluntarily introducing changes in the environment, both social and natural.

Generally speaking, intellectual and political elites in most Latin American republics, concerned with the construction of the state and the modernisation of society, were very receptive of Lamarckism, although many of them also paid lip service to Darwinism (Stepan, 1991). The reading that many Latin American intellectuals and doctors made of psychoanalysis fitted very well into the Lamarckian vision of the evolutionary process. This could explain why, at least in some Latin American countries like Argentina, Brazil, Chile or Mexico, people who became interested in psychoanalysis were also actively involved in education and in the administration of justice, two fields of activity that aim at improving the social environment. The already mentioned Durval Marcondes was for years a health official at the Paulista educational system (the same can be said about Ulysses Pernambucano in Pernambuco, Arthur Ramos in Rio de Janeiro and other intellectuals who, in different states of Brazil, reflected and wrote about psychoanalysis), while in Chile, Mexico and Brazil, there were forensic experts, as well as judges, who believed that educating the population on the principles of psychoanalysis would contribute to the elimination of criminality altogether. Some judges even practised 'wild psychoanalysis' on the suspects brought before them, in order to detect (and eventually correct) the unconscious motivations that led them to crime (see, for instance, Porto Carrero, 1929; for Chile, Ruperthuz, 2015). A case in point was Mexican judge Raúl Carrancá y Trujillo, who corresponded with Freud and who was in charge of judging no one less than Ramón Mercader, the assassin of Trotsky. Mercader had to submit to almost 900 hours of documented 'therapy' and psychological tests administered by judge Carrancá y Trujillo in his own chambers (without even knowing the real name of Mercader, who was in Mexico under a false name!) (Gallo, 2009).

Furthermore, for many Latin American intellectuals, as well as for the general public, psychoanalysis was a key element of cultural modernity. The widely read Buenos Aires newspaper, *Jornada*, for instance, which ran a whole section on 'psychoanalytic' dream analysis in 1930, equated Freud to Henry Ford as paradigmatic characters of modernity and characterised psychoanalysis as a 'cutting edge' medical technique. During the first decades of the twentieth century, urban populations of various Latin American countries went through fast processes of cultural modernisation. Some countries, such as Argentina and, to a lesser extent, Brazil, had received large waves of European immigrants since the last decades of the nineteenth century as a result of an active policy of 'whitening' (both ethnically and culturally) the local population. Moreover, in Argentina in particular, the state played a crucial role in the process of modernisation through an active educational policy. The levels of literacy boasted by the Argentine urban population (particularly in the city of Buenos Aires) by the 1920s easily matched (and in many cases surpassed) those of many European countries.

This rapid increase in the level of literacy was accompanied by a fast expansion of the editorial market. Popular and very cheap collections of books that published translations of fashionable European texts proliferated in Buenos Aires, Rio de Janeiro, São Paulo and Santiago de Chile from the 1920s on. Books by, or on, Freud were among those put out in large (and mostly bootleg) editions at very accessible prices. In the 1920s, Peruvian poet Alberto Hidalgo (then living in Buenos Aires), signing under the pen name of 'Dr Gómez Nerea,' put out a multivolume collection where he discussed—based on fake 'psychoanalytic cases'—aspects of psychoanalytic theory. This collection circulated widely throughout Spanish-speaking Latin America and was soon translated into Portuguese and published in Brazil (Vezzetti, 1996). Moreover, the first version of Freud's 'Complete Works,' published in any language while Freud was still alive, was the Spanish translation carried out by Luis López Ballesteros in the 1920s, which quickly became a best seller in some Latin American countries. The translation was approved by Freud himself, who read some Spanish. One of the earliest biographies of Freud in any language was written (and corrected by Freud) by the already mentioned Honorio Delgado, and published in 1926 in Spanish, and a few years later in Portuguese (Delgado, 1926, 1933; for a discussion, see Plotkin & Ruperthuz, 2017).

All in all, psychoanalysis provided a discourse of cultural modernity that, at the same time, addressed many ancient social and cultural concerns (the mysteries of sexuality and dreams, for instance), thus becoming particularly appealing to populations that were going through what could be characterised as a 'cultural transition' towards modernity. For many, psychoanalysis provided a new language and a novel conceptual framework, legitimised in science, to deal with old preoccupations and cultural obsessions. Discussions about dreams (particularly about premonitory dreams), for instance, had been a standard feature of popular publications since the nineteenth century. During the 1930s and 1940s, these discussions (even those about premonitory dreams) became associated with psychoanalysis in popular publications, including women's magazines and widely read newspapers (Plotkin, 2007).

Unlike in Europe and in the US, the early reception of psychoanalysis in Latin America contrasted with its relatively late institutionalisation.

Until the 1940s, the lack of orthodox psychoanalytic institutions that would establish a canonical version of psychoanalysis—the first officially recognised surviving psychoanalytic association in Latin America is the Argentine one, created in 1942—as well as Freud's own flexibility towards 'deviations' from his theories occurring in areas that he considered as peripheral and exotic (an undifferentiated Latin America was one of those areas)—turned his system into a malleable set of ideas that could be appropriated, reformulated and selectively redefined for different purposes to a larger extent than in Europe (Plotkin & Ruperthuz, 2017). For some, psychoanalysis justified the modernisation of sexual mores, while for others, it could be used as a mechanism for social control associated with pedagogy, or the administration of justice. These unorthodox and divergent readings of Freud's ideas were put forward even by people who were in epistolary contact with the inventor of psychoanalysis, such as the *carioca* doctor Gastão Pereira da Silva, who wrote over one hundred widely read texts (including a large number of novels) discussing psychoanalysis from various perspectives; or, more revealing, Honorio Delgado whom Freud characterised in one opportunity as his first foreign friend. Delgado did establish a personal relationship with Freud and visited him in Vienna a few times. Both Pereira da Silva and Delgado defined themselves as unorthodox psychoanalysts. Delgado would later renounce psychoanalysis altogether.

In general terms, it could be argued that, by the 1920s, psychoanalysis was simultaneously or successively understood in some major Latin American cities as a therapeutic technique and as an instrument for the renovation of psychiatry; as a central component of cultural modernity; as an intellectual instrument to be pitted against positivism; as a set of ideas that confirmed evolutionary theories (particularly those associated with Lamarckism); as an instrument for social control; as an emancipatory theory that promoted sexual liberation; as a theory of dreams; and, especially in Brazil, as a theory that provided instruments to oppose 'racially centred' social ideas, from a progressive perspective. If, as Freud had proved, everybody's self was endowed with a 'wild' dimension, regardless of racial considerations, then the whole idea of the inferiority of black people, which was based on the belief that they were savage beings, fell apart. In Brazil, the discussion of psychoanalysis thus acquired a nationalistic tone: Freud's theories showed that Parisians and New Yorkers were equally likely to have an obscure and uncontrollable unconscious as much as Brazilians (whether white, black or mestizo) did (Castro, 2015; Plotkin, 2011). Therefore, there was no reason for Brazilians to feel diminished vis-à-vis Europeans or North Americans. From what I have said so far, it should be clear that different interpretations of psychoanalysis have become important elements in the urban culture of some Latin American countries—or at least in major cities—at least since the 1920s and 1930s.

How Should We Approach the Social and Cultural Study of Psychoanalysis in Latin America?

Although a lot has been done in different Latin American countries, particularly in Argentina, Brazil, Chile and Mexico, in terms of understanding patterns of early reception and circulation of psychoanalysis, much more is still to be done. Most scholarship originating in Latin America has been successful in identifying who used psychoanalysis and how—and for what purposes—since the early decades of the twentieth century. However, in my opinion, this kind of analysis only provides half (a very important half, for that matter) of the story. This is so, because there is a tendency to focus on psychoanalysis as a set of ideas (no matter how malleable it can be), rather than as a set of practices. Psychoanalysis is a system of ideas and beliefs, but it is also a set of practices that must compete, accommodate, struggle against and articulate itself with other already existent practices that have changed over time.

In its beginnings back in Vienna, psychoanalysis was competing with other medical and semi-medical practices such as hypnotism, different forms of magnetism and somatic psychiatry. In Latin American countries, psychoanalysis was, and still is to a large extent, submerged into a universe of pre-existing therapeutic practices that includes other forms of psychiatric techniques and psychotherapy, but also traditional forms of healing, and magical visions of the world. On this side of the Atlantic, the process of 'disenchantment' of the world described by Max Weber has been probably less complete than in the 'Global North,' where it has remained incomplete.

Looking at the present time, a recent study carried out in Buenos Aires (considered as one of the 'most psychoanalysed' cities of the world) by anthropologist Nicolás Viotti and myself focuses on the universe of therapeutic practices or therapeutic constellations in which psychoanalysis is immersed, in order to see what place it occupies within them. The research reveals a panorama that is far more complex than foreseen (Plotkin & Viotti, 2020). Our quantitative and qualitative data suggest the existence of a large, heterogeneous and hybrid set of practices that could be characterised as therapeutic, that certainly includes psychoanalysis, but as a component of a much richer system of interrelated and competing practices.

Let us start from the well-known facts: Argentina is the country with the largest number of psychologists in proportion to its population in the world. In Buenos Aires, the proportion of psychologists (virtually all of them educated in psychoanalysis) is even higher. Moreover, the expansion of psychoanalysis in Buenos Aires has gone far beyond its utilisation as a therapeutic technique, as anyone who has visited the city can attest. Psychoanalytic terms and concepts have permeated everyday speech. Politicians, artists and even generals regularly use psychoanalytic terms in public appearances. It has been argued that the diffusion of psychoanalysis in the city has generated a particular 'psychoanalytic listening genre' among *porteños* (as those living in Buenos Aires are known) (Marsilli-Vargas, 2016). However, the preliminary results of our study have shown that even in such a city as Buenos Aires, 'modern therapeutic' discourses and practices, including those associated with psychoanalysis, have been integrated into wider well-being constellations that include other types of practices (both secular and sacred), some of which recognise local or colonial origins, such as traditional forms of healing, as well as others which have been imported in more recent times either from the global North—such as New Age practices, self-help literature or charismatic Christianity, among many others—or from other Latin American countries, such as the Afro-Brazilian 'possession' religions Umbanda and Candomblé.

Most current scholarship produced both in Latin American countries and in the 'global north,' as well as what could be characterised as a 'learned common sense,' assumes that the diffusion of psychoanalysis and of other modern forms of psychotherapy is a pervasive—and at the same time unique—feature of 'global' culture associated with the broader diffusion of a 'therapeutic mind.' Therefore, most studies look for examples (historical, sociological, anthropological) to corroborate, at the local level, this a priori assumption. Moreover, for many students of the history of psychoanalysis (both north and south of the Equator), Freud's theories—and the practices associated with them—can only be understood in their own terms, and not as part of a broader system of well-being techniques, or as a situated cultural artefact. This amounts to claiming that psychoanalysis constitutes a therapeutic universe in itself. In part, this is because psychoanalytic concepts (and its own way of self-historicisation) have been internalised by those who study it to the extent that they have become part of their 'world taken for granted' (Plotkin, 2017). However, the place of psychoanalysis within local cultural spaces cannot be separated from other well-being techniques and systems of belief that, in various Latin American cities, include secular, religious, magic and spiritual dimensions, as well as the results of their combination and coexistence. The particular characteristics of these forms of syncretism and hybridisations, and the place that psychoanalysis occupies in them, depend on such factors as social class, gender, levels of education and the cultural specificities of each country or city, as well as on the particular historical moment we are referring to.

In Buenos Aires and its metropolitan area, just to give an example, from a representative survey of more than 700 cases, only 14% of those polled responded that they would seek the help of a psychologist when confronted with distress. Furthermore, 11% of the sampled people rejected the possibility of even referring to a psychologist at all. In contrast, 33% declared that they would approach God and 17% would pray to the Virgin Mary or the saints in order to deal with different forms of distress. Our in-depth interviews and ethnographic observations, nonetheless, show a much more complex situation in which psychoanalytic therapy and approaching God are in fact intertwined within a dense constellation of other practices. We are currently carrying out a similar study in Rio de Janeiro, and the preliminary results show a picture that is even more complex than in Buenos Aires, in part because of the widespread acceptance of Afro-Brazilian religions and other forms of Spiritism across social classes, gender and levels of education. Psychoanalysis, in particular, and what is known as 'therapeutic culture' in general presuppose the existence of the notion of an autonomous self. In Latin America (and in other areas of the world as well), this 'modern' idea of the autonomous self has coexisted and still does, with other, more relational and more heteronomous ideas of subjectivity to a larger extent than in the 'Global North' (for a comparison, see, Losonczy & Mesturini Cappo, 2014; Teisenhoffer, 2007).

In conclusion, I believe that in Latin America a good deal has been done, on the one hand, to study psychoanalysis as a historically analysable cultural phenomenon and, on the other hand, to introduce Latin America into the transnational history of psychoanalysis. Recently, Mariano Ruperthuz and I have shown the place that Latin America and Latin Americans played in Freud's own biography (Plotkin & Ruperthuz, 2017). It is now high time to take a second step and place psychoanalysis within the larger universe of local therapeutic constellations of practices and beliefs or, in other words, to situate psychoanalysis within its various and diverse cultural and social spaces of reception and circulation. In order to do this, we should take a further step back and displace the focus from the supposedly peculiar and unique aspects of the Freudian system in order to return it to the broader constellation of therapeutic practices where the actors place it.

References

Castro, R. (2015). *A sublimaçao de id primitivo em ego civilizado: o projeto dos psiquiatras-psicanalistas para civilizar o país (1926–1944)*. Paco Editorial.

Dagfal, A. (2009). *Entre París y Buenos Aires. La invención del psicólogo (1942–1966)*. Paidós.

Delgado, H. (1926). *Sigmund Freud*. C.F. Southwell.

Delgado, H. (1933). *A vida e obra de Freud*. Marisa.

Freud, S. (1974 [1913]). *Totem and taboo: The standard edition of the complete psychological works of Sigmund Freud* (Vol. XIII). The Hogart Press.
Freud, S. (1974 [1921]). *Psycho-analysis and telepathy. The standard edition of the complete psychological works of Sigmund Freud* (Vol. XVIII). The Hogart Press.
Freud, S. (1974 [1922]). *Dreams and telepathy*. XVIII.
Freud, S. (1974 [1939]). *Moses and monotheism: Three essays. The standard edition of the complete psychological works of Sigmund Freud* (Vol. XXIII). The Hogart Press.
Freud, S. (1987). *A phylogenetic fantasy*. The Belknap Press of Harvard University Press.
Gallo, R. (2009). *Freud's Mexico: Into the wilds of psychoanalysis*. MIT Press.
Gherovici, P., & Christian, C. (Eds.). (2019). *Psychoanalysis in the barrios: Race*. Routledge.
Hale, C. (1989). Political and social ideas. In L. Bethell (Ed.), *Latin America: Economy and society 1870–1930*. Cambridge University Press.
Jensen, U. (2019). *Wie die Couch nach Kalkutta kam. Eine Globalgeschichte der frühen Psychoanalyse*. Suhrkamp Verlag.
Jones, E. (1957). *The life and work of Sigmund Freud* (Vol. 3). Basic Books.
Losonczy, A.-M., & Mesturini Cappo, S. (2014). Ritualized misunderstanding between uncertainty, agreement and rupture. In B. Caiuby Labate & C. Cavnar (Eds.), *Ayahuasca shamanism in the amazon and beyond*. Oxford University Press.
Maffi, C. (2012). *Le souvenir-écran de la psychanalyse: Freud, Klein, Lacan: Ruptures et filiations*. Le félin Kiron.
Makari, G. (2008). *Revolution in mind: The creation of psychoanalysis*. Harper.
Marsilli-Vargas, X. (2016). The offline and online mediatization of psychoanalysis in Buenos Aires. *Signs and Society, 1*(14): 135–153.
Meyer, M. (2017). *Reasoning against Madness: Psychiatry and the State in Rio de Janeiro, 1830–1944*. University of Rochester Press.
Nosek, L. (Ed.). (1994) *Album de familia: imagens, fontes e idéias da psicanálise em São Paulo*. Casa del Psicólogo.
Plotkin, M., & Ruperthuz, M. (2017). *Estimado Dr Freud. Una historia cultural del psicoanálisis en América Latina*. Edhasa.
Plotkin, M., & Viotti, N. (2020). Between Freud and Umbanda: Therapeutic constellations in Buenos Aires, Argentina. In D. Nehring, O. Madsen, E. Cabanas, C. Mills, & D. Kerrigan (Eds.), *The Routledge international handbook of global therapeutic cultures*. Routledge, Taylor & Francis.

Plotkin, M. (2001). *Freud in the pampas: The emergence and development of a psychoanalytic culture in Argentina*. Stanford University Press.
Plotkin, M. (2007). Sueños del Pasado y del Futuro. La Interpretación de los Sueños y la Difusión del Psicoanálisis en Buenos Aires (ca. 1930-ca.1950). In S. Gayol & M. Madero (Eds.), *Formas de historia cultural*. Prometeo.
Plotkin, M. (2011). Psychoanalysis, race relations and national identity. The reception of psychoanalysis in Brazil (1910–1940). In W. Anderson, R. Keller, & D. Jenson (Eds.), *Unconscious dominions*. Duke University Press.
Plotkin, M. (2017). El psicoanálisis como sistema de creencias: un bosquejo de programa de investigación. História, Ciências, Saúde-Manguinhos. Rio de Janeiro: Fiocruz. 2017 vol.24 n°1. P. 15–31.
Porto Carrero, J. (1929). *Ensaios de psychanalyse*. Flores y Mano.
Porto Carrero, J. (1934). A contribuição brasileira á psychanalyse. Anais do III Congresso de Neurologia, Psychiatria e Medicina Legal.
Roudinesco, E. (1988). *La batalla de cien años. Historia del psicoanálisis en Francia. Tomo 1, 1885–1939*. Fundamentos.
Rouquié, A. (1987). *Amérique latine. Introduction à l' Extrême-Occident*. Seuil.
Scheib, M. (2012). *Honorio Delgado und die Frühgeschichte der Psychoanalyse in Peru*. epubli GmbH (kindle version).
Stepan, N. (1991). *The hour of eugenics: Race, gender, and nation in Latin America*. Cornell University Press.
Stubbe, H. (2011). *Sigmund Freud in den Tropen: die erste psychoanalytische Dissertation in der portugiesischprachigen Welt*. Shaker Verlag.
Teisenhoffer, V. (2007). Umbanda, New Age et psychothérapie. Aspects de l'implantation de l'umbanda à Paris. *Ateliers d'Anthropologie, 31*.
Vezzetti, H. (1996). *Aventuras de Freud en el país de los argentinos. De José Ingenieros a Enrique Pichon Riviére*. Paidós.
Zaretsky, E. (2005). *Secrets of the soul: A social and cultural history of psychoanalysis*. Vintage Books.

Part II

Methodological Issues

3

Writing the History of Psychoanalysis in Brazil: Some Questions for Historiographic Research

Carmen Lucia M. Valladares de Oliveira

The psychoanalytic movement has been present in the Brazilian territory for more than a century, where it is firmly established in the most important urban centres, with modules taught in numerous universities across the country. However, historiographic research on the subject is still incipient, despite the long-standing concern with the historical contextualisation of the events.

The first records were written by Julio Pires Porto-Carrero (1929/1932): he was a tireless advocate of the 'cause' and probably the first in Brazil to call himself a psychoanalyst. He was responsible for what is known about the first 15 years of the reception of the doctrine, notably in the medical field, but also in education, as a contribution to the construction project of the Brazilian nation, and was rooted in a positivist style typical of his time. Later, through Virginia Bicudo (1948), these records were given an apologetic reading, mainly around the movement initiated by Durval Marcondes in São Paulo. Since then, several

C. L. M. V. de Oliveira (✉)
Pontifícia Universidade Católica de São Paulo, São Paulo, Brazil

B. Mandelbaum et al. (eds.), *Brazilian Psychosocial Histories of Psychoanalysis*, Studies in the Psychosocial,
https://doi.org/10.1007/978-3-030-78509-3_3

of his followers have contributed to the outline of an official, descriptive, legalistic, triumphalist history, often reduced to an oral, institutional tradition. There is a small difference in Rio, where the production always favoured a more critical approach, which is likely due to the impact of institutional crises and dissidence, especially since the 1980s, when the psychoanalyst Amílcar Lobo was publicly accused of being involved in torture, leading to a crisis in the local psychoanalytic movement (Cerqueira, 1982).

The first methodological rupture with these official approaches occurred only with the inception of academic studies. In 1983, Gilberto Rocha wrote his Masters thesis at the Pontifical Catholic University of Rio de Janeiro (PUC-RJ). Inspired by the Foucauldian model, he used primary and secondary sources to recreate the conditions that allowed the implementation of psychoanalysis in Brazil. Thus, from a tradition reserved only for pioneers or their followers and regarded as a commemorative event, told in the style of a family novel through the heroic acts, myths, and legends which made its implementation possible, we gradually moved on to the more structured, more critical studies, which were generally led by psychologists and psychoanalysts in the Schools of Psychology, sometimes in the Schools of Philosophy, rarely in the Departments of History. Some of these first investigations emphasised regional aspects of the different modes of implementation, while others prioritised acclaimed institutions, personalities or approaches from a more anthropological, cultural or even empirical-conceptual perspective.

However, it is remarkable how, in the last decade, this production has grown in terms of both thematic diversification and emphasis on events and historic characters, either unknown or forgotten, both in Brazil and in the psychoanalytic world. In São Paulo alone, a large number of research projects have emerged since Renato Mezan opened the path with his doctoral dissertation in 1981 in the Philosophy Department of the University of São Paulo, which culminated in the book *Freud, pensador da cultura* (1985). Since then, we had Renata Cromberg's body of research about the work of Sabina Spielrein; the studies on Otto Fenichel by José Henrique Palumbo; the work of Rodrigo Santos, who seeks to retrieve the contribution of Karl Weissmann; Fernando Figueira, who analyses the work of Arthur Ramos; and also the epistemological and methodological questions brought by Rafael Alves Lima.[1] To these, we may add the research done by Josiane Machado on the early days of psychoanalysis in Brazil, and that by Leandro dos Santos, who brings to light the history of the arrival of Lacanianism in the country. Overall, these studies provide an idea of how far the doctrine has penetrated the different segments of social life throughout the twentieth century. It is not by chance that interest in this subject has grown, especially among young researchers and through the events devoted to this theme. After all, the past is always built according to present needs. Nowadays, in face of the theoretical crisis, absence of masters, attacks, and especially cognitive-behavioural approaches, notably on the issue of autism, this returning to the sources and desire to write history—apart from rehabilitating forgotten, overlooked authors and writings—constitutes a chance to update some questions.

This is also the occasion to elucidate the unspoken, the family secrets and repressed events of our history which, as psychoanalysis teaches us, invariably return in a violent way (Freud, 1915). As Marieta Ferreira (2018) rightly reminds us, this forces us to redouble our awareness of the political uses that might follow, under the risk of turning ourselves into judges of history, especially in these times when memory is extremely valued. Writing history must be a precondition for not giving in to the deadly indifference of those who have, for instance, adopted a position of 'neutrality' that did not necessarily entail adherence, but instead, a complaisance with a political situation marked by extreme violence, such as during the military dictatorship in Brazil (Oliveira, 2017). The reaction to the blindness and deafness of those who passively watched or even cooperated with the tragic events can be taken as a passage that allows time to be left behind, negated, silenced, and opens the door to the work of mourning, which can overcome the emptiness which causes feelings of detachment, and perhaps also the journey, however long, towards the production of a story of reconciliation (Hassoun & Waljsbrot, 1991). In any case, we shall reinforce our commitment to the rule of law, as a prerequisite for the unobstructed movement of speech, not only in clinics, but also in social and political life, as another way to mark the

[1] See the chapters by several of these writers in this volume.

presence of psychoanalysis both in what is said in the *polis* and as a knowledge about culture and barbarism (Garner, 2007).

On the other hand, despite the considerable growth in historiographic production, there are many gaps in this writing. We still have a long way to go in terms of document research, through studies of scholarly history, in different epistemological and methodological approaches capable of providing an account of the different ways in which psychoanalysis has been conveyed. In view of its century-long presence in the country and the different fields it has influenced and/or with which it still interacts, such as art, literature, education, sociology, anthropology, psychiatry, and law, which heralds a vast possibility of exploring this history, far from exhausting the subject, here we simply aim to point out some questions and concerns.

Periodisation

The first aspect to be taken into account has to do with this chronological framework, which is always, as Michel de Certeau (1975) suggests, postulated on the basis of an interpretation made in the present. However, any chronology already implies a completed series of individual facts that are rearranged as a set of objects that manifest in the form of events, even if their terms remain uncertain and ever liable to be reconstructed. In addition, we must bear in mind that the event, always incomplete, never definitively established, reflects only a fraction of a forgotten or hindered experience, waiting to be recalled. In this dimension, history is regarded somewhat in the manner of Foucault (1972), through distinct temporalities and spatialities. And the periodisation is established from the internal breakages and discontinuities that have caused ruptures and modifications in the way of producing a certain practice, its materiality, its structure.

From this viewpoint, the framework must consider the events that give meaning to the doctrine in not only the country but also the world, along with aspects of institutional history at the intersection with social medicine, mental health, and the social, intellectual, economic, and political history both in Brazil and internationally. Regarding psychoanalysis in Brazil, it is possible to distinguish six phases:

1914–1937—The arrival and diffusion of Freudian theses in the main urban centres in Brazil, through different routes: social medicine, pedagogy, literature, visual arts, sociology, and law. More often discussed than practised, psychoanalysis, during this phase, has penetrated the social discourse as a knowledge regarding sexuality, children, but mostly culture.

1938–1950—The first generation of analysts graduated under the rules set by the International Psychoanalytical Association (IPA) in São Paulo, Rio de Janeiro, and Porto Alegre, consisting predominantly of medical doctors. This allowed the expansion of child clinical practice through pedagogical methods and dissemination of psychoanalysis in the field of sociology.

1951–1969—Heralded the establishment of four IPA institutions: Brazilian Psychoanalytic Society of São Paulo (SBPSP), Brazilian Psychoanalytic Society of Rio de Janeiro (SBPRJ), Rio de Janeiro Psychoanalytical Society (SPRJ), and Brazilian Psychoanalytic Society of Porto Alegre (SBPPA), concluding its process of implementation with the emergence of psychotherapy practices, along with group therapies, Reichian body therapies, and Jungian therapy.

1970–1990—The boom of psychoanalysis, with the rise of new schools and trends, notably Lacanianism and its different strands. This generation gave priority to investing in private clinics over social ones, characterised by the 'refusal of the political.' The clinic, which had been predominantly run by medical doctors, has been mainly run by psychologists since the mid-1980s.

1990–2010—'Turning towards oneself,' a moment of questioning not only the local production and its relevance to the international stage, but the notion of a Brazilian clinic. Large investments in universities, research, and writing.

2010–present—The psychoanalyst returns to the *polis*. The last decade has witnessed a trend, among analysts, to coordinate the clinic with political and social lives, that is, a concern about the effects of external reality on the psyche, which was predominantly rejected by the generations that preceded them.

Filiations

Another important element to be taken into account concerns the efforts to revisit our most diverse filiations. This was a subject that was close to Freud's heart since the beginning, when, in theorising the Oedipus complex, he turned it into a founding myth that inscribes the subject on the path that leads them to questioning themself about the enigmas of their origin. Filiation, as Granoff puts it, albeit rhythmic by procreation and birth, is 'a fragile and precarious discourse,' for reasons ranging from its origin, to the delimitation of the laws that govern and threaten it, to the determination of its role in the life of individuals, to the 'required separation from this trait which every human bears' (Granoff, 1975, p. 50). As Henri Ellenberger taught us (1954–1991/1995; 1970/1994), in the tradition of long-term history, we must also include a whole line of ancestors and pioneers of the discipline. As a particular form of initiation into knowledge and psychoanalytic practice, this is a journey that operates in the transferential relationship between master and disciple, and in which a third character is introduced, 'the analyst's analyst' (Granoff, 1975), temporarily expanding the different generations that have built and passed on this history in their various statements.

This lineage should also include a fourth character, the 'friends of psychoanalysis,' so dear to Derrida. An important figure, the friend, he used to say, is the one who 'speaks of the freedom of an alliance, an engagement without institutional status.' Simultaneously from within, given their sympathy for the cause, and from the outside, given that they are not a practitioner, the friend 'entertains a reservation, a required detachment from criticism, discussion, and reciprocal questioning, which at times is more radical' (Derrida & Roudinesco, 2001, p. 271).

Thus, in writing the history of psychoanalysis, we must not overlook this particularity of taking into account the different generations and commentators of Freudian work who have formed us in their various translations, languages, and accents, as well as looks and perceptions. A journey that includes comings and goings in Vienna, London, passing through Berlin, New York, Paris, Buenos Aires, Budapest, amongst other places, as well as the inner circulation in countless cities where psychoanalysis is in the process of implementation.

Acknowledging the plurality of modes of transmission is a prerequisite for the researcher to avoid the temptation to restrict psychoanalysis to a single strand, to think of it as a sect, believing that their's is the true way of seeing and observing the phenomena of life, that their background is the only valid one.

The History of the Present Time

Regardless of the approach we adopt, the breakage we would like to emphasise, the events we want to highlight, we must not forget that we are writing a history of the present, of an ongoing chronological period, where the moment being studied and that of its study coincide. This has inescapable implications for the process of documentation.

Of all these implications, it is worth emphasising that, albeit committed to the present, the historian, while working their craft, should perhaps be more open to plurality, to the fragmentation of memory in relation to history, and as Marieta Ferreira (2018) rightly notes, the historian should not 'be associated with a militant movement on behalf of a particular social memory.' Historiographic writing, as Labourie (2001) tells us, should seek to repair the foreignness of a past that both inhabits and shapes the present. Making room for estrangement is the precondition for re-encountering the social actors' different forms of presence in the events of history, and also, we shall admit, for analytic practice. Bearing in mind that, in this specific case, a greater complication is brought about by involving the clinic, as it produces effects on transferential relationships, raising questions such as: How should we write about individuals whose heirs are still alive? Should the historian publish everything they know or have discovered in their research, notably what concerns the intimate history of an analyst?

This is a complex issue which demands a very sensitive approach, for it may have disastrous repercussions, from both omission and excess. This is what Labourie (2001) points out when questioned about a 'guilty complacency' that occasionally occurs in this type of writing, and which pays its price through 'forgetfulness,' 'memorial reconstruction,' and omissions. How can one write history without giving in to the pressure of institutions, characters, and their heirs, while simultaneously preserving the subject's right to privacy? These questions gain another layer of relevance when the researcher is both object and subject. Here, we must create the distance required for dealing with the experience without, nevertheless, succumbing to the temptation of producing a knowledge that aspires to be absolute (Roudinesco, 1994, p. 102) or even omnipotent, which claims to differentiate between true and false, as though the historian were the one holding the 'good word' (Labourie, 2001). The psychoanalyst fulfilling the role of historian, in their need to understand history as an attentive witness, must be less concerned with denouncing than with transmitting, instructing, informing the truth about a past that is traumatic yet constantly being recreated and rediscovered (Labourie, 2019).

Truth and the Construction of History

Freud inaugurated not only the psychoanalytic clinic, but also a branch of social knowledge capable of subverting the image of a perfect world, adaptable to absolute truths (Garner, 2007). Bearing this in mind, Michel de Certeau (1975) noted that history fluctuates between what is told and what is done, between a legible past and a concealed present. It is the historian's responsibility, Jacques Hassoun comments, to navigate between these two poles, starting to open a breach in something that happened elsewhere or in another way (Hassoun & Waljsbrot, 1991, p. 123). In the clinic, he adds, the 'interweaving of the near past, the distant past, the present, and what the analyst can say about it, presents itself as one of the facets, one of the fragments of the subject's truth' (Hassoun & Waljsbrot, 1991, p. 165).

These writers are following Lacan's teachings by seeing the unconscious as 'transindividual,' part of the concrete discourse, a chapter in the censored history of the subject, 'marked by a blank or occupied by a lie' written elsewhere and not at the subject's disposal in reestablishing the continuity of his conscious discourse' (Lacan, 1953/1966, p. 258). Its truth can be found; in most cases, it is still written elsewhere, in different ways, in the subject's symptoms, memories, lifestyle, traditions, and in both individual and collective traces and vestiges (Lacan, 1953/1966, p. 259). The truth in Lacan, according to Garner, is like a mask 'that lies behind the self, and is more dependent on the horror than on the plastic beauty that emerges naked from the well, more so because it is covered with a new skin when it comes to light' (Garner, 2007, p. 116). Unmasking the truth then entails unmasking the self.

When Garner reflects upon the modern myth of Oedipus, he suggests that Lacan appropriated a particular Hellenistic-Heideggerian interpretation of the truth and took it as a revelation, which also entails forgetting, an 'abandonment of memory,' or a hiding place. 'In French Heideggerian, he says, a language that is even more complex than the Lacanian, this "Verbergung," to be hidden, is called "latency"' (Garner, 1994/1997, p. 31). Latency is here used in the sense of a turning towards the safety of oblivion, since, for Lacan, the entire truth is also dangerous, unbearable, for it is 'uncovered, exposed, in a state of insecurity always close to death' (p. 32).

As Foucault rightly analysed, the tragedy of Oedipus, as the first testimony we have of the Greek legal system, 'is the story of a quest for truth,' but whose answers are always lame, incomplete, made up of a series of adjustments to each other. According to Foucault, the ultimate truth in Oedipus—that which leads him to meet his fate—comes from the testimonies, through the multiple wordplays of those who saw, experienced, and remembered what happened (Foucault, 1974/1994).

Testimonial

Similar to the biographical genre, the testimony also expresses the ambivalence that characterises the different registers of the psychic functioning of neurotic subjects: as Freud (1937) taught us, they must be heard in their suffering. By revisiting the past in the quest for truth, remembrance is what enables the work of mourning, of libidinal disinvestment, as the renunciation and resignation which allow them to reconcile with loss (Freud, 1917).

On the other hand, neither the historian nor the psychoanalyst can lose sight of the fact that, although suffering and memory are indicative of exclusion, they do not necessarily mirror external reality. In their writing, they must take into account that memories are not reliable and that what is recalled is not necessarily faithful to the event. In memory, we find oblivion, secrecy, gaps, and feelings of recollection. With its passions, ideologies, and settling of accounts, the testimony, apart from being subjective, unilateral, and partial, is the product of a society and agents of discourse that interfere in the historical process (Rovai & Teixeira, 2016). How not to give in to the temptation of attributing value of truth to memories? 'I was there, I saw it, I know what I am talking about.' How can we challenge the power of testimony from someone who claims to be the bearer of truth?

As historians of the present, we are under permanent 'surveillance,' since, as Voldman states, 'the actors in the period and field analysed may challenge our statements; protest against our interpretations; proclaim, on behalf of their actual presence in the moment when facts unfolded, that, in the best of circumstances, we are mistaken in spite of our good faith, and in the worst, that we are falsifying the Truth' (1992, p. 7).

In addition, how can we deal with this current trend of 'judicialising history' and its potential consequences, through the laws of memorial nature, of victimised positions? Let us not ignore the fact that, according to worldwide trends, it has recently become commonplace to resort to the judiciary to impede the circulation of ideas with which one disagrees, by accusing them of defamation.

In Brazil, this was the case regarding the 'unauthorised biographies' controversy, which resulted in a 2015 Supreme Court decision. At the request of the National Association of Book Publishers, this Court took a unanimous decision against censorship and in favour of freedom of expression and scientific research. This decision stated that the 'consent of the person being biographied'—or their relatives, in case of deceased persons—'is non-required' for the production of literary or audiovisual works. Such was the case in France, when different court actions were filed in 2011 by Jacques-Alain Miller, his family, and the members of the École de la cause freudienne against Elisabeth Roudinesco and her publisher Olivier Bétourné, when they disagreed with passages in the book *Lacan envers et contre tout*.

Whenever possible, testimonies should be recorded to fill their role as oral archives, as an experience of the present in their singularity, as a record of how each gets situated within the psychoanalytic universe. In this respect, a prime example of archival production of this memory is Francisco Capoulade's documentary *Hestórias da psicanálise – leitores de Freud*. If, on the one hand, the witness should not be regarded as a watchdog of history's making, on the other, neither is it a question of writing a neutral history. However, neither sympathy nor familiarity with the subject can be used to conceal or legitimise the memory that reshapes the events in social life. In writing, testimonies must be contrasted with documents, records, and the prevailing perception of the time when the narrative was being produced. Once again, we should not forget Paul Ricoeur's (2000) reminder that it is up to the historian to present the different interpretations of the historical plan, to produce memory, to highlight traces and reminiscences, to investigate enigmas, and to unearth traumas, so as to avoid the repetition of history.

Given that a symbolising identification is impossible, one always runs the risk of a 'settling of accounts' between psychoanalysts in the role of historians and characters from previous generations. Acknowledging the errors of the past is obviously necessary, but it demands great caution when interpreting events, so that historians do not fall into the temptation of becoming judges of history.

Thus, in this effort to construct memory, to give voice to the unspoken, and to update memories as substitute representations of other impressions (Freud, 1901/1973), of a forgotten, masked past, lost in time, and, therefore, of the need to constantly invent it and to symbolise processes, one should maintain the required tension between the true, the credible, the false, and the conjunctural and take into account what Arlete Farge (1997) calls criteria of 'truthfulness and plausibility.'

Repressed Memory

There are in fact still many gaps in our recent past, such as the murky and sketchy relationship between psychoanalysts and the military dictatorship from the 1960s to the 1980s. Although access to public archives has made recent investigations easier, many obstacles still remain in the process of obtaining documents that may confront events and testimonies and, therefore, enable writing that maintains a relationship with justice and the restoration of truth. Ongoing research, such as Rafael Alves Lima's and Aline Rubin's, heavily contributes to shedding light on this period.

Using the Amílcar Lobo case as a starting point, we shall revisit the history of the foundation of psychoanalysis in Rio de Janeiro, to encounter a tragic history of filiations involving the psychoanalyst Werner Kemper and his past of cooperation with Nazism. Even though it has already been analysed by Helena Bessermann Vianna, Gisálio Cerqueira Filho, Chaim Katz, and Nádia Sério, many gaps in the timeline remain. In São Paulo, Adelheid Koch, a Jewish German psychoanalyst who came to Brazil in 1938 fleeing from Nazism, met Kemper—who had never questioned his actions during the war. The two had previously met in Berlin and frequented the local society during the same period. In December 1935, Koch was expelled from the Deutsche Psychoanalytische Gesellschaft (DPG), while Kemper remained in the institution (Oliveira, 2005). The following year, the institute was absorbed into the Göring Institute, where Kemper started working as a teacher and, two years later, as one of its directors. He cooperated with the Nazis until the war ended and later took part in the reconstruction of the Berlin Psychoanalytic Society, backed by Jones, before being sent to Brazil. He arrived in December 1948, as a training analyst, to establish the psychoanalytic movement in Rio, along with Mark Burke—also a newcomer—a Polish Jew who had fought against the Nazi troops with the British army. Although Burke never made accusations about his colleague, they had a difficult relationship from the beginning, with attacks coming from both sides, leading to a rift in the Rio movement and resulting in two psychoanalytic societies. Kemper's concealed past, ignored by his heirs, only began to be unveiled in the 1980s.

The archives of the Brazilian Psychoanalytical Society of São Paulo (SBPSP), accessed during our 1999 research, contained correspondence dating back to the early 1950s, in which Adelheid Koch attested that she had closely followed the disputes between Kemper and Burke, as well as the inquiries made by Rio analysts concerning the legitimacy of Anna Kattrin Kemper's training in Berlin. The Berlin Society's document attesting to Anna Kattrin's training in the 1940s is also included in the collection. As president of SBPSP, Adelheid Koch had even exchanged letters with the IPA board to discuss the case, in which she took the side of Kemper and his wife. During Kemper's sojourn in Brazil, the two maintained cordial relations.

For the testimonial survey, both of Adelheid Koch's daughters claimed to be unaware of this fact. They believed that their mother was not privy to Kemper's collaborative past. And it is highly likely that she had also repressed this memory. Adelheid Koch was very obedient; she would not dare to challenge a decision made by the board of the IPA. She had not even questioned Jones when, in carrying out his disastrous policy known as 'safeguarding psychoanalysis' at that tragic meeting on 4 December 1935, he forced the resignation of all Jewish analysts in the Berlin institution (AIHP, 1987). On that day, while Koch received the title of analyst from the DPG, she found herself banned from the German IPA, with no national filiation. The following year, at the famous Congress of Marienbad, Czechoslovakia, in August 1936, Jones, now concerned with organising the exodus of analysts from Europe, offered her the opportunity to settle in Brazil as a training analyst. There she could count on Durval Marcondes for help, someone who had been dreaming for years of training analysts according to the IPA's guidelines. Her arrival in São Paulo in November 1937, during the Vargas dictatorial era, marked the beginning of the process towards the institutionalisation of this practice in the country, unexpectedly turning her into the founder of the psychoanalytic movement in Brazil, the first training analyst in Latin America.

There still remain many shady areas in the life story of Kemper's wife, Anna Katrin, who, in addition to carrying a controversial title, always remained silent about her husband's collaborationist past, to which she also belonged. This did not prevent her from adopting a left-wing attitude years later, after divorcing her husband during the military regime, and campaigning side by side with Hélio Pellegrino in the project of a social clinic aimed at assisting the dwellers of Favela dos Cabritos in Rio. This project started in 1973 and was inspired by the experience of Abraham in 1920s Berlin, Wilhelm Reich, and Anna Freud (Ferreira, 1986).

There is no doubt whatsoever that both Werner and Anna Katrin played an important role in the history of psychoanalysis in Rio de Janeiro. Yet, a part of that repressed past, which always returns in a violent manner, still leaves deep scars, even on the heirs of the Kemper family—who, until the 1980s, were oblivious to this past. In order to shed better light on this history, institutions would need to open their archives, to be confronted with many other documents as well as primary and secondary sources.

For the Constitution of Archives of Psychoanalysis

In conclusion, from the standpoint of the construction of this collective history, it is worth mentioning the difficulties of an archival nature encountered during the writing of this text. Clearly, this is a problem experienced not only by historians of psychoanalysis, but all those who perform the task of writing history in Brazil, where many are the traumas and the open wounds, the unspoken that needs to be elaborated and repaired—such as the one we have been currently experiencing, regarding our patrimonial, slave-based past, marked by authoritarian tradition and massive social inequality.

Archives are fundamental—necessary, as Le Goff (1990) used to say—to catalogue both the production and its omissions. It is not a matter of encouraging an 'obsession with the past' that can trigger an excess of memory, or of turning it into a place of truth (Ricoeur, 2000). Less so, it is a matter of stimulating a positivist cult of facts and truth in the quest for absolute knowledge, as mentioned above.

In the relationship between truth and power, the archive is more than a tool for registering and organising statements. It is essential as a place of authority, which welcomes both memory as a conscious reserve and writing as a 'Freudian impression,' in the sense proposed by Derrida (2001). For him, the Freudian production can be inscribed in two places: the typographical, which evokes the impression and the feeling, and the circumcision, which refers to a direct mark on the body. The archive is situated between the two. Archives are like meeting spaces for historical vestiges, or an 'instituted space for a place of impression,' where interpretations and assessments of different findings can be both erected and debunked. Archives question history in its gaps, in its forgetfulness, in its voids and blank spaces.

There are significant gaps in the history of psychoanalysis, such as the aforementioned, and archives are meagre. We suffer from a lack of documentary sources and elements that enable the formation of archives, which would be able to cope with the complexity of forms and temporalities in this implementation and expansion. The archives of the first actors in this saga have been practically ignored by the institutions, which until recently showed little interest in them. As an example, it is worth remembering those of the first-generation psychiatrist and psychoanalyst, Mario Yahn, who played an important but little-known part in the field of mental health, and whose records were burned because the family did not know what fate to give them.

The Brazilian Psychoanalytical Society of São Paulo, the first institution founded in the country after the inception of the couch in 1938, disregarded the need to build archives for decades, to the point that, in the 1970s, during times of dictatorship, the board drafted the first project for organising these files, albeit 'with the elimination of confidential documents.' The structuring of documentary sources only began with the creation of the Documentation and Research Division of the History of Psychoanalysis in 2002, although with restricted access (Oliveira, 2005, p. 42).

A great effort is due, therefore, to restore the fragments and elements of this history that have already been gathered in different institutional and researchers' archives. From this perspective, and in conclusion, I believe that historiographic research would have much to gain from the creation of a physical and heterogeneous place that would be able to accommodate both the documentation that each researcher individually compiles in their journey—through recorded testimonies and collected manuscripts—and the archives of the protagonists of this history, who are not being welcomed in their institutions where they belong, and when this happens, their access is restricted, if not denied.

For years, I have argued that the university should develop a project for the constitution of archives of psychoanalysis (Oliveira, 2005), as a field of investigation for 'psi' knowledges, which could begin with the creation of a database.

The university as a space of diversity will be able to welcome the different ways of observing, classifying, and interpreting the history of this knowledge and clinic, which is constantly under construction. In its topo-nomological function and principle of consignment as an attempt to restore the meaning of the archive, the university would be the guardian exercising authority as in the space of *arkhêion*, with the researchers as *archons*, interpreters of the documents that compose it (Derrida, 2001, p. 14).

In fact, this was a dream that Manoel Berlinck had at the Laboratory of Basic Psychopathology of the Pontifical Catholic University of São Paulo (PUC-SP) at the beginning of this century. And there go two decades since that proposition was made, in the International Colloquium Archives of Psychoanalysis (Oliveira, 2005, 2009).

I hope this book, derived from the International Symposium on the History of Psychoanalysis in Latin America, held at the Institute of Psychology of the University of São Paulo, in 2019, can be another step in that direction.

References

Association Internationale d'Histoire de la Psychanalyse. (1987). '*Ici la vie continue* de *manière surprenante*.' *Contribution à l'histoire de la psychanalyse en Allemagne*. AIHP.

Bicudo, V. L. (1948). Contribuição para a história do desenvolvimento da psicanálise em São Paulo. *Arquivos De Neuro-Psiquiatria, IV, 1*, 69–72. https://doi.org/10.1590/S0004-282X1948000100006

Cerqueira, G. (Ed.). (1982). *Crise na psicanálise*. Graal.

de Certeau, M. (1975). *L'écriture de l'histoire*. Gallimard.

Derrida, J. (2001). *Mal de Arquivo. Uma impressão freudiana*. Relume Dumará.

Derrida, J., & Roudinesco, E. (2001). *De quoi demain ... dialogue*. Fayard/Galilée.

Ellenberger, H. F. (1970/1994). *Histoire de la découverte de l'inconscient*. Paris: Fayard.

Ellenberger, H. F. (1954–1991/1995). *Médecines de l'âme. Essais sur la folie et des guérisons psychiques*. Fayard.

Farge, A. (1997). *Des lieux pour l'histoire*. Seuil.

Ferreira, J. B. (1986). Une clinique de la psychanalyse au milieu de la favela de Cabritos. In H. O. Macedo (Ed.), *Le psychanalyste sur la terreur* (pp. 63–84). Matrice.

Ferreira, M. M. (2018). Notas iniciais sobre a história do tempo presente e a historiografia no Brasil. *Tempo e Argumento. Revista de história do tempo presente, 10*(23), 80–108. https://doi.org/10.5965/2175180310232018080

Foucault, M. (1972). *L'Archéologie du savoir*. Gallimard.

Foucault, M. (1973/1994). La vérité et les formes juridiques. In *Dit et écrits, II, 1976–1988* (pp. 538–646). Gallimard.

Freud, S. (1917/1968). Deuil et mélancolie. In *Métapsychologie* (pp. 145–171). Gallimard/Folio.

Freud, S. (1915/1968). Le refoulement. In *Métapsychologie* (pp. 45–63). Gallimard/Folio.

Freud, S. (1901/1973). *Psychopathologie de la vie quotidienne*. Payot.

Freud, S. (1937/1985). Constructions dans l'analyse. In *Résultats, idées, problèmes: Vol. 2. 1921–1938* (pp. 269–281). PUF.

Garner, G. (1994/1997). Sept fragments pour un Œdipe païen. In *Les travaux d'Œdipe* (pp. 21–53). Harmattan.

Garner, G. (2007). *Le psychanalyste infidèle*. Érès.

Granoff, W. (1975). *Filiations. L'avenir du complexe d'Oedipe*. Gallimard.

Hassoun, J., & Waljsbrot, C. (1991). *L'Histoire à la lettre*. Mentha.

Labourie, P. (2001). *Les français des années troubles. De la guerre d'Espagne à la Libération*, Desclée de Brouwer.

Labourie, P. (2019). *Penser l'événement 1940–1945*. Gallimard/Folio.

Lacan, J. (1953/1966). Fonction et champ de la parole et du langage en psychanalyse. In *Écrits* (pp. 237–322). Seuil.

Le Goff, J. (1990). *História e memória.* Campinas: Editora da Unicamp.
Oliveira, C. L. M. V. (2005). *História da psicanálise. São Paulo 1920–1969.* Escuta/Fapesp.
Oliveira, C. L. M. V. (Ed). (2009, March). Dossiê: Fragmentos, traços, marcas da psicanálise. Colóquio Internacional de Psicanálise, 2004. *Pulsional Revista de Psicanálise, 197,* 5–117.
Oliveira, C. L. M. V. (2017, November). Sob o discurso da 'neutralidade': as posições dos psicanalistas durante a ditadura militar. *História, Ciências, Saúde – Manguinhos, 24*(1), 79–90. https://doi.org/10.1590/s0104-59702017000400006
Porto-Carrero, J. P. (1932). A Contribuição brasileira à psychanalyse [Relatório da Seccção de Psychanalyse]. *Annaes do 3º Congresso Brasileiro de Neurologia Psychiatria e Medicina Legal* (pp. 321–325). Typ. Do Jornal do Comércio. (Original work published 1929)
Ricoeur, P. (2000). *La mémoire, l'histoire, l'oubli.* Seuil.
Roudinesco, E. (1994). *Généalogies.* Fayard.
Rovai, M. G. O., & Teixeira, E. A. C. (2016). Batismo de Sangue: literatura testemunhal como ferramenta do reconhecimento histórico da dor. *Revista Eletrônica Literatura e Autoritarismo, 27,* 66–86. https://doi.org/10.5902/1679849X21178. Retrieved June 30, 2019, from http://cascavel.ufsm.br/revistas/ojs-2.2.2/index.php/LA/index
Voldman, D. (Ed.). (1992). Avant-propos. La bouche de la Vérité ? La recherche historique et les sources orales. *Les cahiers de l'IHTP, 21,* 7–9.

4

Wounds of Dictatorship in Brazilian Psychoanalysis: Traumatic Revivals in Research on the History of Psychoanalysis

Belinda Mandelbaum

The reflections I present here are derived from my experience as a researcher of the history of psychoanalysis in Brazil, focusing on the period of the civil-military dictatorship that lasted for 21 years, from 1964 to 1985. In this endeavour, I consider the implications of my subjectivity in the configuration of the field of research, where they affect this field and are affected by it. These implications and the reflections on them will be taken as part of the method of research and the production of knowledge on the subject—a procedure that several authors in the humanities and social sciences call reflexivity (Bourdieu & Wacquant, 2002; Frosh & Baraitser, 2008), and consider ethically necessary to make explicit, as it positions, from the beginning, the perspective from which the researcher observes and mobilises the researched field.

B. Mandelbaum (✉)
Department of Social and Work Psychology, University of São Paulo, São Paulo, Brazil
e-mail: belmande@usp.br

B. Mandelbaum et al. (eds.), *Brazilian Psychosocial Histories of Psychoanalysis*, Studies in the Psychosocial,
https://doi.org/10.1007/978-3-030-78509-3_4

Historical Context

In 1964, a military coup deposed President João Goulart, a democratically elected labour representative who tried to implement basic reforms in the fiscal, administrative, university and, mainly, agrarian areas. His proposals, especially those concerning agrarian reform, were opposed by large landowners and parliamentarians with the support of conservative sectors of Brazilian society, among them businessmen and a significant part of the urban middle classes. In this period of the Cold War, marked by intense political polarisation, the 1964 Brazilian military coup was also supported by the United States, which feared the hegemony of Soviet socialism in Latin America, especially after the 1958 Cuban Revolution. The successive governments of the dictatorial period, that lasted until 1985, imposed a series of institutional acts (*atos institucionais*, AI) that constrained the Constitution and guaranteed the military stayed in power. The first, AI-1, enacted in 1964, ended direct elections; AI-2, in 1965, closed political parties, maintaining only two, the National Renovating Alliance (ARENA) and the Brazilian Democratic Movement (MDB), the latter representing the permitted opposition that gave the government a facade of democratic legitimacy. In 1968, AI-5 was enacted. This was the most terrible of the institutional acts of the dictatorial governments, closing the National Congress, prohibiting meetings and decreeing a state of siege. AI-5 inaugurated the period known as 'the years of lead,' marked by intense repression, persecution, violence, torture, disappearance and the death of those considered to be opponents of the regime. Despite Brazilian society's manifestations of opposition to the dictatorial regime, which emerged in 1968, the years of lead lasted until 1974, when a slow and gradual opening of the regime began. In 1978, a constitutional amendment revoked all institutional and complementary acts contrary to the Federal Constitution, but the military regime remained in power for two more successive government terms. In 1984, the social movement for the restoration of democracy, known as '*Diretas já*' (direct elections now), resulted in universal suffrage for the presidency of the republic. And in 1988 the new Federal Constitution was promulgated, as a result of struggles and consensus between diverse sectors of Brazilian society.[1]

The Research

Our research work, 'Psychoanalysis and social context in Brazil: transnational flows, cultural impact and authoritarian rule,'[2] was concerned with questions of how and why the main institutions of psychoanalysis thrived during the period of the most violent dictatorship in the country, and about psychoanalysis as a site for collusion with, and resistance to, the authoritarian regime. The research focused on institutional practices with reference to political violence, including the effects of authoritarian rule on psychoanalysis, and what happened in the post-dictatorship period in relation to demands to acknowledge, or silence the memory of, complicity. The investigation was carried out through archival research in psychoanalytical societies of São Paulo and Rio de Janeiro, analysis of published Brazilian psychoanalytical literature and extended in-depth interviews with psychoanalysts who lived and worked in the dictatorial period in the cities of Rio de Janeiro, São Paulo, Porto Alegre and London—all with the aim of providing a detailed case study of the impact of political repression on professional and intellectual practices.

After seven years of research, there is much to tell of this story (for some of its results, see Frosh & Mandelbaum, 2017, 2019; Mandelbaum et al., 2019; Mandelbaum et al., 2018; Rubin et al., 2016). First, I shall render account of some aspects mobilised in my subjectivity in the process of research, and the way they determined what

---

[1] Concerning the dictatorial period in Brazil, see: Gaspari, E. (2002/2014). *Coleção Ditadura.* RJ: Editora Intrínseca (Digital Edition, 2017) and Skidmore, T. (1988). *The politics of Military rule in Brazil: 1964–1985.* New York and Oxford: Oxford University Press.

[2] The research work, carried out between 2013 and 2019, was coordinated by myself and Stephen Frosh and received financial support from the São Paulo Research Foundation (Fundação de Amparo à Pesquisa do Estado de São Paulo, FAPESP). Parts of the research project and reflections on the collected data presented here are results of this long-shared research work.

and how I researched. Every research is interwoven, from its conception, with personal aspects of the researcher, of diverse orders: it starts from conscious and unconscious motivations or mobilises them in some way. A research enlaces traces of personal histories and elements of the identity of the researcher. It requires, therefore, as one of the dimensions dynamised in the research process, a true work of psychoanalysis, a 'researcher, know thyself.' This is because, on the one hand, the contact, even if always fragmentary, with the free motivations and associations of the researcher, their reveries and dreams, can allow the emergence of non-manifest elements of the researched field itself, as well as make more explicit and conscious the interests that determine and guide the research, producing choices and blind spots. On the other hand, this (self)reflexive work, by allowing recognition of the participation of the researcher's subjectivity in the determinations of the research field, contributes so that multiple and complex personal elements do not end up preventing the research findings from coming to light in their singularity. Hence, findings can be examined, as far as possible, outside the lights and shadows that the researcher throws on them. The phenomenon under investigation, as part of reality, is always infinite; that is, it is always beyond the work of the researcher. But our methods of knowledge tend to decipher phenomena by enclosing them and reducing them within the limits of our worldviews. 'Know thyself' implies knowing our research motivations and the reading keys we use to understand the world. Thus, I hope to be making it clear that, in this investigation, psychoanalysis is not only an object, but also an important part of the research method itself.

Then follows a part of my 'know thyself' in the research experience, which is interwoven into a personal tangle of many threads involving stories I have witnessed, that I live and have lived, and that constitute who I am. Moreover, as I will try to show, they have been instrumental in the direction of these investigations.

Research Timeline

This research project began in 2013, a year in which popular demonstrations in Brazil began opposing the increase in transport prices, but soon expanded to other demands and criticism of the government for deviations in public spending and corruption. It was also a period when the economy, after a decade of growth that allowed the rise of the so-called 'new middle classes,' began to enter an obvious crisis, threatening the fragile recent social gains. Amidst many protests on the streets throughout the country, voices opposed to democratic institutions began to gain attention among the crowds, calling for the military to return to power after approximately 30 years of incipient democracy, of which for 12 years the Workers' Party (*Partido dos Trabalhadores*, PT) was in government.

In the same year, 2013, the National Truth Commission was operating. This was made up of a group of prominent professionals in the legal, sociological, journalistic and even psychoanalytical fields. In 2011, President Dilma Rousseff had delegated to this group the task of investigating the stories of those persecuted, disappeared and killed by the civil-military dictatorship from 1964 to 1985. The work of this Commission produced an adverse reaction in military sectors, which after all had been pardoned in a broad, general and unrestricted amnesty agreement that marked the transition from dictatorship to democracy in the 1980s.[3]

In the wake of the National Truth Commission, truth commissions have been formed in several Brazilian states and at major universities, such as the University of São Paulo, to investigate crimes related to the dictatorial period. It was amid these tensions—on the one hand, the economic and political crisis and the public re-emergence of banners advocating the return of military governments and, on the other, the constitution of commissions with institutional support to investigate the crimes committed during the dictatorship—that our research project took place. We were, therefore, in resonance with the broader socio-political events underway in the country. Hence, our research could

[3] For the final report of the National Truth Commission, delivered to President Dilma Rousseff on December 10, 2014, see http://cnv.memoriasreveladas.gov.br/.

unfold as a (humble) contribution to the ongoing investigations, given that previous studies (Coimbra, 1995; Russo, 2012; Vianna, 1994) had already shown that the collaboration of professionals in the 'psy' field in general and psychoanalysts in particular, was not insignificant in the construction of theories and practices that legitimised and participated in state repression. In 2013, there was a melting pot of ideological and political struggles in which our research found its moment, motivation and justification.

Nazism and Brazilian Dictatorship

The research work with Professor Stephen Frosh, of the Department of Psychosocial Studies at Birkbeck College, also has a significant background that helps illuminate the whole process. A few years earlier, Stephen had researched the history of psychoanalysis in Germany during the Nazi period, which resulted in the book entitled *Hate and the Jewish Science: Anti-Semitism, Nazism and Psychoanalysis* (2005).

Along the curious paths of the twentieth century, Werner Kemper was one of the German psychoanalysts who worked at the Göring Institute, the key psychotherapy institute in Germany supported by the Nazis (where non-Jewish psychoanalysts from the Berlin Psychoanalytic Society migrated to). Kemper was head of the Berlin Polyclinic, where he treated war neuroses and was in favour of euthanasia for cases considered incurable.

After the war, in 1948 Kemper moved to Rio de Janeiro with the mission of working as a training analyst, thereby facilitating the creation of a psychoanalytic society affiliated with the International Psychoanalytical Association (IPA). In Rio, Kemper was the analyst of Leon Cabernite, who in turn analysed Amílcar Lobo, an army psychiatrist who from 1970 to 1974 served in one of the cruellest dungeons of the Brazilian dictatorship, while doing his psychoanalytic training and being in training analysis with Cabernite. Kemper was never asked about his past in Nazi Germany, and the Psychoanalytic Society of Rio de Janeiro, which he had helped to found, had for years covered up the participation of a psychoanalytic candidate in torture practices. Thus, we perceive a thread of transmission that begins in Berlin in the Nazi period and ends in the co-optation of psychoanalysts by the Brazilian dictatorship. History followed its course, and what Stephen Frosh researched in Germany ended up in Rio de Janeiro. It did not take much to arouse his interest in the relations between psychoanalysis and dictatorship in Brazil. It was, in part, an unfolding of his previous work. Benjamin's thesis on the rubble that accumulates over rubble in a single catastrophe (1940/1987) is a reading that applies to this story.

Dictatorship and Life

In my personal history, Nazism and the Brazilian dictatorship are also interwoven in a singular way. I was born in 1959 into a Jewish family in *Bom Retiro*, a neighbourhood in the city of São Paulo where Jewish immigrant families from post-war Europe have gathered, and I lived through the years of the civil-military dictatorship in Brazil as a child and adolescent. I remember several manifestations of censorship in that period—such as the newspaper *O Estado de São Paulo*, one of the main daily newspapers in the country, which was delivered every day at home with the news interspersed with bizarre culinary recipes in place of information prevented from circulating—and also a censorship imposed by my mother, who frightened at any comment made at home about the political or social reality, even the most banal ones, insisted for years that 'nothing was to be said in the streets,' letting slip into the domestic microcosm part of the micro-fascisms that reverberated across the social context of the period.

This insistence, which she repeated with the same urgency each time, leaning her apprehensive body over us, her daughters, became part of my ambiguous way of being in the world. She did not silence my indignation over social injustices—on the contrary, I believe she educated me to see them. But I did not protest in the streets or take part in strikes, despite having been a student at the University of São Paulo in 1977, a significant time in the student movements, and having a post in the university at a time of major strikes. I see myself then identified with and obedient to my mother, as she was also ambiguous in the face of the terror that had settled in the country. And I wonder if my engagement in this research today, as a psychoanalyst and researcher in the field of Social Psychology, is not also a form of reparation, mobilised by a feeling of guilt for all that I have not done.

Despite playing the role of the censor inside the house, my mother also imbued us with a pride in being from a family identified with the left-wing. Her parents had been from the Jewish workers' movement in Europe, the *Bund*, and my grandfather fled Poland in the early 1920s to avoid serving in the army. She also used to tell that during her youth, in the 1940s, she would sleep with a picture of the communist leader Luiz Carlos Prestes under her pillow. I bring these facts up because, from this experience in my personal history, I can glimpse a rich and, it seems to me, unexplored vein for us, Brazilian psychoanalysts, which is examining how we have been marked, in the most profound depths of ourselves, by the experience of the dictatorship. Because it is not just a question of a socio-political circumstances that shaped a period of our lives from which we would have been freed after the '*Diretas já*' movement of 1984. With this trivial domestic situation, I want to expose how the dictatorship unfolded in our innermost relationships, in the images I have of my mother in my childhood, and which I carry with me as indelible identifying traits, constituents of my personality. Part of my mother's severity—and of my own—as well as her care for us, finds its expressive form in the memory of her leaning body over us as she says: 'nothing is to be said in the streets.'

My mother's ideological affinities also affected the choice of the school I attended from 3 to 10 years old. Throughout the 60s, I studied at the Brazilian Jewish Gymnasium Scholem Aleichem. The *Scholem* was part of the project of a group of progressive Jewish immigrants from Eastern Europe. In the early 1950s, they gathered to create the *Casa do Povo* (House of the People), an institution with ties to secular left-wing Jewish movements in Europe, which were already advocating the preservation of Yiddish culture in the early decades of the twentieth century, within a broad, secular and universalist culture.

The idea for the *Casa do Povo* emerged in 1945, soon after the second great war, and its premises were inaugurated in the *Bom Retiro* neighbourhood in 1953, in memory of those who had succumbed in the

Nazi concentration camps. The project encompassed a newspaper, *Nossa Voz*, a theatre, the Brazilian Jewish Arts Theatre, and a school, *Scholem Aleichem*, pseudonym of one of the greatest writers of Yiddish literature, which also means 'peace be with us.' The *Casa do Povo*, a sort of Jewish cell of the Brazilian Communist Party made up of liberal intellectuals and professionals, had from the beginning, in the 1940s, a role in confronting the dictatorship of the *Estado Novo* (New State) of Getúlio Vargas, in times of exacerbated nationalism and restrictive practices concerning foreign cultures. The defence of Yiddish culture and language, which were taught at school, was part of this confrontation. It was a complex confrontation indeed, because an endangered language was being taught and a culture with an air of obsolescence was encouraged to thrive.

The *Scholem Aleichem* school also played a role in resistance in the years of the civil-military dictatorship during the 1960s and until the1980s, taking in the children of prisoners and politically persecuted persons, whether or not they were Jews (it was during this period that I studied there). In other words, the *Casa do Povo* proposed, as weapons in the fight against totalitarianism, the defence of a minority culture, a Jewish school of universalist ideals and a theatre, the Brazilian Jewish Arts Theatre.

At *Scholem*, in 1969, in the 4th-grade class, I had a colleague who seemed to like to shout in the middle of the classroom: 'my father has the Red Book of Mao at home!' I was amazed at that. Under my mother's orders of silence, I listened in amazement and admiration to the boy's daringness. His name was Marco Antônio Tavares Coelho Filho, and I never heard from him again until, at the beginning of our research, I read the book by the psychoanalyst Helena Besserman Vianna (1994), *Não conte a ninguém: contribuição à história das sociedades psicanalíticas do Rio de Janeiro* (*Don't tell anyone: contribution to the history of psychoanalytic societies in Rio de Janeiro*). Vianna reports the case arising from her denouncement to the Argentinian newspaper of psychoanalysis *Questionamos*, whose editor in the early 1970s was the Austrian psychoanalyst Marie Langer—an activist in Austria and the Spanish Civil War before she fled to Latin America—that there was a candidate in training at the Rio de Janeiro Psychoanalytic Society, affiliated with the IPA, who at the same time as training to be a psychoanalyst was a medical-captain of a torture squad. To support her claim, Vianna sent to *Questionamos* a clipping of the clandestine newspaper *Voz operária* (*Workers' voice*), linked to the Brazilian Communist Party (PCB), which announced that the psychiatrist Amílcar Lobo served as a torturer for the army. Vianna, who belonged to another psychoanalytic Society affiliated with the IPA in Rio, the Brazilian Psychoanalysis Society of Rio de Janeiro, had had access to the clandestine newspaper and recognised her work colleague there. She was also a member of the Brazilian Communist Party and a friend of the editor of the newspaper *Voz Operária*, Marco Antonio Tavares Coelho (my schoolmate's father), the one who had Mao's Red Book at home.

I came to know recently, during this research, that Helena Vianna received Marco Coelho's wife and two children as refugees in her home in Rio de Janeiro, in the period in which he was arrested and brutally tortured in the premises of the Department of Internal Operations (DOI) of the 2nd Army, in São Paulo. Before that, the family lived in Bom Retiro, almost in front of my house, and we studied at the same school. During their childhood, Vianna's children attended a summer camp, the Kinderland, where *Scholem Aleichem* students from São Paulo and Rio met, as there was also a *Scholem Aleichem* school, with the same ideological profile. The disturbing feeling is that the story we are dealing with in this research is not something distant from our spaces and our times. It involves us, and in my case, it has affected my mother, my home, my school and my summer camp holiday. And it unfolded throughout life, not so much as ghosts that haunt us, but as living presences standing beside me. A schoolmate, Olívio Moreira Helou, had his father killed by repression; a collegemate, Vera Paiva, too. Amílcar Lobo confessed in the 80s that he had accompanied, as a psychiatrist of the torture squad, the agony of Vera's father, deputy Rubens Paiva, in the basements of DOI-CODI (Department of Information Operations—Centre for Internal Defense Operations), 'moribund, a single purple ecchymosis from the root of the hair to the tips of the feet.'[4] I currently work with Vera Paiva in the Department of Social Psychology at USP,

[4] Testimony of Amilcar Lobo at the time of his identification. "Lobo gives names of military torturers of the Doi-Codi" (Lobo dá nomes de militares torturadores do Doi-Codi). *Jornal do Brasil*, pp. 18, 28 set. 1986. Pastas de recortes de jornais do STM, n. TGM. Tortura no Governo Militar. https://dspace.stm.jus.br//handle/123456789/130461.

and the theme of her father's disappearance and its various developments in the family and social scene is the subject of distressing conversations until today. I am therefore speaking of a trauma that is a living presence in events that continue to traumatise. As it turns out, the research became entangled in life, and participating in it, publishing its findings, was my late form of denunciation, perhaps at this point in life more free from the censorship motivated by the terror that I shared with my mother.

Research and Trauma

The research into psychoanalysis in the years of the dictatorship is also traumatic: it produces successive traumatising episodes in the form of new findings, new information and, also from the lack of information available. Here are some examples:

1. We searched for the names of psychoanalysts and psychoanalytical institutions in the archives of the Department of Political and Social Order (DEOPS), a former repressive body and prison for political prisoners in the city of São Paulo. These archives are currently maintained by the State Archives, where access to the information is public and open, and many of the datasheets and charts are available online, with the archivists actively assisting in retrieving the information held. However, it is a disturbing experience to leaf through historic processes including enquiries, information and photographs about people and institutions investigated, some of them where I studied, such as the University of São Paulo, where I graduated in Psychology from 1977 to 1981, still during the dictatorship, and the *Sedes Sapientae* Institute, where I did my first psychoanalytical training. But if we look in these archives for agents of repression or who have collaborated with them—in the case of our research, for professionals in the psychoanalytic field who have been part of or acted on behalf of the repressive bodies or had some form of collaboration with them—it is much more difficult to find any information. As one Archive worker told us, 'truckloads of documents were burned.' Having accounts derived from the interviews that pointed to facts about the relations

among psychoanalysts, psychoanalytic institutions and the State in Brazil at the time of the dictatorship, particularly the proximity and collaboration with members of the government, military and press organisations or, on the contrary, resistance to them, we needed to find some documentary evidence. We are aware that the memories of the deponents carry a complex relation to history: it cuts them, deforms them, privileges certain events, exaggerates facts or skips them, according to their ideological and affective dispositions. Also, our elective affinities as researchers, our relations to psychoanalysis and its forms of insertion in Brazil, promote singular manners of reading the facts in these accounts. The material evidence, in its turn, can allow some objective distancing to position the past more clearly, offering plausible and grounded readings. The documents dialogue with the narrated accounts, providing detail and conferring more or less validity on them, but we had to acknowledge that the evidence we were looking for had disappeared. There is evidence that several activities of educational and training institutions in the 'psy' area have been monitored and registered by the repressive bodies. While there is a wealth of information, and charts full of records on opponents of the regime and their victims, nothing remains to indicate the perpetrators.

2. The Truth Commission of the University of São Paulo, which was coordinated by Professor Janice Theodoro da Silva of the History Department, operated between 2013 and 2018. One of her researchers told us that at the time of the dictatorship, there was a DEOPS office operating within the rectory, controlling all the activity of teachers and students, with the power to control who was employed and who was enrolled. Several faculty members who worked during that period were aware of the existence of the office and passed through there, but no material evidence remains. Professor Marilena Chauí, who had been the Head of the Philosophy Department at the time, stated, on the occasion of the launch of the Truth Commission at the university, that she had cause to engage with the DEOPS, as she had encountered difficulties when attempting to hire a Professor of Philosophy who had been approved in a public competition. In the Rectory, she was instructed to enter a small room with

no window where she talked to an authority who told her at the end of the conversation that '...you didn't come here, this place doesn't exist, I don't exist.' In short, it seems almost impossible to accurately reconstruct history and this, in my view, is part of the trauma that continues producing effects to this day.

3. For months, we tried to establish a dialogue with the archives of the Brazilian Psychoanalysis Society of São Paulo (SBPSP) in order to begin our research.[5] There has been a Memory Centre since the 1990s; its webpage used to state that it was open to researchers—until we started the project, but for months we were told that we should wait because the archives were being organised. After some insistent e-mails from us consulting them on the possibility of a first meeting, they replied that the Centre had changed its statute to the effect that only organised archives could be consulted. And as there were none yet organised, none could be consulted. This incident was relayed to Lucia Valladares, who had conducted research on the history of Psychoanalysis in São Paulo between the 1920s and the 1970s (2005), and she told me that in the 1990s, during her research in the same society, she had encountered the same responses. That means that the Division of Documentation and Research of the History of Psychoanalysis of SBPSP existed for over 20 years, with a huge archive about psychoanalysts important to the history of the institution (documents, photographs, libraries, films) and with the public intention of promoting research, but had failed to organise those materials, thus preventing access for research. Some time after our insistent e-mails, the webpage was taken down and substituted with an autographed photograph of Freud, accompanied by the brief history of its acquisition by the division. Cristiana Facchinetti and Carlos Ponte (2003) and Jane Russo (2012), who researched the history of psychoanalysis in Rio de Janeiro, also discuss the active obstruction of access to the archive of the *Sociedade Psicanalítica do Rio de Janeiro* (Psychoanalytic Society of Rio de Janeiro). The institution entrusted to two historians the narrative of its own history and when the document was ready, parts of it were removed.

[5] See Chapter 5 of this volume.

Lack of Evidence and Oblivion of History

It seems, thus, almost impossible to reconstruct history from what remains, but following the recommendation of the historian Carlo Guinsburg (2010), we propose that the obscuring of evidence can work as evidence itself, when documented as a 'witnessing of their own moment' (Guinsburg, 2010, p. 385). This can offer clues towards the construction of a historical account about the relationship between psychoanalysis and the dictatorship in Brazil. Yet the lack of evidence is a fact that demands further interpretation: we understand it as an indication of the presence of the power exercised over the documents created both during and after the dictatorial period. We know how the history of dictatorships in the twentieth century is full of censorship, repression and disappearances, and how the dictatorial forces operate through concealing facts, the murder not only of millions of people, but also the murder of memory (Rossi, 2003). Guinsburg (2010) suggests that 'the obstacles that interpose themselves to the investigation in the shape of gaps and distortions of the documentation are part of the account' (Guinsburg, 2010, p. 383). The destruction of evidence enforces the power operating during the dictatorial period and provides a testimony to its permanence in the present time. Who holds power over the documents related to the history of psychoanalysis in Brazil? The e-mail we have received from the Documentation Division (*Divisão de Documentação*) is signed by two psychoanalysts. Those who prevent access by researchers to the documents at the *Sociedade Psicanalítica do Rio de Janeiro*, or those who censor pages from a historical report about the institution itself, are, most possibly, also psychoanalysts belonging to the same institution. That means, there is a perpetual unease/discomfort produced by the evidence which promotes, on the part of those who hold power over them, its concealment or disappearance. In the specific case of psychoanalytic institutions, this concealment of its own history gains a singular dimension: psychoanalysis has one fundamental path towards the elaboration of trauma that appears as an obstacle to a more fulfilling psychic development, which is the conscious recovering of history and of the patient's manner of operating connected to their lived experiences.

How should we understand, then, the fact that psychoanalytic institutions may activate mechanisms of avoidance of contact with their own histories?

The censorship and destruction of evidence do not, however, make history disappear. On the contrary, it reveals how it operates. We can see an ideology at work, a certain conception of psychoanalysis that makes itself hegemonic, the manifestation of a power that seeks to obscure to the institution and its members the facts of its own history and the motivations for their concealment. It is Freud (1930/1961) himself, nonetheless, who built a strange and surprising hypothesis, yet of deep significance for what we are trying to deal with here: what has lived never disappears; forgetting never means a complete elimination of the traces of memory. He writes, in 'Civilization and its Discontents':

> Since we overcame the error of supposing that the forgetting we are familiar with signified a destruction of the memory-trace—that is, its annihilation—we have been inclined to take the opposite view, that in mental life nothing which has once been formed can perish—that everything is somehow preserved and that in suitable circumstances (when, for instance, regression goes back far enough) it can once more be brought to light. (Freud 1930/1961, p. 69)

In Brazil, the attempt to erase memories and the lack of access to historical evidence are part of the trauma we continue to experience today. Ferenczi (1933/1981) said that trauma occurs in the combination of two times—the time of the traumatic event and a later time of non-recognition by another, by a third, that the event in fact occurred. Only when there is such recognition can the trauma be elaborated. In childhood and adolescence, I lived with experiences of censorship, repression and interaction with children whose parents disappeared, were tortured and died. In this academic research on the history of Brazilian psychoanalysis, I have lived the second time the lack of historical record and memory, the absence or inaccessibility of evidence. This alone is a form of repetition of the trauma, which spreads on the social scene through the reproduction of violence in its various manifestations. There is a recognition of recent Brazilian history that still needs to happen, along with the social instances in which the crimes committed must be judged and punished. In this, I also see the social meaning of our research work, the work of all those who have been focusing on our recent history, to the extent that they can make the records of our history available to the Brazilian society.

References

Benjamin, W. (1940/1987) Teses sobre o conceito de história. In *Walter Benjamin - Obras escolhidas. Vol. 1. Magia e técnica, arte e política. Ensaios sobre literatura e história da cultura.* Brasiliense.

Bourdieu, P., & Wacquant, L. (2002). *Convite à Sociologia reflexiva.* Relume Dumará.

Coimbra, C. (1995). *Guardiões da ordem: Uma viagem pelas práticas 'psi' no Brasil do 'milagre.'* Editora Oficina do Autor.

Facchinetti, C., & Ponte, C. (2003). De barulhos e silêncios: contribuições para a história da psicanálise no Brasil. *Psychê, 7*(11), 59–83.

Ferenczi, S. (1933/1981). *Reflexiones sobre el traumatismo. Obras completas* (Vol. 4). Espasa Calpe.

Freud, S. (1930/1961). Civilization and its discontents. In *Standard Edition* (Vol. 21). Hogarth Press.

Frosh, S. (2005). *Hate and the 'Jewish Science': Anti-semitism, Nazism and Psychoanalysis.* Palgrave Macmillan.

Frosh, S., & Baraitser, L. (2008). Psychoanalysis and psychosocial studies. *Psychoanalysis, Culture & Society, 13*(4), 346–365.

Frosh, S., & Mandelbaum, B. (2017). 'Like kings in their kingdoms': Conservatism in Brazilian Psychoanalysis during the dictatorship. *Political Psychology, 38*, 591–604.

Frosh, S., & Mandelbaum, B. (2019). Psychosocial histories of Psychoanalysis. *Culturas Psi, 1,* 1–13.

Gaspari, E. (2002/2014). *Coleção Ditadura.* Editora Intrínseca (Digital Edition, 2017).

Guinsburg, C. (2006/2010). *El hilo y las huellas: lo verdadeiro, lo falso, lo fictício.* Fondo de Cultura Económica.

Mandelbaum, B., Frosh, S., Rubin, A., & Theodoro, A. R. (2019). Antropofagia e Autoritarismo na Psicanálise Brasileira. *Calibán Revista Latino-Americana De Psicanálise, 17*, 112–125.

Mandelbaum, B., Rubin, A., & Frosh, S. (2018). 'He didn't even know there was a dictatorship': The complicity of a psychoanalyst with the Brazilian military regime. *Psychoanalysis and History, 20*, 37–57.

Rossi, P. (1991/2003). *El pasado, la memoria, el olvido.* Nueva Visión, Buenos Aires.

Rubin, A., et al. (2016). 'No memory, no desire': Psychoanalysis in Brazil during repressive times. *Psychoanalysis and History, 18*, 93–118.

Russo, J. (2012). The social diffusion of psychoanalysis during the Brazilian military regime: Psychological awareness in an age of political repression. In J. Damousi & M. B. Plotkin (Eds.), *Psychoanalysis and politics: Histories of psychoanalysis under conditions of restricted political freedom.* Oxford University Press.

Skidmore, T. (1988). *The politics of Military rule in Brazil: 1964–1985.* Oxford University Press.

Valladares, C. L. O. (2005). *História da Psicanálise – São Paulo 1920–1969.* Ed. São Paulo Escuta.

Vianna, H. B. (1994). *Não conte a ninguém: contribuição à história das sociedades psicanalíticas do Rio de Janeiro.* Imago.

5

Learning from cases—The Problem of Sharing Knowledge in Psychoanalysis

Stephen Frosh

Case Studies

In his posthumously published book *Thinking in Cases*, the British historian of science John Forrester (2017) promotes the value of research based on case histories, with the psychoanalytic case being its exemplary instance. The general argument includes the claim that such case studies offer an in-depth engagement with experience that produces modes of knowledge additional to other types of scientific reasoning. The psychoanalytic case in particular can demonstrate ways of being, feeling and thinking with general implications for the 'human sciences' and yet which tend to be occluded by statistical approaches such as those focused on in psychology. Forrester expresses well the dual dynamic of psychoanalytic discovery, which is that it is concerned with exploring in depth

S. Frosh (✉)
Department of Psychosocial Studies, Birkbeck, University of London, London, UK
e-mail: s.frosh@bbk.ac.uk

B. Mandelbaum et al. (eds.), *Brazilian Psychosocial Histories of Psychoanalysis*, Studies in the Psychosocial,
https://doi.org/10.1007/978-3-030-78509-3_5

the complexity of individual lives *and* making public the findings of such explorations so that they can be turned into more general principles or even theories. These more general versions of the observations of individual cases, which as they find acceptance in the psychoanalytic community gradually become framed as 'discoveries,' guide the development of psychoanalysis in terms of both its theory—its conceptualised way of understanding human functioning—and its application as clinical and (to a lesser extent) extra-clinical practice. Forrester (p. 12) comments:

> psychoanalytic discourse combines two unlikely features: it promises a new way of telling a life in the twentieth century, a new form for the specific and unique facts that make that person's life their life. And at the same time, it attempts to render that way of telling a life public, of making it scientific. The bridge between these two aims is the case history, along with the curious and distinctive narratives of transference and countertransference phenomena that increasingly came to dominate 'clinical writing', as it is called.

There are a number of useful ideas gathered up in this short quotation, aside from the broad problem of the relationship between psychoanalysis and 'science,' which has dogged psychoanalytic epistemology from the start, but which I do not intend to discuss in detail here (see Frosh, 2006). Suffice it to say that whilst that discussion retains some interest, the opening out of the understanding of science in the post-Kuhnian period (Kuhn, 1962)—Kuhn being a major influence on Forrester, who was at one point his student—has removed a lot of its sting. The issue has shifted (or should have done) away from justifying psychoanalysis as 'scientific' and instead towards ensuring that its methods, observations and theoretical claims are well grounded, and that this includes openness to scrutiny and a process of self-questioning that makes it receptive to new ideas and the abandonment, where appropriate, of old ones. This in itself is probably enough to indicate at least that it shares in the scientific 'world view' (as Freud, 1933, was at pains to argue in his 'lecture,' *The Question of a Weltanschauung*). Whether these admirable characteristics reflect the situation or not in practice is still an open question, but the fact that psychoanalysis changes in response to shifts in society and the issues raised by patients—for instance that it is much more heavily ‘relational’ nowadays than it has ever been before, or that there is more interest in an ethical response to race and gender issues than was the case a generation or two ago—suggests that the psychoanalytic edifice is not impermeable to the forces that act on it and that some at least of its adherents are non-defensive enough to keep trying to respond to new cultural currents and indeed to make things better. What is equally significant in Forrester’s comment is how the ‘case’ is seen as particularly appropriate to ‘telling a life in the twentieth century,’ reflecting the domination of psychological narrative and a mode of ‘interiority’ that characterises this phase of modernity. Channelling lives into ‘cases’ helps make sense of them in ways that are culturally communicable (hence, ‘telling a life public’), partly because of psychoanalysis itself, which has made a certain vocabulary and narrative available and comprehensible, so that reference to the unconscious and to developmental conflicts of various kinds is acceptable in accounts that warrant explanatory claims. In addition, the note about transference and countertransference reveals some of the complexities of such stories, to which I shall return.

The idea that ‘thinking in cases’ can be a legitimate way to advance knowledge is fairly widely shared by those who are interested in psychoanalysis as a practice of knowledge. The sociologist Michael Rustin (2019), for instance, who is a long-time supporter of the value of psychoanalysis as both a clinical practice and a social theory, argues that there are systematic ways of doing case study research and that this is a legitimate research procedure not just for psychoanalysis, but for all areas where complex intersections mean that knowledge of the individual case cannot easily be deduced from broad trends across populations. ‘Ethnographers in anthropology and sociology, life-history researchers, organizational researchers, management scientists and consultants all use case-study methods,’ he writes (p.97), ‘even though their “cases” may be communities and institutions rather than individual subjects.’ One might argue that this is as much an ethical issue as a scientific one. Rustin states (ibid.), ‘The practical and ethical reason why attention be given to “cases” in medicine and law is that individuals and therefore “cases” matter in their own right. Individuals receiving medical care, or being tried by the courts, are recognised as of value in themselves, and not only as instances of some larger category.' This perhaps locates a particular reason why psychoanalysis retains its importance in neoliberal times: when so much else is based around a logic of efficiency and productivity, almost always signifying the interchangeability of human subjects as each one wears out its usefulness, psychoanalysis asserts that every individual matters, that therapy for the concerns of complex human subjects might need to be long and intense and hence 'inefficient,' and that whilst understanding one individual might not produce knowledge of all, knowledge of the general can never be confidently focused down on any one person's experience.

This of course does not mean that no generalisations can or should be made, only that the parameters whereby this occurs are always under suspicion. Rustin (2019) notes how when a claim is made for a single case, other analysts who already accept the premises of that claim (for instance, that it includes the unconscious) inspect their own experience to see if it resonates with the case example. This is the main way in which clinical ideas develop and possibly one route whereby theory changes too, though one might also argue that theory has its own dynamic, its own *aesthetic*, whereby something that 'makes sense' and refreshes existing theory comes to have a life of its own as a necessary idea—an argument reasonably in line with Kuhn's (1962) general framework. What is characteristic of psychoanalysis, however, as much as it is of other social sciences and possibly of science more generally, is how much it works with implicit assumptions. Again, this has Kuhnian resonance. As Forrester (2017, p. 9) avers, Kuhn's notion of an 'exemplar' as a textbook way in which scientists learn to do their work gives prominence to a kind of inductive, semi-intuitive knowledge that is hard to counter even by evidence that goes against it. 'One might say,' he writes, 'that a scientific discipline is automatically protected against excessive self-critical and sceptical questioning by its axioms and fundamental tenets being embodied in a set of practices founded in tacit knowledge which cannot be rendered into propositional and thence universal form.' Analysts, like others, know what they are doing because it becomes part of their automatic practice, and it is only at times when something really disruptive takes place (e.g. the clash between Kleinians and Freudians in the British

Psychoanalytical Society that followed Anna Freud's move to England—King & Steiner, 1991) that this knowledge comes into question. And maybe it has to be this way: starting again every day is exhausting, and not necessarily in the interests of patients or analysts themselves; Bion's (1967) famous 'without memory and desire' injunction was never meant to mean exactly that.

Yet everyone also knows there are problems with this, not least because of something intrinsic to psychoanalysis: the issue of transference. Referring to Freud's case histories, Forrester (2017, p.65) comments:

> Analysis of them reveals that the process of their writing obeys the same laws of transference and countertransference as the analytic situation itself. One can show with Dora, or the Wolf Man, or with the rhetorical strategies of the auto-analytic *The Interpretation of Dreams*, how the reader is implicated in Freud's countertransference—his rhetorical mastery or lack of it. Thus, the transmission of psychoanalysis via Freud's clinical writing implies the repetition—or at the very least the remobilization—of the original relations of transference and countertransference evident in the relation between patient and analyst.

Transference and countertransference inhabit the very essence of the psychoanalytic encounter, troubling all attempts at an 'objective' reading and making problematic the generalisation of claims to other situations with different analytic pairs. It is for this reason that Forrester (p.66) dubs all psychoanalytic writing as 'exemplary of a failure': 'Psychoanalytic writing fails to transmit psychoanalytic knowledge because it is always simultaneously a symptom.' Rustin (2019) also acknowledges this, pointing out that the existence of transference makes research that is based, for instance, on transcripts or recordings of sessions dubious as one cannot ever know for sure what a statement from either patient or analyst might 'mean' in the context of the relationship that exists between them. Indeed, even the *absence* of a statement might be highly communicative—an analyst's thoughtful silence, for instance—yet this is very difficult to use as the basis for research and generalisable knowledge claims. For Rustin, this places a responsibility on the analyst to find a way to offer a comprehensive description of the psychoanalytic encounter that includes all aspects of this situation, including what goes on in the analyst's mind. For Forrester, it is as much a matter of recognising how psychoanalysis is what might be called a fully reflexive practice, embodying exactly the theories that it propounds. He writes (Forrester, 2017, p.65), 'Psychoanalytic writing is not just writing *about* psychoanalysis; it is writing subject to the same laws and processes as the psychoanalytic situation itself. In this way psychoanalysis can never free itself of the forces it attempts to describe.'

It will hopefully be clear that this brief account of the issues raised by the idea of 'thinking in cases' is not a critique of psychoanalysis so much as an evocation of the particular contribution of psychoanalysis to the broader psychosocial understanding of what 'reflexivity' might mean in the research process (Frosh, 2019). In terms of research in, or indeed researching, psychoanalysis, reflexivity basically announces that the disciplinary perspective of the 'investigator' as well as her or his 'personal' characteristics impacts upon, and is responsive to, the supposed 'object' of knowledge (the analysand/patient). Put differently, awareness of reflexivity indicates that there is no totally 'objective' knowledge in this field, but rather the existence of human subjects who might take up the position of researcher and researched, but continue with their everyday activities of trying to work out what is happening (the meaning of their encounter) and adjusting themselves to that. It therefore points to a potentially subversive procedure in which there is analysis of the conditions of emergence of knowledge as well as the apparent objects of knowledge themselves. Consistent with this is the vision of research as a mode of knowledge production that directly implicates the *subjective* presence of the researcher within the account of the *object* of study—a position opposed to the traditional objectivism of much social 'science.' To push this to its extreme, we might even say that a truly objective approach *requires* acknowledgement of, and mediation by, the subjective processes of the researcher—a point emphasised in psychoanalytic infant observation procedures as well as psychoanalytic clinical practice. Further practice relevance is generated through the centrality of psychoanalytic *psychotherapy* as the setting for the generation of psychoanalytic knowledge. There is awareness of how the 'patient' comes into being through the activities of psychotherapy as a mode of self-understanding that is saturated with general social assumptions; crudely, we only know ourselves as patients because psychoanalysis exists.

The Impossibility of the Case

The discussion of thinking in cases reveals how powerful this methodology can be in generating forms of knowledge that attend to the complexity of the intense intersubjective process of the psychoanalytic encounter. However, there are some major caveats that are largely to do with the instability of the knowledge produced in this way—how it is highly dependent on the specific circumstances under which it is produced, including the particularities of each analyst-analysand pair. This has long been recognised amongst psychoanalysts interested in what used to be called 'clinical facts.' For instance, Spence (1987, p.112): 'If our hermeneutic position is correct, then it must follow that the meaning of the material is highly dependent on who is listening to it, and that what was true for the treating analyst, at a particular time and place in the treatment, will never be true again.' Or, from a different school of psychoanalytic thought, Edna O'Shaughnessy (1994, p. 941) comments, 'When I make a truth claim, I do not claim to know the truth, or all the truth, but only *a* truth. Other true formulations are always possible.' It might be noted that in essence this is not different from any qualitative research investigation, where the small numbers of participants and reactive nature of the 'measures' used, for example in an ethnography or narrative analysis, place strict limits on generalisability claims. What happens instead is that the 'thickness' of the material generated by the research gives rise to more elaborated understanding of the particular cases being investigated, which then generates new or deepened analysis of other cases in other situations and with other investigators, gradually producing an archive of reputable and repeated findings.

There is an additional difficulty here, however, which has to do with the *quality* of psychoanalytic case reports. Some analysts have themselves been critical about this, doubting the validity of published clinical material because of its low level of objectivity even given the constraints of what might be appropriate to the psychoanalytic situation. Spence

(1987, p.80) is famously scathing on the trustworthiness of the psychoanalytic archive: 'Instead of an archive, we have a literature of anecdotes, a dumping ground of observations which have little more evidential value than a 30-year-old collection of flying saucer reports.' One special problem with psychoanalytic clinical case reports is that they are often *fictitious* in their published form because of the requirements of confidentiality and worries on the part of analysts about what might happen if their patients recognise themselves in the clinical account, or think that they do. The consequence is that the 'archive' of psychoanalysis is an unreliable one not just because of the unconscious investment of psychoanalysts in their material (the wish that it should show their mastery or that the patient will improve or indeed that they will make a great contribution to the literature) but because the conscious, deliberate manipulation of case material interferes with meeting the requirement of full transparency and accountability. If, as sometimes happens (and of course usually for good reason), the gender of a patient is changed or case examples are made up of 'composites,' how can a reader ever be confident that they represent what actually happened in the consulting room? Yet psychanalytic cases often seem to be of this kind—carefully managed to protect the person of the analysand, but in so doing ruining the chance of achieving the level of open scrutiny that makes it possible to determine what can be concluded from such cases. 'Case histories' might still be expressive of an analyst's view and experience and might still offer something to be learnt from and to 'think' with, but they are rarely stable as sources of evidence, creating problems for historical as well as clinical research.

Institutional Histories

The material outlined above is concentrated on the principles of psychoanalytic investigation of individual 'cases' in the major tradition of personal psychoanalysis and clinical writing. However, there is a substantial literature on psychoanalysis applied to organisations and social systems, including ethnographic and historical studies of psychoanalysis itself (e.g. Frosh, 2012; Plotkin, 2001; Schechter, 2014), and some of the same points and concerns arise. In a previous article, Belinda Mandelbaum and I have discussed the effect of the necessary reflexivity of psychoanalytic explorations when considering the histories of the institutions of psychoanalysis, specifically in Brazil (Frosh & Mandelbaum, 2019). There we suggested that psychoanalysis has demonstrated powerfully how institutions have ways of organising themselves that reflect 'unconscious' dynamics, even if what is meant here by 'unconscious' is somewhat different from what is meant by the term when applying it to individuals. Fundamentally, as generations of researchers in the 'Tavistock' open-systems traditions (e.g. Obholzer &Roberts, 1994) have shown, organisations can and do create remarkably inventive mechanisms to defend themselves against anxiety. These often take the form of modes of denial, ways of 'not knowing' that may range between conscious cover-ups and less conscious refusals to acknowledge the truth of the past, or indeed of present-day infelicities. Psychoanalysis consequently offers an entry-point to understand the apparent irrationalities of organisational life, and this includes the organisation of psychoanalysis itself. That is, just as the mental space of *psychoanalysts* is infiltrated and impacted upon by unconscious features of the analytic situation (including transference), so is the social space of psychoanalytic *organisations*. Fear, pressure, egotism, competitiveness, idealisation and professional ambition: these are mobilised in the service of unconscious wishes by people and by the institutional structures which psychoanalysts use to manage their lives.

In the context of the discussion on thinking in cases outlined above, this raises some questions. Do specific 'cases' of psychoanalytic institutional histories, such as those we have been investigating in Brazil, reveal general attributes of psychoanalysis? And to what extent can reports of such 'cases' be trusted when there are often problems about confidentiality and ethical concerns—not to mention conflicts of interest and personal investments—that block publication or wide discussion of their findings? Do the problems of distortion of case material also apply to institutional cases and if so, what can be rescued from them when trying to trace a reliable history of psychoanalysis? There are many issues here, including complex patterns of transference between members of different psychoanalytic generations; preservation of conscious and unconscious ‘secrets’ that develop in all cultures but are perhaps especially potent in societies where there has been authoritarian rule and violent terror; self-protective denial of responsibility for disturbing or shameful events; but also straightforward institutional politics in the sense of one group of analysts seeking to hold sway over others in relation to the development of psychoanalysis as a whole. At times, there have been striking demonstrations of openness that have cast light on the historical functioning of psychoanalytic institutions; the full documentation of the British Psychoanalytic Society’s ‘Controversial Discussions’ (King &Steiner, 1991) and the exhibition put on at the International Psychoanalytic Association Congress of 1985 in Hamburg, documenting the history of psychoanalysis in Nazi Germany (Brecht et al., 1985), are probably the best examples. The latter is a particularly potent instance of an institutional history that was buried for a long time—from the end of the Second World War until the 1985 Congress, to be precise—and which continued to be systematically overlooked even after its details were revealed by the Hamburg exhibition, both reflecting and producing continued enactments of historical denial (Frosh, 2005).

The point here is to ask whether the admirable psychoanalytic notion of ‘thinking in cases’ can be sustained when the ‘cases’ are those of psychoanalytic institutions, if there are pressures at the personal, social and institutional levels to block knowledge of those cases and to prevent communication about them. In relation to historical studies of psychoanalysis itself, this would mean presenting ‘case material’ that is distorted and unreliable. This is indeed the situation, at least in some places. In the context of our research in Brazil, Belinda Mandelbaum and I have had some professional experiences that suggest an institutional temptation towards denial that makes it very difficult to have confidence in the histories of psychoanalysis in the country. Given that our research focused on an especially troubling period—the time of the dictatorship, from 1964 to 1985—this was no real surprise, though we had hoped that the general psychoanalytic impulse towards openness might be more powerful than the contrary defence. A brief list of some of the experiences we have had in our work in Brazil, some of which have been reported elsewhere, includes the following:

1. In a previous article (Frosh & Mandelbaum, 2019), we commented on an official book documenting the history of the São Paulo society, *Álbum de família: imagens, fontes e ideias da Psicanálise em São Paulo*, published by the Sociedade Brasileira de Psicanalise in 1994. We noted that this is a very attractive picture book, but that the 'history' it provides is neither analytic nor critical; rather, it is of a suggestive and evocative, even elusive, kind. The book in fact consists almost entirely of photographs tracing the history of the Society through the figures who dominated it, ranging from its early founders (including photographs of Freud himself, even though he never ventured to Brazil) through to the 1980s, with one highlight being pictures of Wilfred Bion on his visits to Brazil in the 1970s. The situation is compounded by the few written texts that are included in the *Álbum de família*, which studiously avoid any discussion of the social and political meaning of the photographs themselves, or of the Society's actual history. Indeed, in its introduction, the book is accurately described as 'A summary of images, with very little explanatory text. An iconography merely as the raw material for dreams' (p.12). Perhaps ironically, but without any indication of how a reader might act on it, the introduction goes on to hint that these images and dreams could obscure the truth: 'We know how much is hidden in family pictures,' it says. 'They are not true, although not properly lies per se.' This passage ends with a provocation that is enticing but to our minds empty: the texts and photographs in the book are 'suggestions to be taken as remains of the day for us to dream our psychoanalysis, our environment, our history, and finally, our identity' (ibid.; our translation). We argued that this comment is illustrative of a way of conceptualising psychoanalysis that had and continues to have a marked presence in the psychoanalytic community, at least in Brazil and possibly elsewhere. The history of the institution was not *investigated*; that might have shown up numerous issues that would require serious confrontation. In place of the stringent work of memory and reconstruction or working through of history, readers are invited to *dream* the history of psychoanalysis in São Paulo. This means that all the aspects of psychoanalytic history in the region that really demand examination—its high prices, its

elitism, its promotion of conservative family values, its complicity with the civil-military dictatorship of the 1960s and 1970s—and that can be viewed as breaches of the psychoanalytic ethic, are covered over and lost in the mist of dreams. Intriguingly, when a version of our critique was briefly referenced in a previous article (Mandelbaum et al., 2018), we received privately a critical note that had arisen from a reading of the article by a British psychoanalyst in contact with the author of the original introduction to the *Álbum de família*. We were accused in this note of taking the author 'concretely rather than, as I understood it, an invitation to look deeper.' This might be true—except that the 'invitation' is an obscure one, clouded by the language of dreams.

2. We report in our 2019 paper on the difficulty we had in gaining access to the archives in the Memory and Documentation Centre of the Brazilian Psychoanalytic Society of São Paulo, where we were trying to trace a letter written by one of the founders of Brazilian psychoanalysis, Durval Marcondes, which we suspected implicated him in threats against student leaders during the dictatorship, when he was teaching at the University of São Paulo. We were told that this would not be possible and indeed that we could not gain access to any material in the Centre. This was because only documentation that has been organised and catalogued was open to researchers, and the documents we were interested in had not been processed—and there was no timescale for that happening. A year or so later, we were informed that Marcondes' documents were now organised and open for research, although it seems that they had been closed for decades, as was still the case for most of the rest of the archives. Another year later (July 2019) and the website had been reopened (after our initial inquiry, it had been reduced to a paper by Bion), suggesting that it is now possible for research to be carried out in the Centre.
3. The paper we wrote on these institutional issues was initially commissioned and accepted for publication in the *Revista Brasileira de Psicanálise*, which declares itself to be an 'official publication of the Brazilian Federation of Psychoanalysis and linked to the International Psychoanalytic Association groupings' (*Revista Brasileira de*

Psicanálise, 2018). We understood this as part of the gradual emergence within Brazilian society of a willingness to explore the events of the dictatorship, supported by the establishment of the National Truth Commission (2012) and several Truth Commissions in states, cities and Brazilian universities, and by increasingly open documentation of the oppression of that time. Following the paper's acceptance by the commissioning editor of the *Revista* as a 'very important article' with the additional comment that 'It's indispensable that we get contact within history and not only good memories,' the paper was translated into Portuguese and readied for publication. At that point, one of us received a phone call from the overall editor of the journal, who said that she had thought about the article for a week and had decided, on her own, that it could not be published. This was not because of any concerns about quality or accuracy—she had no suggestions to make for alterations and no arguments against the content—but because the Brazilian psychoanalytic societies are 'not ready' for what we were saying. We could interpret this as censorship, but perhaps should more generously understand it as ambivalence towards psychoanalysis' local history and its ethical task. It is in any case consistent with what a psychoanalyst we had approached for an interview at the start of our project told us at that time (2013). He had talked to some people and they all told him not to participate, that there are 'skeletons in the wardrobe that shouldn't be touched.'

4. The most significant prohibition we encountered is also the one most difficult to discuss. In outline, we produced a paper focused on analysis of an interview we had carried out with a Brazilian psychoanalyst who told us a very troubling story about a patient that related to the conditions of social violence in Brazil during the dictatorship and their effects decades later. The psychoanalyst had of course given us permission to use the material and we had done what we could to anonymise and disguise it without losing its force. Our argument in the paper was that unresolved violence constantly returns and we saw this 'case study' as a powerful illustration of this claim. The paper was written, revised and accepted by a journal, but when we sent it to the psychoanalyst for a final check on the grounds of ensuring that research consent was genuinely 'informed,' we were told we could not

publish it and that legal action would be taken if we tried to do so. We therefore recalled it: we would not go against a withdrawal of consent and nor did we wish to do anything that would cause difficulties for the psychoanalyst or the patient. In an email acknowledging this, the psychoanalyst wrote, 'Scientific works are sometimes bound by ethical considerations, even sometimes to a high price for science.'

These experiences are of rather different kinds, but they raise a general issue: how can we carry out genuine psychoanalytically-informed research into the history of psychoanalysis in a context of social tension, both historical and current, when the organisations concerned are involved—for good reasons and, at times perhaps, bad ones too—in obscuring or denying the events concerned or blocking their investigation? History is left to be dreamt rather than examined; archives are closed; papers are not published because it is 'too soon' thirty years after the events they describe; worries over legal action and psychoanalytic ethics require the non-publication of a detailed analysis of a specific 'case.' Under these circumstances, and whether or not the concerns are justified (sometimes they clearly are not and seem more like a conscious cover-up than an unconscious denial; at other times, the issue of protection of individuals might legitimately come into play), one wonders if it is indeed possible to learn from cases in the way that Forrester, Rustin and others suggest; and hence whether in the socio-historical plane, there is a significant reduction in what psychoanalysis can offer to the uncovering and understanding of its own history and that of the surrounding culture. Can we trust the information we have, or do we have to become detectives as well as researchers, suspicious of everything we come into contact with and willing to become unpopular with our colleagues in the interests of some kind of psychoanalytic and historical 'truthfulness'? I have to say that despite the obvious reputational dangers, I would prefer to be in the position where I can defend the psychoanalytic method on the grounds that intense case investigation offers the most open, detailed and complex, and therefore 'valid,' account of experience that is available, and that nothing is turned away from, however troubling it might be to consciousness—which I take to be part of the psychoanalytic 'ethic.' But the problem of distortion at the individual level and—as we have found in our work—resistance of various kinds at the institutional level suggests as yet this is not possible. Maybe one day, when there is no need for fear, it will become so.

References

Bion, W. (1967). Notes on memory and desire. *The Psychoanalytic Forum, 2*, 272–280.

Brecht, K., Friedrich, V., Hermanns, L., Kaminer, I., & Juelich, D. (Eds.) (1985). *'Here life goes on in a most peculiar way': Psychoanalysis before and after 1933*. Goethe Institut.

Forrester, J. (2017). *Thinking in cases*. Polity.

Freud, S. (1933). New introductory lectures on psycho-analysis. *The standard edition of the complete psychological works of Sigmund Freud, volume XXII (1932–1936): New introductory lectures on psycho-analysis and other works*, 1–182.

Frosh, S. (2005). *Hate and the Jewish science: Anti-semitism, Nazism and psychoanalysis*. Palgrave.

Frosh, S. (2006). *For and against psychoanalysis* (2nd ed.). Routledge.

Frosh, S. (2012). The re-enactment of Denial. In A. Gulerce (Ed.), *Re(con)figuring psychoanalysis: Critical Juxtapositions of the philosophical, the sociohistorical and the political* Palgrave.

Frosh, S. (2019). Psychosocial studies with psychoanalysis. *Journal of Psychosocial Studies, 1–2*, 101–114.

Frosh, S., & Mandelbaum, B. (2019). Psychosocial histories of psychoanalysis. *Revista Praxis y Culturas PsiSantiago De Chile, Enero, 1*, 1–13.

King, P., & Steiner, R. (1991). *The Freud-Klein controversies 1941–45*. Routledge.

Kuhn, T. (1962). *The structure of scientific revolutions*. University of Chicago Press.

Mandelbaum, B., Rubin, A., & Frosh, S. (2018). 'He didn't even know there was a dictatorship': The complicity of a psychoanalyst with the Brazilian military regime. *Psychoanalysis and History, 20*, 37–57.

Obholzer, A., & Roberts, V. (Eds.). (1994). *The unconscious at work*. Routledge.

O'Shaughnessy, E. (1994). What is a clinical fact? *International Journal of Psycho-Analysis, 75*, 939–948.

Plotkin, M. (2001). *Freud in the Pampas: The emergence and development of a psychoanalytic culture in Argentina.*. Stanford University Press.
Revista Brasileira de Psicanálise. (2018). http://pepsic.bvsalud.org/revistas/rbp/iaboutj.htm. Accessed 24 July 2019.
Rustin, M. (2019). *Researching the unconscious: Principles of psychoanalytic method*. Routledge.
Schechter, K. (2014). *Illusions of a future: Psychoanalysis and the biopolitics of desire*. Duke University Press.
Sociedade Brasileira de Psicanalise. (1994). *Álbum de família: imagens, fontes e idéias da Psicanálise em São Paulo*. Casa do Psicólogo.
Spence, D. (1987). *The Freudian metaphor*. Norton.

6

Clinical Cases in the History of Brazilian Psychoanalysis

Christian Ingo Lenz Dunker
and J. Guillermo Milán-Ramos

Introduction

This chapter provides an overview of the history of psychoanalysis in Brazil from the perspective of clinical cases. By examining the functions of psychoanalytic casuistry[1] within the psychiatric, anthropological and

C. I. L. Dunker (✉)
Universidade de São Paulo, São Paulo, Brazil
e-mail: chrisdunker@usp.br

J. G. Milán-Ramos
Universidad de La Republica, Montevideo, Uruguay

[1] Casuistry is a process of reasoning that seeks to resolve moral problems by extracting or extending theoretical rules from a particular case, and reapplying those rules to new instances. This method occurs in applied ethics, medicine and jurisprudence. Casuistry dates from Aristotle (384–322 BC), yet the zenith of casuistry was from 1550 to 1650, when case based reasoning arose, particularly in administering the Sacrament of Penance. The term casuistry became pejorative with Blaise Pascal's attack on the misuse of casuistry. The 'case by case' approach to personal moral decisions ultimately developed and accepted a casuistry (the study of cases of conscience) where at the time of decision, individual inclinations were more important than the moral law itself.

B. Mandelbaum et al. (eds.), *Brazilian Psychosocial Histories of Psychoanalysis*, Studies in the Psychosocial,
https://doi.org/10.1007/978-3-030-78509-3_6

literary discourse, we can better understand the path of assimilation and autonomy of psychoanalysis in Brazil.

This process begins in the years 1909–1949 when psychoanalytic ideas were introduced in anthropological and literary debates in Brazil. When we look at clinical cases through the psychoanalytical analysis of discourses (Dunker et al., 2018), significant traces of class, race, gender and ethnicity emerge. Between 1950 and 1984, the function of the clinical case changed in the context of the institutionalisation of psychoanalysis. This occurred during a new wave of social development that was marked by modernisation, development and urbanisation, but also by the military dictatorship from 1964. Clinical cases began to integrate the training devices of psychoanalysts, giving them proof of pertinence and affiliation, resulting from the domination of a linguistic and conceptual universe. The role of the author in these cases seems to be to demonstrate that Brazilian suffering has adjusted to European diagnosis, rather than demanding recognition of native categories.

By the end of the military dictatorship in 1984 and throughout the years of re-democratisation of the country until 2000, a new development in casuistry became evident, which could be seen in the context of expanding consumption of psychoanalytical ideas and practices. This involved overcoming the tension between psychotherapies and psychoanalysis; the arrival of Lacanianism; the gradual decline of other psychotherapeutic tendencies (such as psychodrama, Reich, Jung, phenomenology and Gestalt); culminating in the opposition between psychoanalysis, which began to include psychodynamic tendencies, and new cognitive-behavioural therapies. The clinical case came to represent the visible form of psychoanalysis. The discussion of the 'truth of psychoanalysis' and its 'impure or illegitimate' combination ran across all levels of Brazilian psychoanalysis. New studies emerged around Brazilian colonisation, conducted through imported psychoanalytic ideas, new modalities of practice (such as group analysis) and a growth in the number of new authors translated. Study groups, autonomous institutions, associations and many other fora were created. Psychoanalysis sought to integrate with new critical tendencies drawn from deconstructionism, post-Marxist and feminist studies. In terms of clinical cases, clinical activity became separated from descriptive rhetoric, scientific aspirations, diagnostic rationality and incorporated aesthetic exemplification of best practice and excellence in conducting treatments. Psychoanalysis combatted its own representation as an elitist institution, as middle-class and working-class people gained access both to treatment and to psychoanalytic training. The standard form of construction of clinical cases was stabilised through enunciation of the subject; establishing the circumstances of the subject's history and the demand for treatment; the development of crucial therapeutic events; and ending with a statement of the problem with the available concept. This is not a description of all varieties and kinds of clinical writing, but a '*form*' taken as '*literary form*' as described by Lukács (2009). A form is neither poor nor rich, since it only describes a recurrence and an iteration of writing strategies.

After 2000, signs of revitalisation within Brazilian psychoanalysis become apparent through audience expansion, both as a way of reading and interpreting culture, and by facilitating access to treatment. It was no longer only a sign of upper social class, but also of an alternative or culturally critical attitude. There were increases in psychoanalytical activity in Brazil before 1984, but when compared to other psychoanalytical cultures, where psychoanalysis was more focused on training and medical institutions, the Brazilian 'psychoanalytical uprising' gradually came to prominence. The size of the country presented difficulties in the dissemination of information, in addition to the well-known social inequalities in the distribution of material and symbolic capital. Nevertheless, the expansion particularly of Lacanianism, its spread into university and health institutions, brought with it a conceptual hypertrophy as well as the appreciation of the personal experience of analysis, known as the 'pass.' The clinical case, as a teaching method, essentially linked to supervision, acted as a collective sharing of the ethics of healing, or as a rational justification for doing therapy. It acquired new functions in the formation of the psychoanalyst, as part of self-authorisation in the Lacanian field.

This new cultural and moral environment, designed by neoliberalism, demanded greater social recognition, whereby old personological forms of authority were replaced by theoretical diversity and conceptual indeterminacy; instead of an institutional certificate, the style of an author;

instead of long trainings with close supervision, the new idea of 'transmission'[2] within the field of psychoanalysis. Until the turn of the century, even the most progressive, open and democratic spaces, such as the Instituto Sedes Sapientae in São Paulo, the Iracy Doyle Psychoanalytic Society in Rio de Janeiro and the Círculo Psicanalítico in Pernambuco, which had been developing since the 1970s, still demonstrated an enormous disparity between the extensive number of candidates and the small number of notable figures. This evolved into a pyramid scheme of power distribution, with systemic divisions between zones of influence and affiliations. After the 2000s, with the decline of the 'Schools Age' (Figueiredo, 2003), there were increased opportunities for transversal and hybrid training, through the reduction of institutional control and the creation of self-made analysts who 'authorised themselves' as entrepreneurs.

By exposing what is essentially a private practice, the clinical case was then required to respond to the demand for political transparency and the distribution of symbolic capital, as well as acquiring a critical dimension in the face of institutional opacities. This brings us back to the demonstrative function of the concepts within the context of the wider debate on Brazilian identity, where the clinical case has emerged as a discourse increasingly addressed to specialists. The concepts and terms provide access to a particular language which has restricted use assuring institutional affiliation. Through this institutionalisation, the function shifts from the descriptive and normative paradigm of reporting events. In its place comes the model of the short story or poem. The fragment becomes the preferred form for the clinical case, no longer the novel. We return to the discourse of aesthetic pertinence and the standard form of the clinical case, but now to criticise or clarify the enigmatic character of Lacanian concepts, both preserving and derogating their aspirations as science.

[2] Lacan proposes the concept 'transmission' of psychoanalysis to contrast the Freudian idea of formation (*Bildung*). Transmission focuses on the receiver, the candidate as he or she recognizes the effect on them of psychoanalytic discourse. The idea is connected with the concept of 'matema,' as the model of an 'integral transmission,' deprived from imperfections of speech.

Discursive Hybridity

The publication of the 1919 newspaper article '*Do Delírio em Geral*' by Franco da Rocha was followed a year later by *Psicanálise e pansexualismo* (*Psychoanalysis and Pansexualism*) in 1920 (Franco da Rocha, 1920). These articles are considered to be an inaugural milestone in the arrival of psychoanalytical ideas in Brazil, but the use of clinical cases in these articles does not go beyond the idea of illustration and the clinic is restricted to observation:

> This observation illustrates very well the general description of paranoia. Here the main content of the delusional ideas is evidently born from the sexual instinct: it is love. Well, now I appeal to some considerations about Freud's doctrine. (Franco da Rocha, 1914, p. 18)

In 1914, Genserico Aragão had presented the first Brazilian thesis in psychoanalysis, including five clinical cases. The first was a case of a 30-year-old Spanish widow who had presented symptoms such as 'cross-eyed breathing,' sensations of heat and light-headedness. She was determined to be in a '*light hallucinatory state*,' with restless sleep and numerous afflicting dreams. She reported getting up during the night in constant restlessness and presented '*pain of all sorts*' through her body, anorexia and amnesia, in addition to episodes of hysteria.

> We isolate ourselves several times with the patient in a silent room and little by little capturing her confidence and her sympathy, we are able to take away her detailed history of life and the cause of her evil. (Aragão, 1914, p. 97)

The story of her life and the story of her ills were stories of passions. First for her husband who died eight years after their marriage. Then she moved in with a violent man, and the first hysterical symptom appeared. Finally, she fell in love with a fellow Spaniard, until someone took charge of '*instilling in our patient's spirit that there was no sincere love on the part of her fiancé, but a low interest*' (p. 98) in her savings. She was already suffering by this time with what Freud called '*the anguish of the bride and groom*' (p. 101). When they said goodbye, he launched '*two or three solemn and terrible sentences*' (p. 99) and after two days he fell ill with pneumonia. She was very shaken by the news and '*spent a few hours lying there unable to speak and cry*' before further episodes of hysteria began.

These attacks belonged to a line of symptoms that should not be confused with the symptoms coming from the concomitant anguish neurosis. The Spanish widow thus suffered from the same mixed neurosis that Freud had diagnosed in most cases of his *Studies on Hysteria.* There was a certain degree of intimacy among the engaged couple that allowed them to drive to distant corners and deserts of the city, where they practised what would be, according to Freud, '*frustrating acts*' (p. 99). The crises were, therefore, a combination of hysterical episodes and attacks of anguish marked by scrupulousness:

> 'I have the impression,' the sick person said, 'that this world is over for me. I no longer have the right to enjoy what the earth produces; the heat of this sun that is there, I no longer feel the brightness of the day, I no longer see it; everything in me is shadow'. (Aragão, 1914, p. 100)

She refused to eat and drink and understood that all this was a punishment for '*my horrible sin.*' The neurosis paved the way for psychoneurosis. The treatment therefore required '*even greater patience than the analysis of the symptoms. The suppression of sexual practices, the honest environment of the hospital were the auxiliaries of the treatment*' (p. 100). Ten to twelve days later, the patient appeared significantly improved, but when '*positive affective transference*' was verified, the relatives removed her from the treatment to '*our displeasure.*'

In the second case, the patient was a 32-year-old Portuguese widow, a seamstress. She suffered from joint, muscle and bone pain, respiratory crises, '*a great weight in the heart*' and lack of gastric and motor coordination completed the picture. She had suffered from mistreatment since childhood and heard '*voices that spoke to her from the inside.*' She did not love her husband, but was faithful to him, and when he died, she took refuge in the home of family friends and lived there for years in poverty. She had stomach pains linked to hunger and the memory of hunger. She reported the thought that '*If someday I can't eat when I'm hungry, my headaches will be so big that I, for sure, will go crazy*' (p. 102). The hysteria is triggered when the household did not '*have the delicacy*' to invite her to eat; she waited for a fruit vendor to pass, and offer food, but he didn't pass. The hunger came, and with it the headache, followed by the hysteria, which she was unable to medicate.

However, after some time listening to the symptoms, the doctor elicits another narrative. She was deeply in love with a married man with whom she had frequent and intense sexual encounters, but developed symptoms of shortness of breath, pressure in the chest and craving when she realised that he intended to reduce the number of meetings. In one month, she shows great improvement and leaves the hospital.

The third case is reported by Juliano Moreira, a black psychiatrist and introducer of psychoanalytical ideas in Brazil (Oda & Dalgalarrondo, 2000). As director of a great asylum that would later receive his name, he fought against the scientific racism of the time, which was represented by Nina Rodrigues. Medicine had a strong presence in the Brazilian modernisation process, mainly through psychiatry and epidemiology, which reflected the changes in habits and mentalities that were necessary for progress. Moreira explored the triggering of hysteria in a woman following her travels in Europe. She had a gynaecological operation and was required to avoid sexual intercourse. As a result of her abstinence, her husband found a lover, which resulted in the patient hastening her return to Brazil. However, the mistress followed on the next ship and appeared, driving through the streets of Rio de Janeiro with the patient's husband.

Case number four was a French woman who was unhappy with her husband's sexual performance. Her suffering of a melancholic type, combined with anorexic symptoms and insomnia, began when she was 28 years old. She reported that '*from a while back she no longer found any sexual pleasure with her husband*' (Aragão, 1914, p. 111) since the husband, busy with his work, had neglected intimate relations with her. In a conversation, 'with great ability not to hurt him,' the doctor exposes the situation to her husband, who returns to the '*normal and very regular practice of coitus*' (p. 107). The case finds a complete cure, whereby the patient became '*free of all her moral tortures, without insomnia, much fatter and in a good mood, is completely cured, in short*' (p. 107).

The fifth and last case described in Genserico Aragão's thesis is that of a 24-year-old Brazilian who suffered from nocturnal pollution. He was completely weakened, with constipation and dyspepsia; the diagnosis was neurasthenia, with the cause determined as excessive study and masturbation between 17 and 18 years. The effect was great shame and great hesitation in everything he did.

> The treatment of this case, although a little long, was not difficult for us. We showed the patient the great inconveniences and the enormous danger of onanism; we advised him with affection and kindness; we gave him the normal practice of genitality. (p. 109)

It is notable that of the four cases only one is really from a Brazilian. With the changes brought by modernisation before the turn of the twentieth century came social and institutional transformations, including the end of slavery in 1888, and the establishment of the republic in 1889, the necessary sanitation of cities, creation of accessible education and health care, stimulation and suppression of rebellions. Cultural realignment with the European powers (France, England and Germany) also took the country away from Portuguese colonial influence. In this context of internationalisation and whitening, former slave labour is beginning to be replaced by new waves of immigrants (Italians, Spanish, Germans and Japanese).

This growth in internationalism does not only point to the increased migratory flows, it also suggests how 'modern' psychoanalytic patients are. All cases presented some variation of current neurosis, in the woman the neurosis of anguish, or in the man, the neurasthenia. It is in the elucidation of these cases that Genserico can exert his practice of delicate persuasion and can use sympathy as a means of persuasion. Even if the theoretical discourse that underlies it resonates strongly with the medical pedagogy of coercion, in practice this means benevolence, patience, care and listening. Even though there were still no psychoanalysts in Brazil, psychoanalysis was anticipated as a generic approach to treating patients.

All of these cases comprise of impasses within personal relationships and they are presented according to a repetitive strategy: first identification of the symptoms, then the diagnosis, then the 'family romance' not without the details of the 'unconfessable practices,' culminating in treatment through discussion and reporting of its eventual result. The use of the word 'onanism' for 'masturbation,' rather than the use of a Latin or medical term, indicates the presence of a more practical approach and understanding within the clinical context. It also highlights how the cases seem to approach difference in social class: identification of those able to travel abroad is contrasted with those who suffer from hunger; several of them express themselves by insomnia and anorexia, but hysteria remained the most diffuse, superimposed, underlying circumstance in relation to masturbatory practices or abstinence.

These cases present a distinct shift away from magical, religious and animistic views, which were prevalent in discussions of mental health at the time, and a move towards valuing new and modern ways of describing suffering. Even when guilt is discussed, a term with overt religious ramifications, no mention of religion is made. On the other hand, the doctor appears as a Foucauldian figure of the family counsellor and guardian of good intimate practice between couples. With regard to identification of social class, the cases of Genserico are upper class; even the hungry woman came from a formerly rich family. In addition, the identification of links from Europe and of travel to Europe also firmly suggests a specific class. Genserico Aragão's thesis, along with the requirements of title and university, states that the author was born in Ceará (a north-eastern Brazilian state) and that he is a 'legitimate son of Guilherme Augusto de Souza Pinto and Amalia de Aragão Pinto.' There is an overlap between the moral theme of origins, the exercise of sexual practices and sexuality remembered as a universe of fantasy and forgetfulness from childhood. But the most interesting character of this discourse is that it indicates the capacity of Brazilians to suffer as Europeans do.

Genserico Aragão's accounts can be compared with the way Nina Rodrigues' anthropological school listed symptoms to describe the paranoia of a black man:

> *Religious paranoia in a light-degenerate mulatto. Delirium of grandeur and persecution. Erotic ideas. Visual and auditory hallucinations, verbal impulses.*
>
> P. C. da Rocha Pitta, light mulatto, forty-five years old. Unknown hereditary background as stigma of physical degeneration accuses a

> marked degree of acrocephaly. Lush temperament; has always been very inclined to venereal excesses. He confesses to having forced his wife, now dead, to lend herself to acts of pederasty and recognizes having deflowered, before being widowed, one of his sisters-in-law, whom he made his mistress. (...) Pitta's delirium is partial, and this allows the Asylum Administration to use him in services that he is able to render. (...) God commanded Pitta to go from Pirajá to Imbassaí, telling him that on the road he would find a rider on a white horse, whose dung he would carefully keep in a bag; that this rider would give him three coins of $30,000 réis each, and that as for the price of his train ticket, he would not have to pay anything. The trip happened, and Pitta reported it in a manuscript where he says: 'I did everything the God-Snail commanded me, but in vain; my trip had no result. Strange thing!' After having filled him with grace, God betrayed him and had him locked up like a madman in an asylum; this caused him to break off his relations with God. It is this struggle that provides the matter of delirium. (Rodrigues, 1903, p. 123)

There is nothing specifically 'black' that may be determined in the paranoia of this patient, except the fact that the case unfolds during the time of the abolition of slavery, and that his delirium may be seen to capture the betrayal imposed by promises of benefits and land to newly freed slaves. Note the emphasis on the relevance of race and then sexual practices, ending with the circumscription of delirium, but the criterion of compatibility with work is also notable.

Nina Rodrigues used Morel's theory of degeneracy, applying it to black Brazilians, trying to describe situations created by the family, but determined by race. He was particularly interested in Freudian ideas of contagion and identification in hysteria, looking for their correlation in groups and psychic epidemics (such as those registered in Bahia and Maranhão during the establishment of the republic). Here, we find the theme of the moralisation of origins. It fell to his student Arthur Ramos to employ psychoanalysis as a method to criticise his teacher's racialist anthropology, by showing that the 'primitive' in psychoanalysis was represented by children, madmen and certain neurotics, but not 'backward peoples' or races. Black people who were brought to Brazil as slaves suffered from colonialism and dislocation from their origins. The syncretic manifestations in Brazilian culture, art and religion express a hybrid of conflict and resistance, in the Freudian sense of the word (Gutman, 2007).

In this way, the clinical case is a means of allowing the experiences of the individual to speak and not rely upon the racial category or ethnic group to determine the diagnosis. Alongside the clinical moral hybridisation of Genserico Aragão and the anthropological hybridisation of Nina Rodrigues, literary hybridisation may be found among the precursors of Brazilian psychoanalysis.

Febrônio Indio do Brasil was born in 1895 in the small town of Jequitinhonha, three years before the abolition of slavery in Brazil. He was abandoned at 12 years old after successive mistreatments and left to wander the streets of Rio de Janeiro committing petty theft. He accumulated dozens of police arrests, after which he dedicated himself to reading the Bible. He experienced a vision of a blond saint, who told him that Christ did not die, because he was the true 'son of light.' He subsequently tattooed the letters D (God), C (charity), V (virtue), S (holiness), V (life) and I (magnet of life) onto his chest and created a new surname for himself: Indian of Brazil.

During a time of general illiteracy of the black population, Febrônio wrote a book that narrates his events, which became a prototype of Brazilian surrealism: *As revelações do príncipe do fogo* (*The Revelations of the Prince of Fire*) (Indo do Brasil, 1926). The book was sold in bookstores without the author's permission and then was confiscated and burnt by the police. Febrônio dropped out from completing a degree in dentistry and opened a clinic where he practised massive extractions in an attempt to purify the clients' mouths. He also pretended to be a doctor and delivered babies. He travelled through several states in Brazil, taking on different names and professions; after being arrested for causing the death of a pregnant woman, he was interned for the first time. Following his release, he began tattooing the initials (DCVSVI) on children and adolescents before raping them. His crimes acquired increasing levels of notoriety after he was reimagined as a villain in children's stories. His mestizo, black and indigenous origin is captured by the debate about whitening, and in 1929, he became the first patient of the Rio de Janeiro's Judiciary Asylum, where he died in 1980.

> 'I cannot fight with you, my species is weak, but behold, the army of Light comes to my rescue. I, Febrônio, do not give you glory because I have a thief's soul. And to a certain extent, you ask: what is the greatest power He, LUCIFER, or the Light? Answer: I must be true, even though I am one of his countless victims.' In the final analysis, the drawings of Febrônio and the inscriptions that accompany him, like his book and his acts, reflect well the unconscious struggle of primitive instincts and possible sexual complexes repressed with liberating or substitutive ideas. The mystical ideas that are revealed in him, and the very tattoos which he used, are satisfactions that replace these perversions, if not an unconscious attempt at liberation. In this regard, it is worth recalling the concept of Freud in his '*Introduction á la psychanalyse*' (French translation), who believes that paranoia itself 'results rigorously from an attempt at defense against very violent homosexual impulses' (p. 33). His book is a revelation in this sense. (Carilho, 1930, p. 23)

Heitor Carrilho's psychiatric report for the 1928 trial shows how psychoanalysis, even in the early days of its assimilation by psychiatric circles, was already linked to the appreciation of the patient's own words. It was not his successive acts, nor his violence, much less his popular repercussion, that required the trial. To re-categorise Febronio from the black, wandering, diabolical and violent individual to that of someone suffering from a mental illness, we need the hybridisation of psychiatric and judiciary discourse. Febronio became a kind of national hero or anti-hero for modernist writers, such as Mario de Andrade and Oswald de Andrade,[3] who saw in him the prototype of the social outcast, who had denounced the unresolved contradictions of our 'civilising' process.

Clinical cases, in this first period, adjust Brazilian suffering to adapt to a European concept, but they are centres of individual differences, examining the abnormality of the patient, and removing the art or geniality of the writer. These 'tropical cases' are paradigmatic examples of Brazilian strategies of individualisation: crime, family origins, ethnicity or race capture the allegory of the difference they represent.

---

[3] 'The [money] which, through inheritance and theft, is kept in the closed hands of the rich… (…) I know you, loose beast, capable of the worst purposes. Febbrônio dissimulated from the streets of Brazil!' (De Andrade, 2000, p. 151).

Normative Descriptivism

In 1927, Durval Marcondes, together with Franco da Rocha, wrote to Freud to inform him of the foundation of the Brazilian Society of Psychoanalysis, which was the first in Latin America. In the same year, the *Revista Brasileira de Psicanálise* appeared. The Society was renamed the São Paulo Psychoanalytic Group in June 1944, and in 1951, during the International Psychoanalytical Association Congress in Amsterdam, it became the Brazilian Psychoanalytical Society of São Paulo. Durval Marcondes was the Director between 1944 and 1969 and he was succeeded by his student, the psychoanalyst Virgínia Bicudo. As a black woman of rural origins and a background in sociology and politics, she was subjected to considerable racial prejudice (Braga, 2016). When Durval Marcondes was defeated in the competition for the Chair of Psychiatry at the University of São Paulo, pamphlets were circulated saying, '*If you are neurotic and you want to become psychotic, look for Dr. Virgínia Bicudo. Talk to Dr. Virgínia Bicudo*' (Bicudo, 1994).

Bicudo had trained in London with Melanie Klein, Bion and Winnicott and returned to Brazil in 1962, where she became accepted as a leader in psychoanalysis. The authority of the European element allowed a level of protection against the prejudice of origins affecting Bicudo, who encouraged the process of international recognition of Brazilian psychoanalysis and dedicated herself to promoting psychoanalysis within Brazil. She was known and respected in political circles and in the Ministry of Health, where she sponsored the definitive incorporation of psychoanalysis into the Brazilian public space, the effects of which are still felt today.

Milton Zaidan was a student of Virgínia Bicudo and Durval Marcondes, who participated actively in one of the first unofficial institutes for training psychoanalysts in Brazil, *Sedes Sapientae*. Zaidan published a small clinical case of no more than two pages in the first issue of the *Jornal de Psicanálise* in 1966 (Zaidan, 1966). The article is divided into four parts, reflecting a university format in section '*II. Material and Method*,' where it is reported that there are 187 sessions with an adult patient at the rate of four sessions per week (p. 1), and in section

'*III. Evolution*,' where he divides the treatment into two periods. In the first:

> He feels that he has obligations and wants to fulfil them, but he also complains that I am 'bossy', being reluctant to accept the situation, having stayed most of the first session standing, not lying down. (...) In the transference I am idealized, giving myself all the expectations of healing. (...) The ego and superego are felt as weak and impotent in the face of the id, greedy and insatiable requests, because they overuse the split. (...) Idealization increases his envy of me and persecutory fears. (...) As a defense against his anguish of emptying and fear of losing his individuality, he went into acting out, competing in various situations with friends or strangers. (Zaidan, 1966, p. 1).

In the second period, the analyst reports his own feelings of envy and his anger at not being understood by the patient in his interpretations. The patient remained fixed in the report of his daily life. The patient's words were 'said without affection,' which caused a counter-transferential displeasure, which made the analyst feel that the patient had disconnected and separated from him. Realising that this came from the counter-transference, it was possible to 'get rid of the feeling of displeasure and then interpret.' The objective of the work '*has no other pretension than to add a confirmatory data to a fact already known and demonstrated*.' The counter-transferential feelings must be 'captured and understood, after which the interpretation is elaborated' (p. 2). The private life of the analyst, including his friends, relatives and feelings, must be strictly separated from public and professional activity. The old hybridism between public and private, together with all forms of syncretism and mixing, becomes sign of insufficient modernisation or lack of 'professionalism.' This creates the expected social image of a psychoanalyst who resembles a combination between a scientist and a doctor: distant, self-controlled and evasive.

The conflict is referred to traces of moral discourse and a competition between analyst and analysand, but demonstrates a struggle between describing the facts and living the events at a distance or letting oneself be enveloped by the analysand's narrative. The patient does not speak as he should for the analysis to function satisfactorily. Hence, the tacit element of the conflict is precisely this contradicted norm, although this is not fully recognised by either party.

The discourse is full of psychoanalytical concepts, but there is no diagnostic discussion: this is the beginning of the process of autonomation of psychoanalytic diagnosis in relation to psychiatric nosology. It is as if from then on the notion of diagnosis was created from a psychodynamic viewpoint, culminating in the idea of a psychodiagnosis. The pychodiagnosis progressively annexed the use of psychological tests, particularly tests inspired by the notion of projection, that were adopted by the increasingly important university psychology courses. This marks the Brazilian psychoanalytical drift from psychiatry to psychology making construction of clinical cases part of the process of formation and legitimisation of the candidate as a psychoanalyst, so the *author* becomes the one being evaluated.

There is a great overlap of concepts, with a decrease in expressive narrative. To confirm the demand for synthesis, objectification and data, the clinical case plays an important role in the semantic adjustment and stabilisation of the candidate as a psychoanalyst. By mimicking aspects of the scientific-university discourse, such as *Material and Methods*, this also indicates the search for legitimacy: *the counter-transference exists, and I was able to witness it*. The conclusion is procedural: first capture-understand, then interpret. It is clear that the author was experiencing counter-transference, but the text suggests that this is in itself a discovery and a revelation. This confirmed that concepts described in a European language of psychoanalysis could translate into the Brazilian 'subtropical' reality. This view was corroborated by the difficulty that the psychoanalyst demonstrated in front of a patient, who in other aspects does not behave as he should, according to the network of expectations formed in the description of European cases. It is as if in the face of a different sociability than the one foreseen, what needs to change is reality and not concepts. This corroborates the great discursive obedience, which is compatible with the process of institutionalisation of psychoanalysis, but also with the country's processes of censorship and silencing at the height of the military dictatorship.

The hardening of the story, the formalisation and depersonalisation of the relations of recognition converge on the idea that it would be especially important to 'speak the same language,' resulting in ambiguities and indeterminations of meaning being carefully reduced and controlled. The psychoanalytic casuistry under the military dictatorship of 1964–1985 reflects the effort of discursive self-justification, as well as the construction of border security between psychoanalysis and psychotherapy, between psychoanalysis and religion, between psychoanalysis and the university. The great expansion of psychology courses during that period sought to take advantage of psychoanalysts to organise their practical courses and supervision, in such a way that after a moment of joint aspiration with the Brazilian educational and civilising project, psychoanalysis gradually created its own separate entity. As it moved forward in its own process of institutionalisation, it moved away from the common public space, constituting itself as a good example of what some authors call Brazilian regressive modernisation (Faoro, 1992).

Canonical Form of the Clinical Case

Thirty-three years later, in the same *Jornal de Psicanálise*, we find a somewhat different format for the construction of clinical cases. Let us now take for reference the eleven-page article: '*No Jogo dos Afetos; quando Rapunzel não joga suas tranças*' by Gina Levinzon, which was published in 1999. This account is structured in a way that repeats itself in numerous clinical cases, to the point of suggesting that these are variations of an elementary structure. This form is characterised by a declarative opening about a theme and its theoretical references, in this case affection. After that, we find the residue of the traditional scientific-university discourse that announces a problem or obstacle: '*the affect is immutable, even after long periods of analytical work*' (Levinzon, 1999, p. 22). The presentation of the case begins with a profile of the patient, her family circumstances and the particularities of the demand for treatment: '*I have no conditions to do analysis.*' She did not want to discuss her family history; even so, we learned that she was separated from her mother early due to the birth of a brother. After this initial assembly of the situation, we find at least two series that are repeated in the treatment: the silent adversity and the previous abandonments. Among them are the analyst's interventions: asking, silencing, sharing, suggesting and interpreting.

The patient, about 40 years old, lies down on the couch in silence for long periods while she undresses some lint: '*I will never start talking spontaneously*' and this will be so '*forever*,' because '*she had no way*' (p. 408). At first, she justified herself by saying that '*she would only say nonsense*,' because she knew that the analyst '*had no interest in her*' and that she expected '*to be sent away like the previous analysis*,' where a similar procedure ended with the statement by the analyst that she '*was not fit to do analysis*.' Here, a curious observation appears in the text, assuring the reader that the former analyst '*was not a Lacanian*,' that is, suggesting that if he was a Lacanian such procedures would be more understandable.

The analyst felt that her patient had '*borrowed her vitality*' (p. 409). She simply waited for her initiative to be able to derogate from it, whilst moving her feet like '*a little dog wagging its tail*.' One wiggles her foot, and the other gives way and asks a question. Whoever speaks first loses. When she invested in the counter-transferential report, the patient agreed saying: '*That's right, but what does it change?*' When she is forced to recognise the progress made in her life, during the time under analysis, she responds with months of mutism. Silence after silence, which led to crying and despair.

After presenting the scenario, delimiting the series that composes it, delineating the structure of repetition, we are offered the presentation of the transforming event. Years go by like this with the patient indicating improvement but showing intense repetition in the transference, until the analyst makes a bold move; the patient declares that the analyst is right and that she has no way forward. The analyst in turn declares herself defeated and proposes interrupting the analytic work; the analyst is disturbed and realises that she has arrived at a limit situation. Despite all this, the patient does not want to interrupt the treatment.

After that, the text tries to symmetrise the experience with the concepts: projective identification (Klein), negative therapeutic reaction (Freud), transferential envy (Rosenfeld), pathological organisations of the personality (Steiner), fear of collapse (Winnicott), dead mother complex (Green) and near-death addiction (Betty Joseph). In these successive conceptual descriptions, the impasse of the case is gaining ground, until it is formulated as a contradiction or paradox:

> If the mother is lost to the subject, dead, at least she is present in this way, 'dead present'. However, if the mother heals herself, wakes up, cheers up, and lives, the subject loses too, because she abandons him to take care of his occupations and to invest in other objects. (pp. 412–413)

Vitality and lack of vitality, transference and counter-transference would thus be the most important measure of this analytical situation. When the affections of this critical situation, though paradoxical, can be shared, the case evolves. It is justified not only as part of the institutional ritual, or as a clinical exercise in psychopathology, but also as an extension of the very transference that made it possible. The writing of the case is part of the transference that animates it, by involving the process of separation from the analyst, counterpart and equivalent of the passage of the experience from the oral and private space, to the public and common space.

The case closes with one of the canonical features of writing clinical cases: the literary effigy. It is employed to provide unity and connection of the case with other languages, such as a passport, which authorises its migration to other universes of speech:

> Rapunzel is at the top of the castle, inaccessible. There is a request for help. Underneath is a cry: Throw down your braids, and I'll get in there and try to help you. Nothing happens. If I turn my back and resign myself to this situation Rapunzel cries in despair. If I ask her for the braids, she says she doesn't feel like throwing them. Rapunzel's desperation touches me. I try to climb the tower in other ways, but Rapunzel throws stones. (p. 415)

The literary openness counterbalances the translation from experience to concepts, and from concepts to experience. Now, it is no longer just about proving the mastery of psychoanalytical discourse, nor of access to the multiplicity of authors and schools, but of bringing uncertainty, doubt and the discordant affections of the analyst as a resource for generalising the experience to other cases.

There are many variants of this format, with varying degrees of commitment to normative descriptivism, or with less narrative compression. The coherence or dispersal of problems can give the whole case a more ordered or worse finished aspect. There may be more than two transformative series, besides those we have seen in this case, which are exemplified by the history of real abandonment and perpetual virtual abandonment in transference. The transformative event can be described through a decisive act, event or interpretation, but also through a strategy, regular and constant, that guides the interventions.

Cases are not always built to show great transformations. Sometimes it is a successful failure; in others, it can provide the local reversion of a symptom and even the overcoming of a repetition. Small advances can generate great reports. There are some cases where the transformation seems to occur only on the psychoanalyst's side, and in others, it occurs exclusively with a particular analyst, many times, but without it being clear why and how. This canonical form offers the ease of solving, directly or indirectly, the problem of the mode of belonging or affiliation to the psychoanalytical schools. The mode of distribution, or the spectrum of quotations and references, works as the geography of the institutional space to the author and the moment of his or her formation.

The constant element in this canonical form of construction of clinical cases in Brazilian psychoanalysis is that the clinical dimension, as we show elsewhere (Dunker, 2011), determined by diagnosis, by semiology and by aetiology, seems secondary to the therapeutic dimension. The psychodynamic history, the psychodiagnosis and the various ways of organising clinical cases gradually migrate towards their conceptual adjustment. Gradually, the psychoanalytic diagnosis becomes independent and sometimes indifferent to the psychiatric diagnosis. The location, description and semiology of the symptoms become less important than the narrative of the family novel, psychic reality and the transference. The psychiatric reform in Brazil between 1978 and 2001, and the role occupied by psychoanalysis during this time, contribute to cut psychoanalysis and its former alliance with psychiatry (Kyrillos Neto et al., 2015).

The authority of the clinic acquires another sense: one that is less public, comparative and scientific, and more closely linked to the authority constituted by the established analysts. This can be attributed to the increasingly complex and potentially conflicting coexistence between different generations of psychoanalysts. It is also the period in which the importance of the history of psychoanalysis begins to be perceived, and where discursive endogeny begins to be seen as a problem. The return to novel form, with greater authorship and greater personalisation of the story, also suggests incipient criticism of those who 'merely reproduce ideas and practices out of place without proper cultural appropriation' (p. 12). This process is also linked to the cultural dissemination of psychoanalysis: this can be interpreted as a listening practice for the middle classes, as a discourse of interpretation of culture, as a theory of European rather than North American reference, for the nascent university courses in psychology (Dunker, 2008). Moreover, the therapeutic and clinical dimension both seem to be subordinated to the ethical or aesthetic experiences of cure.

The Lacanian Inversion

Since the 1980s, but gaining ground since the turn of the twenty-first century, the Lacanian movement has spread throughout Brazil, appearing in numerous schools, institutes and formative associations. The writing of cases ceases to be a condition of registration or part of the candidate's agenda and becomes, along with the device of the 'pass,' a way of presenting the practice. Let us take as a paradigmatic example the seven-page work published by Rita Vogelar in the journal *Livro Zero* of the School of the Lacanian Field in São Paulo in 2011, entitled *Sintoma e fenômeno psicossomático: letra e número?* (*Symptom and psychosomatic phenomenon: letter and number?*).

Vogelar (2011) begins with an enigmatic passage from Jacques Lacan's 1975 text entitled: *Conference in Geneva*, in which he asks himself about the status of jouissance in psychosomatics, associating it with the metaphor of freezing and the fixation on the order of number. Here, we have the first characteristic inversion of the construction of clinical cases in the Lacanian universe: the cases are brought to clarify the conceptual or textual indeterminations promoted by theory and not the opposite;

that is, the concepts are tested by being deployed to understand the clinical obstacles.

To clarify the question about psychosomatic jouissance, the author mobilises two cases marked by the taking of hands. In the first case, the hands hurt and 'don't let go,' and in the second case, the hands are stained with vitiligo. A first theoretical contrast is interpolated between the letter and signifier, or between the real and the symbolic, between the object a (and its hole) and the lack.

> After that we return to the clinic. The pain in the hands appeared in the moments: '(...) that I was distressed, or in which I did not know what to do or in which I felt lost ... but that it hadn't done any good to know about it. (...) and having reached all the conclusions I had not made the pain go away (...) I look at my hand and it hurts'. (p. 192)

The analyst retains the presence of this look associated with the hand, but at that time this seems irrelevant to the patient. Months later, when talking about the dying grandmother, she will say again: '*I was looking at my mother who was looking at Oma* [grandmother's nickname in German] *and I was suffering*.' That is, instead of saying '*sofria*' (suffered),' she says '*Sofia*,' her own name. Again, we find the theme of looking. All that is missing is finding the location of the mother, which is easily produced by the anagram of 'Oma,' that is, 'm-ma-o,' but to do this we need to corrupt the signifying dimension and transform it into an exercise of reading letters.

This operation of 'po(a)tisation' (see below) has made it possible to clarify both the concept and the case: it represents an advance of knowledge for the analyst and a reversal of the symptom for the analysand. It can be interpreted as a kind of rule of action, of direction of the treatment, healing, towards the creation of a sense hole. For Lacan, psychosomatic phenomena have a similar structure to what linguists refer to as 'holophrase,' that is, the same word which simultaneously identifies the object, the context of enunciation and the relationship to the other. When children are developing their capacity for speech, they may designate with the same word many different contexts and objects. When the author points to the emergence of a master signifier (S1), as a way to separate it from the signifier of knowledge (S2), she is demonstrating some progress in treatment, but typically, detailed descriptions of dynamics and transference deadlocks disappear.

At this point, the first case is compared with the second, where similar operations are proposed but with different outcomes. In this second case, the significance was not in the series and the letter, but instead it was the number and frequency, through the widening of vitiligo by the hand of the patient. The hand continues to show no associations at all: neither a lapse, nor a dream, nor a faulty act, nor any significant substitution or succession. What had apparently been discovered with the first case, by means of '*writing a hole*,' had no equivalent in the second case.

The quotations of two commentators (Soler and Valas) maintain an allusive relationship with the case, where it is suggested that there would be a difference between the phallic jouissance (between the symbolic and the real) present in the first case and the Other jouissance (between the imaginary and the real) acting in the second. Both are resistant to the sense (or jouissance of sense), between the imaginary and the symbolic, but both have different incidences in relation to the body: this indetermination between the clinical case and the concepts works as a closing point of the text.

We find a new regime of textual authority, in which the enigmas foreseen by the different moments of Lacan's work end up replacing the previous theme of the development of the case. Authorship manifests itself in a more fluid way, in the first person, with high doses of narrativity and including the dialogue used, but the traditional introduction based on the family scene is absent. A stylistic of the invention of terms such as 'po(a)tisation' (by allusion to object a) instead of 'poetisation' appears. However, the failure of symmetry between concept and signifier will appear displaced to the theme of the irreproducibility of the feeling of the symptoms: both linked to the hand, but with diverse aetiology and therapeutics. The aspiration of science remains indicted by the Borromean schemes and the writing of mathematics, but the normative weight and the effort to prove the expertise and rectitude in the clinical use of the concepts are absent: the entire text is dominated by diagnostic or aetiological discussion.

Conclusion

The four initial trends of psychoanalytical casuistry, in its context of assimilation to Brazilian culture, have progressively lost their strength over time. The undisguised concerns surrounding social class, gender identity and issues surrounding sexual practices, that were described by Genserico Aragão, in combination with the groupings of indifferent forms of suffering, defined by race or ethnicity, in the school of Nina Rodrigues, and the literary-criminal fusion represented by Febrônio Índio do Brasil, have been gradually abandoned as formative prototypes of psychoanalytic casuistry.

Perhaps this oversight of Brazilian issues was a secondary effect of the internationalisation and the circumstances which allowed a specific, imported vocabulary and diagnosis of suffering to take hold. In the 1960s, the persistence of the ideal of science and descriptive austerity dominated, but this was replaced in the 1990s by the combined resource of concept and literature in the construction of clinical cases. The arrival of Lacanianism seems to have reactivated the tension between literature and science, at the same time as it deflated the normative context of case writing.

Historians of psychoanalysis have marked the importance of the modernisation process and hygienism as a condition for the greater implementation of psychoanalysis in Brazil (Valladares de Oliveira, 2006). This requires consideration of the inflexion points of modernity, as well as its devices of moralisation and control, as points of transformative impact on its history. In this sense, the 1960s and 1990s neatly bookend this, with a period of military rule at the beginning and then a process of re-democratisation of the country in the midst of the emergence of postmodernity, making these eligible as critical points of change and discontinuity. It is possible that the 2016 coup will bring a new influx to this process, but until then it is understood that the 1980s/1990s are associated with the spread of Lacanianism in the country, as a process that has already been synthesised by the tension of '*the body against the word*.' Thus, we also need a more careful evaluation of the participation of psychoanalysis in the current and ongoing nationalist modernisation project of the military dictatorship (Lima, 2017) and of the effects of the 'anarchic self-taught tendency characteristic of the Brazilian' (Nogueira do Vale, 2003, p. 234) to think of the years 2000–2016.

The impact of Lacanianism is representative of the discontinuity that we want to point out in Brazilian psychoanalysis (Bezerra, 2018). Many other authors, such as André Green, Jacques André, Roussilion, Kaës and Joyce McDougall, plus the Italian Antonino Ferro, joined the Brazilian debate on psychoanalysis, making it less 'vertical' when it comes to conceptual affiliation. The same can be said of the expansion of the presence of psychoanalysts in institutions of health, education and assistance. However, besides being more diverse and less vertical, it turned again to France, persisting in the pattern of low penetration of North American ideas and practices, such as relational psychoanalysis.

We hope to have shown that the use of clinical cases by Brazilian psychoanalysis has never been a merely extensive or imitative practice of medicine or psychiatry, but instead has involved dialogue with literature and anthropology from the beginning. Casuistry has acquired increasing normative force in the context of the descriptive fixation of psychoanalysis, most notably between the 1950s and 1984s. This can be attributed to the strong desire for institutional legitimisation of Brazilian psychoanalysts in a context of chronic failure and patrimonial excess in the occupation of public space, which is a concept of Max Weber applied by many Brazilians in order to understand historical long-range processes. Since there are some families that have so much capital, land and influence, they can impose their interest and occupy the State so that there is no genuine separation between public and private interests.[4] The discourse of development and progress, before and after the military

[4] 'In Brazil, it can be said that we have only exceptionally had an administrative system and a body of employees purely dedicated to objective interests and founded on these interests. On the contrary, it is possible to follow, throughout our history, the constant predominance of private wills that find their own environment in closed circles and are little accessible to impersonal ordering. Among these circles, it is undoubtedly the family that has expressed itself with the greatest strength and resourcefulness in our society. And one of the decisive effects of the undeniable, absorbing supremacy of the family nucleus [...] is that the relationships that are created in domestic life have always provided the obligatory model of any social composition between us that is based on patrimonialism' (de Holanda, 1927, p. 121).

dictatorship, contributed to a decline in clinical narrative in favour of clinical description.

The context of chronic failure and mistrust of institutions in general, as well as of their sociological assumptions, such as the separation between the public and private spheres, has gone through a process of critical revision since 1984, with the re-democratisation of the country. Writing a case was not only proving authorship and clinical mastery, but it showed that it was possible to understand and recognise the processes of individualisation and forms of psychic suffering considered analogous to Europeans. Hence, the writing of the case became fundamental proof of the discursive affiliation to psychoanalysis and a condition of access to the full exercise of the profession.

Between 1984 and 2000, the construction of clinical cases acquired an increasingly critical content, with the gradual intrusion of concepts that transform it into a kind of illustration or variation of the theory. We distinguish here an allegorical use of the clinical case, which groups metaphors and discourses to create a new unit, which can be seen through the illustrative use of the case, when it is considered in terms of concepts; and the authorial use of the clinical case, when it serves for the authorisation, recognition and legitimisation of the psychoanalyst. Lacanianism in Brazil reverses these uses, by substituting the direct account for cultural pieces available to all; fulfilling the allegorical function; creating texts where the concepts and theoretical formulations are completely imposed on the narrative form, as if the concepts were their own illustration; and valuing the authorial function, where the case is worth the difference, to the singular mark. We have seen that this has gone through a kind of inversion, congruent with the critique of traditional formative mechanisms brought about by the Lacanianism of the 1990s. Connected with leftist resistance, supported in many cases by Argentinian exiled analysts, readers of Marie Langer and the Plataforma Group, who openly criticised IPA psychoanalysis, there is a kind of equivocation in the Brazilian reception of Lacan. Whilst he attacked ego-psychology, represented by New York psychoanalysts such as Lowenstein, Hartman and Kris, the absence of this kind of psychoanalysis moved Brazilian Lacanian critique against Bion, Klein or Winnicott, as they were compromised with the same old hierarchical power relations. So, the reversion of the clinical case strategy follows the logic of the inversion in power relations on the analyst in training (Dunker, 2015).

If in the first moment the cases were part of the impersonal discourse of psychiatric medicine, in the second period they become part of the master narrative of formative institutions, then this authority seems to have migrated to the stylistic individuality of each psychoanalyst, consecrated to his or her unique process of formation and authorisation. Now, perhaps, it is time to give voice to the patients themselves.

References

Aragão, G. (1914). *Da Psicoanalise: a sexualidade nas nevroses*. Pap Modelo (44).

Bezerra, D. (2018). *Lacan para Historiadores*. Appris.

Bicudo, V. L. (1994). Já fui chamada de charlatã. (Testimony to Cláudio João Tognolli). *Folha de São Paulo*, São Paulo, *Caderno Mais*, p. 6, 5 de jun. de, p. 6.

Braga, A. P. M. (2016). Pelas trilhas de Virgínia Bicudo: psicanálise e relações raciais em São Paulo. *Lacuna: uma revista de psicanálise, 2*, 1.

Carrilho, H. (1930). Laudo do exame médico-psicológico procedido no acusado Febronio I. do B. *Archivos do Manicômio Judiciário do Rio de Janeiro*. Rio de Janeiro: Papelaria Globo, Ano 1, n. 1., 1930.

De Andrade, O. (2000). *O Rei da Vela*. Companhia das Letras.

De Holanda, S. B. (1927). *Raízes do Brasil*. Companhia das Letras.

Dunker, C. I. L. (2011). *Structure and constitution of psychoanalysis: Cure, treatment and therapy*. Karnac.

Dunker, C. I. L. (2008). Psychology and psychoanalysis in Brazil: From cultural syncretism to the collapse of liberal individualism. *Theory & Psychology, 18*(2), 223–236.

Dunker, C. I. L. (2015). *Mal-Estar, Sofrimento e Sintoma: uma arqueologia do Brasil entre muros*. Boitempo.

Dunker, C. I. L., Paulon, C., & Milán-Ramos, G. (2018). *Análise Psicanalítica de Discursos*. Letras e Cores.

Faoro, R. (1992). A questão nacional: a modernização. *Estud. av., 6*(14) [cited 2021-01-07], 7–22.

Figueiredo, L. C. (2003). *Psicanálise: elementos para a clínica contemporânea*. Escuta.

Franco da Rocha, F. (1914). Paranoia e Syndrome Paranoide. In *Annaes Paulistas de Medicina e Cirurgia,* Março – Anno II – vol. II – nº 3 – páginas 65–75.
Franco da Rocha, F. (1920). *O pansexualismo na doutrina de Freud*. Typographia Brasil de Rothschild & Cia.
Gutman, G. (2007). Raça e psicanálise no Brasil. O ponto de origem: Arthur Ramos. *Rev. latinoam. psicopatol. fundam., 10*(4).
Indo do Brasil, F. (1926). *As revelações do príncipe do fogo.* Pap. e Typ. Monteiro & Forrelli.
Kyrillos Neto, F., Moreira, J. de O., & Dunker, Ch. I. L. (2015). DSMs and the Brazilian psychiatric reform. *Frontiers in Psychology, 6*, 1–6.
Levinzon, G. K. (1999, November). No Jogo dos Afetos: quando Rapunzel não joga suas tranças. In *Jornal de Psicanálise, 32*(58/59): 407–417.
Lima, R. A. (2017) Análise Reparável e Irreparável: o Conceito Psicanalítico de Reparação na Agenda da Transição Brasileira. *Psicol. cienc. prof., 37*, n.spe.
Lukács, G. (2009). *Teoria do Romance*. Companhia das Letras.
Nogueira do Vale, E. (2003). *Os Rumos da Psicanálise no Brasil*. Escuta.
Oda, A. M. G., & Dalgalarrondo, P. (2000). Juliano Moreira: um psiquiatra negro frente ao racismo científico. *Rev. Bras. Psiquiatr., 22*(4) [cited 2021-01-21], 178–179.
Rodrigues, N. (1903). A paranóia nos negros: A paranóia nos negros: estudo clínico e médico e médico-legal (Parte 2). *Rev. Latinoam. Psicopat. Fund., VII*(3), 131–158.
Valladares de Oliveira, C. L. M. (2006). *História da Psicanálise: São Paulo (1920–1969).* Escuta.
Vogelar, R. B. (2011). Sintoma e fenômeno psicossomático: letra e número? In *Livro Zero- Revista de Psicanálise do Fórum do Campo Lacaniano de São Paulo, 2*, 191–198.
Zaidan, M. (1966). Evolução de uma análise: transferência e contra-transferência. *J. psicanal., 1*(1) [citado 2021-01-06], 21–22.

7

Politics of Secrecy in the History of Psychoanalysis

Rafael Alves Lima

We are faced with the challenge of making some contributions on the matter of truth in psychoanalysis during a time when revisionism, negationism and fake news are spreading and undermining long-established criteria for validation. In present-day Brazil, revisionism and negationism are used to constrain several areas of common knowledge, but it is not incidental that one of its favourite methods of dissemination is through historical studies on the dictatorial period, which will be discussed later in this piece. Those who devote themselves to the study of psychoanalysis and its history must inevitably turn to reflection about the archive. The most famous instance is probably the story of Jeffrey Moussaieff Masson, who had been in charge of editing the letters exchanged between Freud and Fliess, under the auspices of Kurt Eissler and with authorisation from Anna Freud. Masson had been guaranteed free access to the Freud archives in the Library of Congress, containing letters and all

R. A. Lima (✉)
Laboratory of Social Theory, Philosophy and Psychoanalysis, University of São Paulo, São Paulo, Brazil

B. Mandelbaum et al. (eds.), *Brazilian Psychosocial Histories of Psychoanalysis*, Studies in the Psychosocial,
https://doi.org/10.1007/978-3-030-78509-3_7

kinds of documents that had so far been kept secret. At the same time as researching and compiling the letters in the 1980s, Masson wrote the boisterous *The Assault on Truth* (Masson, 1992).[1] His hypothesis was that Freud may have been reluctant to admit that child sexual abuse genuinely existed in *fin-de-siècle* Vienna. This would be the ultimate proof of Freud's conformism: the supposed refusal to accept the factual truth of child sexual abuse might have been dissimulated behind a theoretical device (the abandonment of seduction theory) and justified by the fear of scandalising the scientific community of which the father of psychoanalysis sought to be a member.

The Masson chapter[2] could have been merely one among countless others in the long history of revisionism in psychoanalysis, which received many names, including 'anti-Freudianism' and 'Freud-bashing' (Grubrich-Simitis, 1997), and continues up until the present day. Indeed, Masson's career as a prodigy of the history of psychoanalysis was completely ruined after *The Assault on Truth* (Gay, 1985), and from the 1990s onwards, he devoted himself to exploring themes of questionable value, such as the loving behaviour of house pets. By having access to documents that were secret up to that point, the researcher granted himself the right to pass moral judgements on the author of the archived manuscripts, mixing up the order of concepts through alleged controversies that are biographical in nature.[3] Peter Gay sums up the revisionist strategy in a rather pedagogical formula: 'These historians have made things easy for themselves: by making nonsense of Freud, they have had no trouble demonstrating that Freud is talking nonsense' (Gay, 1985, p. 31). For no other reason than that, Elisabeth Roudinesco qualifies Masson's hypothesis as a 'delirium of archive' (Roudinesco, 1995), given

[1] It seems to us that the word *assault* was not an incidental choice: the polysemy of the term points at meanings such as mugging, attack, physical violence, rape and violation.

[2] For more details, cf. Malcolm, 2004.

[3] The historian Paul Robinson makes a detailed analysis of the arguments in *The Assault on Truth* and the Jeffrey Masson case as a whole. According to his analysis, *The Assault on Truth* and Masson's following books are infused with the anti-sexual rhetoric of the New Puritanism, a moral reaction typical of the North American conservative sectors in the 1980s to the Freudian-Marxist libertarianism which had set the countercultural agenda during the previous years (cf. Robinson, 1993).

that the work of interpreting and 'revealing the truth' through the archive may intentionally confuse *who* is accessing and *what* is being accessed.

It is because of such chapters in the history of psychoanalysis that we are led to highlight the category of the 'secret' within the historiographical debate in psychoanalysis. We consider two aspects of the secret: (1) its social dimension, understood as an elementary operator of power relations, and (2) its subjective dimension, capable of answering and clarifying certain metapsychologically described phenomena. Thus, from the combination of these two aspects, we see the secret as a category that coordinates metapsychology and politics. In this first moment, we shall devote ourselves to the metapsychology of the secret.

For a Metapsychology of the Secret

In 1906, in the text 'Psychoanalysis and the establishment of the facts in legal proceedings,' Freud proposed an unusual contrast between the hysteric and the criminal. They both keep or hide a secret; the difference is that the criminal knows and hides the secret from the other, while the hysteric is unaware of the secret they keep, i.e. the secret is hidden from themself:

> In the neurotic the secret is hidden from his own consciousness; in the criminal it is hidden only from you. In the former there is a genuine ignorance, though not an ignorance in every sense, while in the latter there is nothing but a pretence of ignorance. Connected with this is another difference, which is in practice of importance. In psycho-analysis the patient assists with his conscious efforts to combat his resistance, because he expects to gain something from the investigation, namely, his recovery. The criminal, on the other hand, does not work with you; if he did, he would be working against his whole ego. (Freud, 1906/1959, pp. 111–112)

Based on this fragment, we are able to outline some premises for a first schematic draft of the secret's metapsychological aspirations:

1) The secret is always secret in relation to something or someone, even if this someone is the subject themself—the secret is, therefore, relational, and its unveiling depends on the kind and quality of the relation which is established;
2) The secret depends on an exchange between knowing and not knowing—thus, it depends on whether it is, or is not, accessible to the conscious mind;
3) After the secret is available to the conscious mind, the subject still has the opportunity to deliberate, to choose whether or not they will share the secret—which makes both the negotiation around the secret and the economy of symbolic exchanges founded on the secret even more complex.

From the viewpoint of the clinic, any and all subjects undergoing analysis will submit themselves to the fundamental rule of free association. Whether or not they are conscious of the secret they bear, the patient who speaks freely reveals their intimate secrets, their own logic of understanding things and their personal history. That is, when surrendered to the condition of suspending previous moral judgements and speaking whatever comes to mind, both the criminal and the hysteric are subjected to the 'incidents' of deliberation and conscious will. Freud illustrated the fundamental rule of psychoanalysis through this example:

> I once treated a high official who was bound by his oath of office not to communicate certain things because they were state secrets, and the analysis came to grief as a consequence of this restriction. Psychoanalytic treatment must have no regard for any consideration, because the neurosis and its resistances are themselves without any such regards. (Freud, 1913/1959, p. 136)

Free association elevated to the condition of a fundamental rule would represent, in a way, a certain ritual of power conversion, similar to the episode of hospitalisation of King George III that was described by Foucault in 'Psychiatric Power' (Foucault, 2008): when admitted into an asylum, the King will be stripped of his monarchic powers to become a patient like every other.[4] Up to a point—since the subject under analysis will always be free to interrupt the process or change analysts, to give everyday examples from the clinic—the fact is that the fundamental rule of the psychoanalytic clinic aims to be unavoidable. It is interesting to observe through this that Freud is aware that certain unspeakable secrets are not necessarily of the sexual order. Even when it is 'imposed from the outside,' the restriction on free association will inevitably hinder the analysis' development: if an analysis is to be satisfactorily experienced, not even State secrets should be acceptable exceptions to the fundamental rule of psychoanalysis.

Against the backdrop of the theory of sexuality, Freud has been heavily criticised, notably by Foucault (whose criticism, we may note in passing, does not resemble Masson's revisionism): intimate sexual secrets, either conscious or unconscious, might be the most 'valuable confession' for a treatment whose ultimate criterion lies within sexuality (Foucault, 1998). Whether we agree or not with well-founded, non-revisionist criticism, such as Foucault's, we must take into account that even if the secret told in the clinic involves confession and sexuality, it is not limited to that. In fact, within the field of psychoanalytic theory, there is a perspective that radicalises the metapsychological understanding of the conditions of possibility for the points raised here (the relational character, the transition between the conscious and the unconscious mind, and the decision of sharing) that seems impervious to the criticism of psychoanalysis: the perspective of trauma.

In relation to trauma, the recurrence of the idea of secrecy as a metapsychological category revisits a debate between Freud and Ferenczi. It is not my intention to reconstruct this debate here, but we should keep in mind that, roughly speaking, if for the former the traumatic experience has been translated as one of unbearable excess for the psyche, for the latter trauma implies a divisive experience that operates as a strategy for psychic survival. By this means, Ferenczi opens up an important front of reflection about trauma, which had been encouraged by

[4] The George III case has been minutely examined in Macalpine & Hunter, 1995.

the Freudian metapsychology,[5] but not examined in all its radicalism or multiple possibilities: comprehending, first of all, how the traumatic experience is mainly an experience of dissociation, fragmentation, and pulverisation of the psyche. In other words, not all contents are unknown to the subject and made unconscious by a direct action of repression—there might be other psychic mechanisms responsible for the destinies of trauma in psychic life. Dissociation is the mechanism responsible for the experience of disconnecting from the traumatic content, in an attempt to make it 'tolerable.' The classic Ferenczian analogy is that of the lizard that detaches its tail when feeling threatened by a predator (Ferenczi, 1968); the psyche similarly dissociates itself when threatened by the unbearable nature of the traumatic experience. Therefore, reflecting upon the fate to which these fragments are subjected in the relational and metapsychological aspects requires complementary reflections on silencing, on traumatic elements that cannot be metabolised in the psyche and in culture, on the transgenerational aspects of the familiar unspoken, and many other issues. This requirement, which permeates a whole Ferenczi-inspired psychoanalytic tradition, is of particular interest.

When considering the metapsychology of secrecy in the Hungarian tradition of psychoanalysis, Nicolas Abraham and Maria Torok's *The Shell and the Kernel: renewals of psychoanalysis* (1994) must be considered. Abraham and Torok propose a distinction between introjection and incorporation with regard to the grieving process. If introjection points to the good prognosis of grief, in the sense of restoring the capacity of the self to reconnect with the objects in the world,[6] then incorporation refers to a state of unprocessed grief, an assimilation of losing the object that gets confounded with feelings of shame, with disparate affections leading to a painful experience of hallucinatory realisation that I have called 'impossible reparation' (Lima, 2017).

---

[5] This is not to deny that there is a theory of splitting in Freud. From *Studies on Hysteria* up to the unfinished manuscript 'Splitting of the Ego in the Process of Defence,' from 1938, it is possible to observe the notion of division, or splitting, as well as the development of such ideas (Nobus & Quinn, 2005, p. 41). We would merely like to emphasise here that a reflection on how an experience of splitting may be appropriate to the dimension of trauma is something best developed in the intellectual programme by Ferenczi and his followers.

[6] This is a particularly original interpretation of the Ferenczian concept of introjection (Ferenczi, 1994b).

> *Incorporation results from those losses that for some reason cannot be acknowledged as such.* In these special cases the impossibility of introjection is so profound that even our refusal to mourn is prohibited from being given a language [...]. The words that cannot be uttered, the scenes that cannot be recalled, the tears that cannot be shed – everything will be swallowed along with the trauma that led to the loss. Swallowed and preserved. Inexpressible mourning erects a secret tomb inside the subject. (Abraham & Torok, 1994, p. 130)

Thus, the unrevealable secret of a traumatic experience pulverised in the psyche is transmitted through a complex web of incorporations, whose naming processes are reproduced through what Abraham and Torok (2005) call 'cryptonymy.' That is, following on from the later Ferenczian theory of trauma, which is based on the perspective of language confusion (Ferenczi, 1994a), the idea of the crypt makes it possible to read trauma as an unnameable secret. The generational transmission, by means of what the authors call 'preservative repression,' concerns what is preserved as an intrapsychic tomb (Abraham & Torok, 2005, p. 159); it is disseminated like a text that happens in secret, like a fossil of 'defunct words,' as interpreted by Derrida (Derrida, 2005, p. xxxv). The course of inoculation and irradiation of secrets is perpetuated as concrete experiences of 'hauntings' (which is not simply a metaphor), recalling Frosh's reflections on individual and collective memories, such as phantoms (past traumas, catastrophes, colonial inheritances), which return as uncanny experiences (Frosh, 2013). In fact, the authors of *The Shell and the Kernel* claim: 'The phantom is therefore also a metapsychological fact: what haunts are not the dead, but the gaps left within us by the secrets of others' (Abraham & Torok, 1994, p. 171).

To this, we add the idea of the enclave. This geographical metaphor indicates a territory entirely contained within another, where crossing the borders confirms the perception of insulation, which seems to be quite appropriate to illustrate the isolated parts of the psyche that are separated from the condition of what may be elaborated:

> The crypt marks a definite place in the topography. It is neither the dynamic unconscious nor the ego of introjections. Rather, it is an enclave between the two, a kind of artificial unconscious, lodged in the very midst

> of the ego. Such a tomb has the effect of sealing up the semipermeable walls of the dynamic unconscious. Nothing at all must filter to the outside world. The ego is given the task of a cemetery guard. (Abraham & Torok, 1994, p. 159)

In order to decipher the encrypted code capable of putting an end to the uninterrupted cycle of traumatic violence, it is a matter of, firstly, recognising the impossibility of seeking to apprehend the secret content as a text that can be read in the light of consciousness, and afterwards, of creating, above all, the psychic conditions required to overcome the enclave that is transgeneratively reproduced in the repetition of traumatic violence. Such conditions are, first and foremost, relational conditions of symbolisation, of sharing and naming of the trauma. Abraham and Torok underline the social dimension to which the elaboration of trauma is subordinated: 'We must not lose sight of the fact that to stage a word [...] constitutes an attempt at exorcism, an attempt, that is, to relieve the unconscious by placing the effects of the phantom in the social realm' (Abraham & Torok, 1994, p. 176).

How can the material field of intersubjective relations be organised in such a way as to make the conditions for symbolising trauma sustainable? Françoise Davoine and Jean-Max Gaudillière, in a luminous book called *History Beyond Trauma*, affirm:

> Every catastrophe in the social order [...] sets in motion a loss of trust, limited or radical, in the safety of the laws governing men, the universe, or the body. Otherness undergoes an abrupt change of status. From guarantor of the good faith from which issue speech and the permanence of physical laws, the other becomes a surface of signs and forms to be deciphered against a background of devaluated words. (Davoine & Gaudillière, 2013, p. 64)

Here, we have one of the most sensitive aspects of the effects of trauma: the damage caused to trust in the Other. How is it possible to trust something or someone again after a traumatic experience? One can understand how serious is the degradation of trust through what the French psychoanalyst Piera Aulagnier (2003) calls 'the right to secrecy.'

Without resorting necessarily to transgenerational artifices, Aulagnier underlines a rather important difference that is worth explaining briefly here: the difference between primary and secondary violence. Primary violence refers to the moment when the mother names the affliction of which the baby complains (sleep, hunger, etc.); she becomes the spokesperson for that which the baby expresses without being able to name. Such a maternal gesture is fundamental for structuring the psyche of the baby, but it is not performed without a remarkable degree of violence, albeit involuntary. In secondary violence, the excess of such a maternal position becomes more dynamic in that the naming of the complaint becomes a demand for answers. In more advanced moments of the subjective constitution, when the child feels in charge of their own thoughts, they tend to benefit from the secret as a defence against secondary violence.

Acknowledging that certain contents may be kept secret by the child's deliberate and conscious action recognises a fundamental psychic recourse in the process of subjective constitution. Thus, this moment, when the processes of alienation and separation of the child from its mother are further elaborated, starts with the experience of violence. According to Aulagnier, the secret emerges in this way, in the context of secondary violence, as a kind of right to subjective life. It is, therefore, a mechanism for preserving the individuality of thought, as a strategy for separating from the mother, as a perception of the self and, above all, as *disalienation*, a conquest of autonomy and emancipation with regard to the violence of the mother's interpretation in its broadest sense. According to Aulagnier, in order for the pleasure of 'thinking secretly' to happen, there must be a pact signed between the parties:

> It is a pleasure that is reinforced by the unexpected discovery that, despite the little real power possessed at this stage in terms of bodily autonomy, despite one's state of dependence for the satisfaction of one's needs, despite the vital demand for love to which one is subjected, *in the register of thinking the Mother may be just as much at your mercy as you are at hers.* (Aulagnier, 2003, pp. 152–153)

Finding that certain elements need not be revealed, that certain omissions, deceptions or lies challenge the parental figures' fantasy of omnipotence and omniscience, promotes a real revolution in the child's subjective experience. In other words, a secret, when conscious, becomes an instrument of emancipation and liberation from the judgement of the other. Therefore, such a discovery can never be a strictly individual prerogative: it will always be relational.

What is interesting about this incursion into Aulagnier's 'right to secrecy' is the consent between the parties, which gives consistency to the experience of trust: only by a tacit agreement to curb the unlimited reproduction of violence is it possible to positively acknowledge the child's discovery, that they can carry a secret and challenge maternal omniscience. The devastating effects of breaking the trust pact between the parties appears to rediscover something of the traumatic experience: with the subject being left to individual solutions for elaborating raw violence, the right to secrecy is lost as a right to subjective life. The subjective achievements of emancipation and autonomy regress to incorporation, that is, to forms that are not psychically metabolisable.

Nevertheless, I believe at this stage that we have been able to list examples that are sufficiently expressive and which confirm the power of the category of secret as an articulator between metapsychology and politics. Unfortunately, here we are not able to examine other theorisations that point to rather similar problems, such as the concept of 'cumulative trauma' in Masud Khan (Khan, 1996), a concept later expanded by Ilse Grubrich-Simitis (1981) in order to reflect upon the experiences in the concentration camp and extreme experiences. There is also a proposal for a characterological typology of psychopathological relations with secrecy and forms of politics (Young-Bruehl, 2010). On the Lacanian side, there is an abundant tradition of trauma as the unassimilable Real (Lacan, 1977), also clinically understood in its therapeutic function (Dunker, 2011)—this tradition is so extensive in itself that it would require another entire text dedicated to the theme. In any case, these all underline the relational and metapsychological aspects of the secret that go directly towards the reflection upon the social and the political.

Politics of Secrecy

In *The Secret and the Secret Society* (Simmel, 1950), the eminent sociologist Georg Simmel writes about the 'reciprocal concealment' implied in any social bond. This dimension becomes more complex within organisations sustained by some sort of common purpose, with secrecy being a key element in group cohesion. Through direct reciprocity among the organised members, the lie is interpreted as a response to the pressing need to keep the secret:

> Every lie, even if its object were of a factual nature, is by its inner essence a generation of error outside the lying *subject*, for it consists in the liar hiding from the other the true conception that is treated. That the one lied to has a false ideal about the *matter* does not exhaust the specific essence of the lie—it shares that with simple error—but rather what one will accept about the inner opinion of the *lying person* in a deception. Truthfulness and falsehood then are of the most far-ranging importance for the relationships of people with one another. (Simmel, 1950, p. 311)

Although Simmel does not resort to any concept of unconsciousness, he interprets secrecy in a way that is close to the Freudian view, in that the secret is always a secret in relation to another. When the other has an attitude of respect for what is being concealed—that is, an attitude which includes and accepts the secret—we have what Simmel calls 'discretion.' The stranger who 'gets too close,' however, disturbing the other's personal value, infringes upon the honour of the other—the invader is understood as a 'personality violator,' whose disrespect is motivated by curiosity and goes beyond the bounds of discretion in raising suspicion about the qualities of the other. In this case, there is a restoration of the dimension wherein secrecy requires negotiation between the parties involved. The question is whether the intention to conceal finds in the other the intention to discover; thus, the intention becomes a central element in the process of negotiation. In an argument that evokes Aulagnier's right to secrecy, Simmel resorts to an analogy. It is like when a child, for example, learns that they can say to the other 'I know something you don't know.' Whether or not this is true—for as soon as they find out they will exhaustingly repeat the formula with everyone around them—they will quickly learn its effect, which is to produce a sentiment of inferiority and humiliation in the other (Simmel, 1950, p. 327). This would, according to the sociologist, be the matrix that explains the common feeling that everything that entails secrecy 'must also be profound and important,' something that expands into the social bonds as a whole and their respective power relations. That is, according to Simmel, since it is impossible to verify all the results obtained by others, we organise a system which 'rests on faith in the honesty of others' in a 'credit economy'[7]: 'life stands on a thousand presuppositions the causes of which the individual cannot at all trace and verify, but which must be taken on faith' (Simmel, 1950, p. 312). This is precisely why it is possible to call it a sociology of secrecy, as it is possible to describe and analyse how communities of either simple or complex reliability can be constructed upon this system. 'The secret is a general sociological form that stands completely neutral over the value-relevance of its contents' (Simmel, 1950, p. 326). Secrecy being an articulator of everyday sociability,[8] whose relationship with the content that is kept secret is one of relative independence, 'the use of the secret as a sociological technique' (Simmel, 1950, p. 326) is what allows us to elevate it to the status of an articulator of power relations. The lie expresses a power relationship, insofar as 'the deceived—hence those harmed by the lie—will always be in the majority in relation to the liar who finds advantage through deception. Therefore, "enlightenment," which aims at the elimination of falsehood at work in social life, is thoroughly democratic in character' (Simmel, 1950, p. 313).

By going beyond the understanding of sociology of secrecy in Simmel, the political philosopher Norberto Bobbio takes this reasoning of the use

[7] The idea of a 'credit economy' is not postulated here fortuitously. In the sociology of Simmel, it connects with the reasoning explored in another famous book by the author, *The Philosophy of Money* (Simmel, 2004).

[8] It is worth mentioning the paper written by the sociologist and psychoanalyst Michael Rustin which discusses Simmel's sociology of secrecy, which sees psychoanalytic institutions as secret societies. Cf. Rustin, 1985.

of secrecy a step further[9] by interpreting it in terms of what he calls 'invisible power.' In a series of books and essays published between the 1970s and 1980s, Bobbio (1987, 1989, 2015) explores a subject that is utterly meaningful, yet underutilised in contemporary psychoanalytic literature: the continuum between totalitarian or dictatorial regimes and modern democracies, maintained through State secret services. In other words, whether in democracies or in states of exception, the State depends upon an institutional policy of generating and managing secret information. Due to its opaqueness, this 'invisible power,' which acts as a false background for democracy, comprises the denial of a democratic principle par excellence, so-called 'transparency.'

Here, we revisit the issue of trust in order to amplify it: whether directly or indirectly, every citizen is, in theory, safeguarded by trust in their relationship with the hidden operations of the State. Although citizens recognise the opaque background of democracies' secret intelligence services, and although they are unaware of the information they generate, the cohesion of the social fabric depends on the credibility and legitimacy entrusted to the State by the very citizens upon which the invisible power acts to maintain public security, protect the population, defend national borders and so forth. In the same way that trust requires intelligence services not to encroach on their constitutional prerogatives, it also demands in return that their professional agents observe strict and incorruptible secrecy. As seen in the example of Freud's patient, it is an imposition of secrecy of such legal value that not even free association in an analysis would prove feasible.

Nevertheless, in 'flawed' modern democracies, it is a recurring feature that constitutional intelligence departments make alliances with civil society sectors. Finally, we move towards the fine line that simultaneously unites and divides dictatorships and democracies by means of the cover-up of State secrecy, 'which in the modern constitutional state is allowed

[9] Indeed, if we wanted to adhere to a strictly Simmelian perspective in order to discuss the function of secrecy in the democratic system, this would be possible through conceptual mediations such as the differentiation between secrecy as an institution and secrecy as an organization, or more specifically, by devoting ourselves to the transition from the microsociological to the macrosociological perspective (Nedelmann, 1994). We ask the reader to trust our 'epistemological leap' towards Bobbio's perspective, hoping that it will be explained by the forthcoming discussion on the politics of secrecy as an archival policy.

only as an exceptional remedy' (Bobbio, 1989, p. 18). These alliances are responsible for the formation of a truly subterranean government, typifying what Bobbio calls 'crypto-government,' which he defines as 'the totality of actions carried out by paramilitary political forces which operate behind the scenes in collaboration with the secret services, or with sections of them, or at least with their connivance' (Bobbio, 1987, p. 95). We are, therefore, facing a contradiction, in which the State coexists with its antagonist, an uncompromising denial of the Weberian maxim which ascribes to the State the legitimate monopoly of violence, the use of force or coercion [Gewalt in German] (Weber, 2004). The State secret services thus configure a kind of 'modern democratic anomaly' in resorting to the support and collaboration of civil society, crossing the fine line between democracy and dictatorship where often 'the principle of official secrets was used to protect the secrets of the "anti-state"' (Bobbio, 1987, p. 95).

Now, we have come to this point where we can build a conceptual platform by connecting some elements. The postulation of a 'crypto-government,' which suggests an association with Abraham and Torok's idea of a 'crypt,' seems to grant an unmatched intelligibility to the scenario of Latin American dictatorships. In the particular case of the Brazilian military dictatorship at least, which lasted from 1964 to 1985, the anti-State overcame the State in the unmeasured exhortation of the intelligence apparatus, to such an extent that its inventor, General Golbery do Couto e Silva, later regretted having—in his words—created a 'monster' (Stepan, 1988, p. 16).

Secrets that have never been deciphered, traumas that have never been named or processed, crimes committed by the State that have never been prosecuted or punished, cooperation with political persecution that has never been revealed, authoritarian corruptions of democratic institutions that have never been restored, bonds of trust that have never been re-established, vulnerabilities to revisionism and negationism that have never been overcome: here is a small but representative collection of the pernicious consequences of Brazilian military dictatorship, which, on the one hand, directly challenges us when we study its history and, on the other, attests to the frailty of Brazilian democracy since the transition days in the 1980s up to (evidently) the present. Having said that, let us finally devote ourselves to the historiographical reflection that such a challenge brings to the history of psychoanalysis in Brazil.

Secrecy and Archive: Historiographic Consequences for the History of Psychoanalysis

Invariably, the debate on a policy of secrecy in the archives of psychoanalysis will lead to questions regarding the ethics of research concerning the disclosure of patients' names, for example (Fichtner, 1997). At the same time, research within the history of psychoanalysis increasingly demands a theoretical and methodological reflection that is written about (or by means of) clinical cases (Borossa, 1997; Lima, 2015).[10] I find that this is one example among several that comes close to expressing the range of problems that we have sought to highlight so far, for it inspires an analysis that is diagonally political: the history that should be known and that which should not; the one that will be made public and that which will remain private; the convenient and the inconvenient narrative; the respect for privacy within clinical practice; and the urgency to clarify historical facts of relevance to the field.

Extending the argument slightly, that is why we should not be naïve: *archives are never neutral*. It is true that the organisation and systematisation of historical documents respond to fundamentals (which are both technical and scientific) of recording and cataloguing. In practice, however, a hypothetical technical-scientific neutrality of the archive unfailingly bows to the *very intention of archiving*. In the psychoanalytical field, the archive seems to be subject to a unique principle, in which *institutional secrets are levelled with personal or private secrets*. Whether it is due to a mix-up with the sensitive point of clinical secrecy in case inventories, or for protecting against revisionist 'assaults on truth,' such

[10] The posthumous publication of *Thinking in Cases* by John Forrester brings up a highly sophisticated reflection on what is the case—in the author's words, it expresses an intellectual programme of 'History and Philosophy of the Case' (Forrester, 2017). In this regard, see the Chapters 4 and 5 in this volume.

an artifice focuses on theses about what the archive ultimately represents for a historiography of psychoanalysis.[11]

In passing from intimate secrets to the realm of State secrets, the history of psychoanalysis in Brazil is quite exemplary: for example, it is known that a relative lack of commitment to the ordinary reality of social life in Brazil led to a mix-up between clinical and political neutrality under the Brazilian military dictatorship (Oliveira, 2017; Rubin et al., 2016).[12] Thus, following this line, a provocation remains: in a context like this one, could anyone 'believe' in such a thing as 'archival neutrality'?

As it is not a matter of faith, but of method, we are faced with an academic responsibility of the highest degree: to resort to documentary research. Consequently, it is not a mere coincidence that in accessing the archives we find closed doors, blocked accesses and unfair negotiations between the parties involved.[13] I therefore contend that this is a true policy of archival secrecy, which takes place at different levels simultaneously. As previously discussed, it is widely known that the intelligence services of the Brazilian dictatorial regime relied on the support of sectors of civil society in order to go beyond their institutional prerogatives and to provide information to the military sectors responsible for political persecution, imprisonment, torture, murder and the disappearance of political opponents. For example, the archives of the Brazilian dictatorial 'crypto-government,' in which both the military and paramilitary coexisted, mention the use of 'shame management' to protect State secrets from the archives of the dictatorship, a ploy to sustain falsified narratives and to build up a certain political memory of the country in an attempt to make it seem, perhaps, less hideous. We revisit Simmel here through a historical perspective: the deceived will only inherit misconceptions

[11] This is certainly not the only possible definition. In this ongoing debate, among the most renowned authors in the psychoanalytic field, there will certainly be Foucault in *Archaeology of Knowledge* (2002) and Derrida in *Archive Fever* (1996). There is a more thorough discussion about these authors in Lima (2015).

[12] It is worth mentioning Nancy Caro Hollander's very interesting article on the Argentine case as a basis for comparison. Cf. Hollander (2006).

[13] See this volume, Chapter 4.

about the liar's true intentions. We were compelled to legitimise authoritarianism, to naturalise the atrocity of missing bodies, to believe that the dictatorship was a 'necessary evil' to contain the 'advance of communism in Brazil.' Under the proselytising of those who aligned themselves ideologically with the capitalistic Western hemisphere in the context of the Cold War, we have been indoctrinated—speaking in broad terms—to live with the traumatic ghosts of our own history.

As for the sensitive issue of 'shame management' in the private Brazilian archives of psychoanalysis (i.e. the documentation sections of psychoanalytic institutions), academic research units in psychoanalysis committed to collecting historical documents are still quite rare in Brazil. With regard to research devoted to dark periods in politics, such as the military dictatorship,[14] although absolutely fruitful in general Brazilian historiography, academic research gathered from the 'public' archives of the State is rare. To credit such scarcity to a supposedly 'widespread ontological discredit' of Brazilians towards their own history seems to be a rather worrying misconception: the rhetoric manufactured to contend that Brazilians are 'naturally' uninterested in their own history is nothing but the rhetoric of the dominant ideology and, as such, must be confronted. In fact, the problem seems to be of another sort.

While the archives of psychoanalytic institutions have insisted for decades on maintaining, as the norm, a policy of non-transparency as a 'credit economy,' in Brazil there has been in recent years a policy of openness and wide dissemination of the so-called 'archives of the secret services of the State,' belonging both to the National Intelligence Service (SNI, in its Portuguese acronym) and to the regional intelligence services of the Armed Forces and various documentation departments from the military regime. Since the process of democratic transition began in 1985,[15] it has become imperative as part of the political agenda to understand a historical past through the undisclosed secrets and repressive

[14] To be fair, we must underline here Nadia Sério's exceptional research through the archives of SPRJ, a Rio de Janeiro institution linked to IPA. The research with institutional archives had the merit, for instance, of bringing up previously unpublished documentation on the Amílcar Lobo case. Cf. Sério, 1998.

[15] The year 1985 also marks the publication of the book *Brasil Nunca Mais* (Brazil Never Again), which disclosed several documents from the SNI and strengthened the fight for the right to truth, memory and justice in our country. Cf. Arns, 1985.

actions of the State, in order to have the chance not to repeat it in future. After all, should not diligence over repetition (of the mistakes, the afflictions, the barbarities) be what makes the ethics of psychoanalytic treatment coincide with the craft of history? Even when psychoanalysts and their institutions may potentially appear in State archives, the standard response is to revert to the reactive discourse of the 'out of debt, out of danger,' so as to confuse 'authentic ignorance' with 'simulated ignorance,' as seen in Freud. Perhaps the intention of such a policy of secrecy may even be to emulate the slow pace at which Freud's archives have been opened in the Library of Congress over the years. In any case, the rhythmic mismatch between the opening of the archives of psychoanalysis and that of the Brazilian State seems like a sensitive and inescapable comparison at this point. The anachronism of this policy of secrecy fosters mistrust in alliances with the 'crypto-government,' but this mistrust will be a hindrance to rigorous research insofar as, in the absence of documentary evidence, it will ultimately disorientate historians of psychoanalysis beneath the haze of mystery. Thus, one can only believe that such a policy of secrecy is based on some 'secondary benefit,' such as the anachronism of a symptom: one only needs to find out what is the advantage in being methodically aware to counter the argument that not everything that is secret is fatally profound and important.

Conclusion

In 'Questions for Freud,' Nicholas Rand and Maria Torok affirm that: the 'history of psychoanalysis is comparable to a vast mental organisation that includes, among other features, areas of silence, secrets, and crypts' (Rand & Torok, 1997, p. 99). In fact, this sentence is a well-rounded synthesis of what has been preliminarily and rudimentarily inferred: that the secret, relational by definition, would be a defensive recourse against the interference of the other against ourselves. The metapsychology of psychoanalysis invites us to a conceptual journey through the nooks and crannies of psychic life, deepening the first impression of the secret through the incidence of trauma and the right to subjectivity. The secret is therefore valued and elevated to the condition of a general sociological form, which has allowed us to approach it: whether it is when one hands over the word to the other—in psychoanalytic listening and ordinary sociability—or when one hands over the archive to the historian, each in his own way, the truth that is intended to be intimate or under some control becomes subject to interpretation and resignification.

From a historiographical position, truths that are intimate or shared among the few constitute a certain 'narrative fortress,' whose domain is restricted (i.e. 'safer') within officialdom, with its internal networks of pre-selected officials. However, we must also bear in mind the psychic and social dimension of trauma: even the most official secrets are cryptic and are likely to propagate and repeat the traumatic experience continuously unless they find objective conditions for being deciphered, re-signified, nominated, elaborated and, finally, overcome. Therefore, the challenge for the historians of psychoanalysis cannot be less than this: to renegotiate the work relations between researchers and archives within the framework of a relationship of trust.

Every historian knows how necessary it is to find creative solutions and explore multiple primary sources (including, of course, all kinds of State archives), whose material surface reveals what should have been hidden. Resourcefulness and scientific research are urgently needed in present times, since it may take too long for us to establish the truth. To give an example, if the scope of a particular historical research includes a period of dictatorial rule, then criticism ought to be greater than ever with regard to the interpretation of content derived from interviews and testimonies. If the politics of secrecy in the history of psychoanalysis lay in the unlimited terrain of dispute over versions of history, then imposture, bluffing, fraud and lying will be the very raw material of research work. However, the archive alone does not subtract the predictable lie from the oral testimony. We should not be naïve: archives are products of human activity, they are constructed according to their own intentional logic and, therefore, their contents also lie, bluff and deceive.

I believe that the solution to this gridlock lies in the accumulation of documents and their respective interpretations. Forgive our recourse to such a 'quantitative' notion, but we must promote the confrontation of contradictory data and incongruous versions of similar facts. Perhaps this is another Freudian lesson for the historian of psychoanalysis: in the quest for truth, one of the most consistent psychoanalytic concepts is, precisely, conflict.

Therefore, I also believe that it will not be an intimidating and incriminating attitude towards the archon (of the archivist, the librarian, the secretary of the institutional sections of documentation), when searching for the 'secret truth they are hiding,' that will open the archive. It would be more effective to assert that a policy of transparency for the archives of psychoanalysis in Brazil is nothing more than a responsible way of engaging the psychoanalytic field in the political struggle for truth, memory and justice through access to information. To this end, all parties involved in this pact must sign the supra-institutional (should we say, 'supra-psychoanalytic'?) agreement to ensure that the archive is available for strengthening the principle of transparency. Even if this may, at first glance, undermine the system of 'faith in the honour of others' (after all, the defensive argument of threat to personal honour is an expedient which is par excellence aversive to historical research in psychoanalysis), it is worth remembering that every shake tends to be transitory. Historians themselves will be ready to reject revisionisms and their respective contempt for truth, as seen in the first few paragraphs of this text. Historical facts tend not to accommodate themselves well in rigid packaging, in definitive and static versions, as psychoanalysis itself teaches: to historicise is, first and foremost, to mobilise. In a country such as Brazil, whose current political culture encourages revisionism and negativism of all kinds, from both the dictatorial period and the present time, doing science (in our case, doing historical science dedicated to psychoanalysis) is a mobilisation of an urgent civilising vocation.

References

Abraham, N., & Torok, M. (1994). *The Shell and the Kernel: Renewals of psychoanalysis.* University of Chicago Press.

Abraham, N., & Torok, M. (2005). *The wolf's man magic World: A cryptonymy.* University of Minnesota Press.

Arns, D. P. E. (1985). *Brasil Nunca Mais.* Vozes.
Aulagnier, P. (2003). *The violence of interpretation: From pictogram to statement.* Taylor & Francis.
Bobbio, N. (1987). *The future of democracy: A defence of the rules of the game.* University of Minnesota Press.
Bobbio, N. (1989). *Democracy and dictatorship: The nature and limits of state power.* University of Minnesota Press.
Bobbio, N. (2015). *Democracia e Segredo.* Editora Unesp.
Borossa, J. (1997). Case histories and the institutionalization of psychoanalysis. Em: *The presentation of case material in clinical discourse* (pp. 45–63). Freud Museum Publications.
Davoine, F., & Gaudillière, J.-M. (2013). *History beyond trauma.* Other Press.
Derrida, J. (1996). *Archive fever: A freudian impression.* University of Chicago Press.
Derrida, J. (2005). Foreword: Fors: The anglish words of Nicholas Abraham and Maria Torok. Em: *The wolf's man magic words: A cryptonymy* (pp. xi–xlviii). University of Minnesota Press.
Dunker, C. (2011). Logic and politics in psychoanalytic healing. Em: *The constitution of the psychoanalytic clinic: A history of its structure and power* (pp. 345–364). Karnac.
Ferenczi, S. (1968). *Thalassa: A theory of genitality.* W. W. Norton & Company Inc.
Ferenczi, S. (1994a [1933]). Confusion of tongues between adults and the child. In: *Final contributions to the problems and methods of psychoanalysis* (pp. 156–167). Karnac.
Ferenczi, S. (1994b [1909]). Introjection and transference. In: *First contributions to the theory and technique of psychoanalysis* (pp. 35–93). Karnac.
Fichtner, G. (1997). Professional secrecy and the case history. *The Scandinavian Psychoanalytic Review, 20*(1), 97–106.
Forrester, J. (2017). *Thinking in cases.* Polity.
Foucault, M. (1998). *The history of sexuality: The will to knowledge* (Vol. 1). Penguin.
Foucault, M. (2002). *The archaeology of knowledge.* Routledge.
Foucault, M. (2008). *Psychiatric power: Lectures at College de France, 1973–1974.* Macmillan.
Freud, S. (1913). On beginning the treatment. Em: *The standard edition of the complete works of Sigmund Freud - Volume XII (1911–1913).* The Hogarth Press, 1959, pp. 123–144.

Freud, S. (1906). Psychoanalysis and the establishment of the facts in legal proceedings. Em: *The standard edition of the complete works of Sigmund Freud - Volume IX (1906–1908).* The Hogarth Press, 1959, pp. 97–114.

Frosh, S. (2013). *Hauntings: Psychoanalysis and ghostly transmissions.* Palgrave Macmillan.

Gay, P. (1985). *Freud for historians.* Oxford University Press.

Grubrich-Simitis, I. (1981). Extreme traumatization as cumulative trauma: Psychoanalytic investigations of the effects of concentration camp experiences on survivors and their children. *The Psychoanalytic Study of the Child, 36*, 415–450.

Grubrich-Simitis, I. (1997). *Early Freud and Late Freud: Reading anew 'Studies on hysteria' and 'Moses and monotheism.'* Routledge.

Hollander, N. C. (2006). Psychoanalysis and the problem of the bystander in times of terror. Em: *Psychoanalysis, class and politics: Encounters in the clinical setting* (pp. 154–165). Routledge.

Khan, M. M. R. (1996). The concept of cumulative trauma. Em: *The privacy of the self* (pp. 42–58). Karnac.

Lacan, J. (1977). *Seminar XI: The four fundamental concepts of psychoanalysis.* The Hogarth Press.

Lima, R. A. (2015). *Por uma Historiografia Foucaultiana para a Psicanálise: o poder como método.* Via Lettera.

Lima, R. A. (2017). Análise Reparável e Irreparável: o Conceito Psicanalítico de Reparação na Agenda da Transição Brasileira. *Psicologia: Ciência e Profissão,* 37(spe), pp. 116–132.

Macalpine, I., & Hunter, R. (1995). *George III and the Mad-business.* Pimlico.

Malcolm, J. (2004). *In the Freud archives.* Granta.

Masson, J. M. (1992). *The assault on truth: Freud's suppression of the seduction theory.* Harper Perennial.

Nedelmann, B. (1994). Secrecy as a macrosociological phenomenon: A neglected aspect of Simmel's analysis of secrecy. Em: *Georg Simmel: Critical assessments,* vol. 3 (pp. 202–221). Routledge.

Nobus, D., & Quinn, M. (2005). *Knowing nothing, staying stupid: Elements for a psychoanalytic epistemology.* Routledge.

Oliveira, C. L. M. V. d. (2017). The discourse of neutrality: Attitudes of psychoanalysts during the military dictatorship. *História, Ciências, Saúde - Manguinhos, 24*(1), 79–90.

Rand, N., & Torok, M. (1997). *Questions for Freud: The secret history of psychoanalysis.* Harvard University Press.

Robinson, P. (1993). *Freud and his critiques.* University of California Press.

Roudinesco, E. (1995). *Genealogias*. Relume-Dumará.
Rubin, A., Mandelbaum, B., & Frosh, S. (2016). 'No memory, no desire': Psychoanalysis in Brazil during repressive times. *Psychoanalysis and History, 18*(1), 93–118.
Rustin, M. (1985). The social organization of secrets: Towards a sociology of psychoanalysis. *The International Review of Psychoanalysis, 12*, 143–159.
Sério, N. M. F. (1998). *Reconstruindo 'Farrapos', a trajetória histórica da S.P.R.J.: instituição e poder.* Universidade Federal Fluminense (UFF).
Simmel, G. (1950). The secret and the secret society. Em: *The sociology of Georg Simmel* (pp. 307–378). The Free Press.
Simmel, G. (2004). *The philosophy of money*. Routledge.
Stepan, A. C. (1988). *Rethinking military politics: Brazil and the Southern Cone.* Princeton University Press.
Weber, M. (2004). Politics as a vocation. Em: *The vocational lectures* (pp. 32–94). Hackett Publishing Company.
Young-Bruehl, E. (2010). Characterological secrecy. *Journal for the Psychoanalysis of Culture and Society, 15*(2), 189–203.

Part III

Specific Histories of Psychoanalysis in Brazil

8

Between Race Degeneration and the Primitive Unconscious: The Circulation of Psychoanalytic Theories in Brazil

Cristiana Facchinetti and Rafael Dias de Castro

This chapter focuses on the founding of psychoanalytic thought in Brazil during the first decades of the twentieth century. To this end, the narrative follows historiographic approaches that consider the sociocultural force and autonomy of the different contexts in which psychoanalysis was developed. Identifying these differences and valuing them is particularly important in the context of Latin America, which is traditionally relegated to the margins of the centres of science and culture. Regarding the *circulation* of ideas, there is no longer a need to frame reception as being from the centre to the periphery. Rather, we can focus on local values and interests that emphasise the activities of agents when choosing psychoanalytic practices from a vast repertory of knowledge that could have been assimilated by that generation of physicians. Thus, we follow Kapil Raj,

C. Facchinetti (✉)
Departamento E Pesquisa Em História das Ciências E da Saúde, Fundação Oswaldo Cruz (FIOCRUZ), Rio de Janeiro, Brazil

R. D. de Castro
Universidade Estadual de Montes Claros, Montes Claros, Brazil

B. Mandelbaum et al. (eds.), *Brazilian Psychosocial Histories of Psychoanalysis*, Studies in the Psychosocial,
https://doi.org/10.1007/978-3-030-78509-3_8

for whom statements, objects and scientific practices only spread from their origin at the expense of adjustments made in the places where they are incorporated. The scientific procedures are reconfigured in order to adapt them to the social context in which they are integrated (Raj, 2007, p. 155).[1]

Geographically, this study is restricted to Brazil, with a focus upon Rio de Janeiro, which was the federal capital during the first decades of the twentieth century. In particular, we concentrate on the *Hospício Nacional de Alienados*[2] (HNA) [National Hospital for the Mentally Ill] and on the *Sociedade Brasileira de Neurologia, Psiquiatria e Medicina Legal* (SBNPML) [Brazilian Society for Neurology, Psychiatry and Forensic Medicine]; these were founded and operated at the same location. It was in this environment, among a group of German-speaking psychiatrists, that the concepts of psychoanalysis began to circulate during the 1910s, among other theories of a psychodynamic nature (Muñoz, 2015). It was also from this centre of theories and practices that psychoanalysis began to radiate out to fields such as forensic medicine (Russo, 2000), mental hygiene (Reis, 1994) and education (Castro, 2016). This period was also marked by bio-deterministic, racialist and/or degenerationist theories in local psychiatry. These other theories of the psyche–which were not always in opposition—sometimes also appropriated psychoanalysis, creating very specific polyphonic discourses and practices (Ponte, 1999).

Our starting point is the first thesis published on psychoanalysis at the *Faculdade de Medicina do Rio de Janeiro* [Rio de Janeiro School of Medicine] (FMRJ) and, after that, medical or psychiatric periodicals, published minutes of the SBNPML, texts published during the period and psychiatric manuals written by physicians at the HNA and/or FMRJ during that period who participated in the process of institutionalisation of psychoanalysis. Our investigation ends during the period between

[1] Studies on the history of the circulation of psychoanalytic ideas in Latin America have expanded in recent decades through narratives highlighting their appropriation by medical, legal and behavioural sciences, in addition to by the arts and culture. See, among others: Russo (2000); Castro (2014); Plotkin and Ruperthuz (2017), Facchinetti (2018).

[2] The HNA had different names over the years: *Hospício de Pedro II* (1852–1889), *Hospício Nacional de Alienados* (1890–1911), *Hospital Nacional de Alienados* (1911–1927), *Hospital Nacional de Psicopatas* (1927–1937) and *Hospital Psiquiátrico* (1938–1944). The most common name is *Hospício Nacional de Alienados*. Therefore, we use its initials here.

the World Wars, when psychoanalysis was already widely disseminated within scientific circles and embedded in Brazilian society (Marcondes, 2015).

With the support of primary sources from different periods—dissertations, minutes of meetings, specialised periodicals and books for the general public—we contend that the key points that led the psychiatrists of the period to become interested in psychoanalysis were the way Freud's theory provided new options for the old problems of race and the mentality of the local population, and also represented innovations in terms of outpatient practices. These psychiatrists were hoping that, with the support of this knowledge, they could contribute more substantially to the development and evolution of the 'Brazilian race' (Stepan, 2004, pp. 368–369).

From Degeneration of the Race to Physical and Situational Factors: The Diseases of Brazil

Various theories relating to concepts of race and evolution, and their impasses, circulated during the second half of the nineteenth century. In the case of Brazil, according to Skidmore (1976), the race question reached its peak between 1880 and 1920, stimulated by the end of slavery. Abolition had a big impact on the nationalistic proposals for a modern Brazil and stimulated considerable intellectual output on the problems arising from local miscegenation.

In the specific case of psychiatric medicine, the link between degeneration and mental illness proposed in 1857 by Bénédict Morel (1809–1873) and in 1870 by Valentin Magnan (1835–1916), led to the question of the problematic relationship between multiracial composition and the construction of a collective 'soul,' of a national identity, that would be able to forge the future of the young nation as modern. It was during this period that Raimundo Nina Rodrigues (1862–1906), a professor of Forensic Medicine at the *Faculdade de Medicina da Bahia* [Bahia School of Medicine], sought to contribute to the 'work of individuation of the nation' (Nina Rodrigues, 2006, p. 214). Supported in large part by deterministic theories, such as those by the physical anthropologist Cesare Lombroso (1835–1909), and racialist theories such as Magnan's, Nina Rodrigues became a professor of the Bahia School of Medicine, highly respected among his national and international peers. He believed that the existence of non-white races refuted fundamental principles of liberalism, such as free will and the capacity for discernment.[3] This was, according to Nina Rodrigues, because the 'pure Negroes' coming from Africa were primitive people, physically and mentally marked by innate, practically fixed characteristics (this position is known as 'fixist racialism') that caused them to believe in mysticism and superstition, and to have little ability for abstraction and a lack of intelligence. Additionally, their primitivism made them impressionable, emotional and instinctive, little accustomed to reason. Conversely, the European, white race had reached the highest level of evolution of the species. Mixing of these two peoples, with such different degrees of evolution, would produce physiological instability in individuals and would result in the degeneration of the 'Brazilian race' (Oda, 2003; Facchinetti & Muñoz, 2013). From Nina Rodrigues' point of view, there was no means for this population to develop in a way that would allow the country to keep up with modern nations. Blacks, due to their primitivism and racial stability, would progress, but over a much longer time frame. Brazilian mestizos, predisposed to instability though functional when they lived on the 'fringes' of modernity, were doomed to fall ill given the high demands of the process of modernisation (Oda, 2003; Venancio & Facchinetti, 2005).

Despite their strong, long-term impact on local society, during the early twentieth century racialist theories began to compete with hypotheses more in line with the experimental requirements of the biomedical sciences of the time, and also with preventive actions. The task force implemented during the Presidency of Rodrigues Alves (1902–1906) to reform the Federal District (Rio de Janeiro at that time) in order to make it modern and hygienic (Benchimol, 1992), included not only physical changes to the city, but also brought together a group of physicians linked to the experimental and laboratory work of Louis Pasteur

[3] On the debate between polygenists and monogenists in Brazil and abroad, see: Schwarcz (1994). On the influences of Nina Rodrigues and his interlocutors in São Paulo and Rio de Janeiro, see: Oda (2003). See also Chapter 9 of this volume.

(1822–1895) and Robert Koch (1843–1910) to address the epidemics that had spread throughout the city and to prevent future diseases. The same occurred in the field of psychiatry. When seeking new 'solutions' for treating mentally ill patients, José Joaquim Seabra (1855–1942), then Minister of Justice and Internal Affairs, appointed psychiatrist Juliano Moreira (1873–1933) to direct the HNA, and to lead and support the reorganisation of the Mental Health Service in the Federal District (Facchinetti & Castro, 2015) on the basis of scientific assumptions more appropriate for the twentieth century.

When he became director of the HNA (1903–1930) and director general of the Mental Health Service (1911–1930), Juliano Moreira, who was himself the son of a free black woman and a white Portuguese father, sought in the theory of Emil Kraepelin (1856–1926) not only greater adherence to the scientific model of the period, but also a more positive and effective solution for local racial multiculturalism than the degeneration-madness combination (Muñoz, 2015). Through an emphasis on health and education as prophylaxis and treatment, Moreira adjusted psychiatry to better fit the broader proposals of public health practices during the first decade of the twentieth century. Insisting on the idea that mental disease was a biological exception, and that the idea of degeneration of people was just a sign of 'ridiculous prejudices based on colour or caste' (Moreira 1922 cited in Oda & Dalgalarrondo, 2000, p. 178), the director of the HNA sought to redefine the discourses and practices of Brazilian psychiatry. Although German theories were not unanimously accepted at the asylum, since they competed with the French and Italian ideas circulating there, the former slowly gained prominence at the HNA (Penafiel, 1913, p. 121). Psychoanalysis was one of the theories appropriated in that context.

The First Contours of the Appropriation of Psychoanalysis in Rio De Janeiro

The ideas of psychoanalysis began to circulate in Rio de Janeiro as early as the first decade of the twentieth century, demonstrating that local physicians became aware of international theories remarkably quickly, especially when we consider that, according to Freud himself, it was only beginning in 1907 that the Viennese psychiatric community became interested in psychoanalysis, and only from then on did his ideas attract the attention of a larger number of individuals in different fields throughout Europe (Freud, 1916). However, as we will see, Brazilians learning about the most recent ideas and having access to a broad repertoire of psychoanalysts and their texts did not mean that they uncritically accepted everything that came from Europe. On the contrary, in the first years of the twentieth century, rare references were made to the ideas of Freud, and when they occurred, they were frequently with great reluctance.[4]

Juliano Moreira was one of the first Brazilian psychiatrists to promote psychoanalysis in Brazil, introducing it at the HNA and at the SBPNML as early as the 1910s (Facchinetti & Castro, 2015). Given that Freudianism was being accepted 'little by little, not only in Austria but also in Germany, England and especially in the United States,' Moreira thought that Brazil also should not overlook 'the extremely rich contributions of the many disciples of Freud, whether orthodox or not' (Moreira, 1920, p. 366). However, although he discussed Freud in classes and at conferences (Porto-Carrero, 1926), used the technique in his psychiatric clinic (Castro, 2014) and was the founder of the Rio de Janeiro section of the *Sociedade Brasileira de Psicanálise* [Brazilian Psychoanalysis Society] in the 1920s (Facchinetti & Ponte, 2003), he never wrote articles or books on the subject, nor called himself a psychoanalyst. As he himself explained several times, psychoanalysis did not need to be treated as a discipline (Cerqueira, 2014), nor was it 'indispensable to be an orthodox follower of Freud's ideas' in order to selectively use those ideas that were 'usable' (Moreira cited in Austregésilo 1922, p. 113).[5]

Antônio Austregésilo (1876–1960) was a psychiatrist and professor of neurology at the FMRJ who worked with Moreira at the HNA and the

---

[4] Reservations regarding psychoanalysis were not limited to Brazil. According to Roudinesco, 'the attacks [against psychoanalysis] were due essentially to Freud's "pansexualism" in France too' (Roudinesco, 2000, p. 104).

[5] The SBPNML was founded by Juliano Moreira and Afrânio Peixoto in 1907, two years after the creation of the periodical *Arquivos Brasileiros de Psiquiatria, Neurologia e Ciências Afins* (1905) —the first periodical for disseminating Brazilian psychiatric research—by the same physicians (Facchinetti & Muñoz, 2013, p.247).

SBPNML, and is also a good example of the gradual appropriation of psychoanalysis in Brazil. Looking into the specificities of this appropriation allows us to consider the negotiations and adjustments that were required for psychoanalysis to finally be accepted by the local medical community at that time.

In 1908, in an essay on the subject of hysteria, Dr. Austregésilo demonstrated that he was already aware of the new ideas introduced by psychoanalysis. However, he stated that the sexual theory of hysteria put forth by Freud and Breuer was 'absurd,' since 'in hysteria there is more sexual coldness than eroticism' (Austregésilo, 1908, p. 64). According to him, psychoanalysis was just 'another theory' (Austregésilo, 1908, p. 65) among many. Nevertheless, in an article published in 1919 entitled 'Sexuality and psychoneuroses,' Austregésilo stressed that 'Freud's ideas are so clear and philosophical that reason cannot fail to accept them.' Furthermore, 'the absurdity of the concepts is only apparent' (Austregésilo, 1919, p. 87). Thus, after 11 years of constant adjustment, psychoanalytic theory and the centrality of sexuality in human life finally seemed settled to him. Austregésilo even went so far as to say that 'the good and the bad in humans originates from the sexual instinct' (Austregésilo, 1919, p. 89) and 'at first glance, it is curious that psychology tangles sexuality with love of country, and maternal love or filial love with certain repulsions or aversions…[but]…sexual life is not good or bad: it is a biological fact of life' (Austregésilo, 1919, p. 86).

Austregésilo's assertions call attention to certain important translation choices. When translating *Trieb* as 'instinct' and calling human sexuality a 'biological fact of life,' Austregésilo linked the psychological to the organic, and to biological determinism, despite the opinion of his peers that 'evidently, translating [*Trieb*] as "instinct" would be unwise' (Porto-Carrero 1932 as cited in Castro, 2015, p. 1465). Nevertheless, the version of psychoanalysis appropriated by Austregésilo circulated widely during that period. This was, in part, because that reading simultaneously contributed to the organicist and determinist perspective that was already established during that period, despite suggesting that psychoanalysis was an important development that could expand the effectiveness of psychiatric diagnosis and therapy.

Another early reader of Freud was FMRJ Professor of Psychiatry and Mental Illness, and director of the *Pavilhão de Observação* [Observation Pavilion], Dr. Henrique Roxo (1877–1969). His first reference to Freud was made in a text written in 1916, when he addressed the diagnosis of 'nervousness.' Roxo discussed some authors who helped frame the category of 'nervousness' more fully, and listed Freud among them. According to Roxo, malaise was a symptom of the Freudian 'neurosis of anguish' and was the basis for the *nervousness* category. He concluded by stating that, in Freud's approach, there was a strong preoccupation with analysing intrapsychic phenomena (Roxo, 1916).

Here we see another interpretive variation, now at the content level: Roxo saw psychoanalysis as a technique for diagnostic exploration through which the physician could access a patient's 'internal' phenomena, allowing him, in his words, to detect probable 'psychic degeneration' that might accompany the diagnosis of 'nervousness' (Roxo, 1916, p. 77). Thus, Roxo adhered to psychoanalysis through an appropriation that subordinated it to degenerationist logic, which continued to fascinate him and other physicians during that period. In agreement with Freud, he believed that, in the presence of degeneration, frequently 'ideas of a sexual nature are buried in the depths of the patient's consciousness' (Roxo, 1919, p. 338). Roxo even stated that exact knowledge of the intimate secrets of mental patients would help clarify the reason for some apparently insignificant acts, and that they could represent a reaction to complexes situated in the unconscious (Roxo, 1919, p. 348). However, despite approving of psychoanalysis as a means for diagnosis of neurotics and psychotics, Roxo continued to reject the central role of sexuality in psychic life, stating that 'one of the exaggerations in Freud's doctrine is the emphasis on sexual occurrences in childhood' (Roxo, 1933, p. 131) and Freud's belief that it was 'impossible for someone with a normal sexual life to have a neurosis' (Roxo, 1919, p. 338).

Despite interpretive variations, these physicians who began to include psychoanalysis in their discourse were important leaders at the HNA, FMRJ and/or SBPNML. It was precisely through the weight of their combined influence that, beginning in 1914, they decided that the

SBPNML should support the Freudian cause, seeking to attract new physicians to defend psychoanalysis.

The first reference to psychoanalysis occurred during the presentation of a case study by Dr. Pedro Pernambuco Filho (1887–1970), who had recently returned from studies in Paris and Vienna (Cerqueira, 2014). In this, he described to members of the Society a case of epilepsy in which self-mutilation phenomena occurred in place of attacks. Austregésilo used the opportunity to introduce psychoanalytic theory into the debate, questioning if the patient's behaviour, like any other self-mutilator, was unconscious, subconscious or conscious. On the same occasion, Juliano Moreira and Henrique Roxo also spoke, discussing similar self-mutilation cases from the psychoanalytic point of view.

In the course of the debate, Austregésilo proposed that the next session be dedicated to psychoanalysis. Following up, he proposed that those members who were already employing psychoanalysis (there were already members devoting themselves to this method!) should present some of their case studies, in addition to providing details of the methods used and the results obtained (Atas, 1914, pp. 268–269). It seems that there was a strong synergy between his talk and that of Juliano Moreira, since the latter asked to speak and said that he had been writing up his experiences with psychoanalysis and that he would present them during another event. His talk occurred during the next session, on 24 September 1914 (Atas, 1914, p. 275).

A few years later, Moreira returned to the topic of psychoanalysis at a meeting of the Society, calling attention to the fact that, in 1914, psychoanalysis was already being practiced at the HNA and at the Santa Casa da Misericórdia Hospital, and that it was, additionally, the subject of research at the School of Medicine (Moreira, 1920). To highlight this development, he mentioned the thesis of Genserico Aragão de Souza Pinto, entitled *Da psicanálise: a sexualidade nas nevroses* [*On psychoanalysis: the sexuality of neuroses*]. The thesis was defended in December 1914, and presented the results of a series of studies of clinical cases analysed since 1911 and a study of psychoanalytic theory. Austregésilo supervised the research, and during the doctoral defence the PhD student, Genserico, also thanked Prof. Juliano Moreira 'for his great interest in the work' (Pinto, 1914, p. 1). In fact, Moreira's interest seems to be related to the fact that he had given the student some of his case studies, analysed using psychoanalytic techniques and theory.

It is worth noting that Moreira stated in 1920 that the dissertation was sufficient for psychoanalysis' first steps in Rio de Janeiro (Moreira, 1920), but according to Pinto, Freud's methods were not that easy and given their complexity, the need to explain their assumptions was increasingly essential, since only after fully understanding the theory could it be disseminated and become acceptable to Brazilian psychiatrists and available in practice (Pinto, 1914, p. 93).

Juliano Moreira's opinion in 1920 was that psychoanalysis was already far from the phase of 'almost absolute condemnation, akin to the early years when the Viennese Professor's statements were repudiated' in the country (Moreira, 1920, p. 366).

Prevention: Psychoanalysis and Mental Hygiene

Based on the appropriation of Kraepelinian theory, especially his emphasis on longitudinal study of a disease, the local collective of psychiatrists began to believe it was possible to identify mental illnesses based on early signs, and established protocols for early intervention. The idea of intervention was also spurred by the creation of mental hygiene scientific networks around the world.[6] Wrapped in an appropriation of Kraepelin's theories and public health, and combined with mental hygiene proposals, the normalisation of the population through health education and healthcare, with the support of psychiatrists, began to be imagined as a feasible process (Reis, 1994).

Contrary to the degenerationist theories that, as we saw above, underlined the progressive, transgenerational character of disease and predicted a sad future for individuals and their descendants, the hygienist perspective provided an opportunity for the development of psychiatric

[6] For constant, longitudinal observation of patients and the course of the disease, Kraepelin developed an analysis instrument he called diagnostic maps (*Zahlkarten*), with which he constructed statistics for nosological purposes and to support early intervention (Engstrom 2003).

medicine. Previously limited to hospitals, mitigating the suffering of mentally ill patients and dealing with their 'degenerative defects,' psychiatric ideas began to circulate in schools, factories, weekly magazines and etiquette manuals, with the objective of preventing predisposed individuals, or even normal people, from becoming degenerate due to the physically or mentally unhealthy environment (Russo, 2000). The shift from determinism to scientific education meant that the State itself, in its biopolitical processes, began to depend increasingly on the expertise of psychiatrists to treat the mentally ill and to shape the model of the modern/healthy Brazilian, who would be capable of increasing the speed of modernisation of the country (Facchinetti, 2018).

While expansion of prevention increased the reach of psychiatry, it also brought new problems. Mental hygiene, so fundamental for prevention and mental health, translated into actions to fight venereal diseases, to prevent premature illness, and the development of measures against excesses that disturbed the spirit. But the question of how people could be convinced to support the new models of normality remained. How could physicians contribute to formal, social and even sexual education? How could hearts and minds be influenced? In the 1920s, psychoanalysis became the response to the question of how this internal 'hygienisation' could be produced, with a view to progress and evolution. Moving from the individual to the collective, the psychodiagnosis formulated by the group whose members began to call themselves psychoanalysts indicated where work should be done, based on the observation of what needed to change so that the individual and the country could modernise and progress. Laziness, roguery, the lack of ideas, surrender to impulses and passions, none of this was now a sign of degeneration, but rather a sign of the juvenile, the primitive, and these traits could mature or evolve.

The psychiatrist Júlio Porto-Carrero (1887–1937), one of the most active members of the first Brazilian psychoanalysis society (SBP-Rio de Janeiro section), was responsible for the Psychoanalysis Clinic of the *Liga Brasileira de Higiene Mental* [Brazilian League for Mental Hygiene] where he sought to work towards changing the standards of predisposed Brazilians:

> Psychoanalysis, by investigating the repressed complexes that predispose neurotic children to be the most likely to be dependent on drugs, to be timid, to have 'peculiar' characters, etc. — you could say that it disperses the fringes of madness. (Porto-Carrero, 1926, pp. 27–28)

In his view, psychoanalysis could also influence 'primary education, and primary companies' (Porto-Carrero, 1926, p. 28), supporting a prophylactic project through education, thus avoiding the emergence of future offenders and/or deviants:

> Given the profound influence of sexuality on the formation and operation of a child's psyche, it is not fair that education avoids the sexual side of life and simply rejects sexual manifestations and knowledge as immoral. There is an urgent need for sex education. (Porto-Carrero, 1927, pp. 58–59)

Another crucial point was that psychoanalysis could be taught to educators and parents, expanding its potential exponentially and putting an end to the 'art of perverting' (Porto-Carrero, 1929). It was psychoanalysis that could provide a way to implement sexual education, which was one of the most important guides for educating children, parents and teachers, as it represented the core of actions for prophylaxis of neuroses and various anomalies.

Generalising individual conclusions to the entire nation, Porto-Carrero showed that the local model of social organisation was one of the factors contributing to the 'backwardness' of Brazil, when compared to countries with 'superior civilisation' (Porto-Carrero, 1933). He believed that the problem of civilising the nation derived from the fact that most of the population was 'mediocre.' The 'mediocre' were those who, with a 'primitive id,' were incapable of controlling their impulses and tended to act unreasonably, due to their lack of self-control (Porto-Carrero, 1933). Acting in this way, they would be always irresponsible in terms of civilised values, inconsistent in their attitudes and guilty of degeneration of the species and the backwardness of the country.

If the Brazilian people, like children, were primitive, acting like the horde in *Totem and Taboo* (Freud, 1913), the psychiatrists proposed encouraging their maturation or civilising processes by using psychoanalytic tools. The pedagogical plan to influence the impulses of each child thus became the way to transform Brazil.

Modernising the Country by Analysing Individuals

We see that psychiatrists indicated their belief in social development and in individuals through the use of psychoanalytic tools: through psychoanalysis, they focused on forming 'good habits,' building 'normal men,' 'men for the country,' and 'Brazilians useful to the country' (Porto-Carrero, 1933, p. 144). In this sense, psychoanalysis also provided insights for greater comprehension of the environment and for society to be improved, leading to the possibility of understanding the collective psychology of Brazilians, their 'totems and taboos' (Porto-Carrero, 1933) and their most peculiar characteristics, all from the perspective of a prophylactic mental hygiene programme.

In fact, *Totem and Taboo* (Freud, 1913) was essential reading for Rio de Janeiro psychiatrists when they were developing an intimate relationship between the Brazilian people and the primitivism of the primordial horde, marked by direct access to the unconscious. As is well known, in *Totem and Taboo* Freud recounts a mythical narrative of the beginning of civilisation, based on the ethnology of the period and addressing the myth of the primitive horde and the death of the totemic father. When read by Brazilian psychiatrists, *Totem and Taboo* showed that Brazilians, due to the lack of well-established repressed feelings, had not overcome the Oedipus complex, with the id driving behaviour in society. According to self-described psychoanalyst Carneiro Ayrosa (1903–1969), one must accept that this society, like an organism, needed growth and evolution to perfect itself:

> Taboos, that is, the ambivalent situations that accompany certain facts and objects, dominate the mentality of the non-civilised (...). We observe those around us and we will surely find identical situations. They are nothing more than a current state, reminiscent of a form of primitive

> thought from which our society has not yet emancipated itself. (Ayrosa, 1932, pp. 56–57)

In this reading, one could compare the 'mental development' of all civilisations: 'Australians, Europeans, Americans, their dominant traits are governed by common lines that, in turn, coincide with the childish traits of our civilised children' (Ayrosa, 1932, p. 56). Imagining the initial similarity of the evolution of all societies, it was assumed that all of them had once been primitive, including the 'countries with more advanced cultures.' Thus, Brazil could become civilised too:

> It is almost worth saying that in each of us, now civilised, there sleeps an aboriginal, our ancient predecessor, baring his poorly hidden nails under the lacy disguise that civilization seeks to weave. What is the origin so resistant and rebellious to the effects of progress and of civilisation? What are the seeds of these attitudes that force conscious adults to resemble, in a single step, the primitives, children, and some mental patients? (Ayrosa, 1932, p. 58)

Psychoanalysis provided a new nosological framework for what had been seen as Brazilian defects and stigmas: excessive sexuality, laziness and lack of initiative were now simply proof of their primitivism, as guided by the unconscious, the source of all members of the species, since even the most developed cultures had passed through this stage. The possibility of educating them, through ideals, could be introduced, allowing them to adapt to modern times: 'each of us could retroact and recall the evolution of these remote periods, it would certainly shed light to avoid so much misunderstanding, the roots of much human unrest and adversity' (Ayrosa, 1932, p. 68). The characteristics that had until then determined the population's inability to be civilised came to be understood as available for sublimation through educational work and, as Facchinetti (2018) pointed out, this representation of drive and of excess came to be understood not only through its negativity, but also as an energetic source of the most elevated goals of humanity.

This was the raw material that the erudite intellectuals thought was available for analytical work capable of modernising the national identity. For this reason, repression of impulses—a sign of a backward, immoral education—was seen as an error and as producing criminality, prostitution, alcoholism and venereal diseases, among the many deviations in the sexual and moral behaviour of Brazilians (Roxo, 1933, pp. 19–20). These tendencies could only be redirected through sublimation for the betterment of society; sublimation was a psychoanalytic tool that would be able to lift Brazil to a civilised stage through balanced, harmonious foundations for the normal development of citizens. A 'universally Brazilian' modernising and civilising programme needed to be established that sought 'through reasoning, the causes of our failures, the reason for our defects' (Porto-Carrero, 1928, p. 38), guiding this 'primitive id' for purposes consistent with the modern ideal.

Partially based on Freud's second structural model (Freud, 1923) and partially founded on the ideals put forward in the first model (Freud, 1908), Roxo proposed the ego as the instance that could ensure a harmonious relationship between the primitive interior of an individual and the moral norms of society:

> The Ego is the part that acts and wants. It also feels. The essential objective of the Ego is to safeguard the individual. The Ego results from a modification, an evolution of the Id, and in fact maintains ties with the unconscious, from which it originated, and is sometimes able to reach the unconscious through psychic phenomena [like dreams]. The most numerous and strongest impulses in life derive from the Id, the foundation of our unconscious. The Ego, that forms the majority of the conscious personality, is a defence organ that monitors that which will be done with respect to the environment, which develops the impulses of the Id, which stores the memories that have not yet been linked to deep, primitive instances. (Roxo, 1938, p. 498)

The challenge for these authors at the time was to transform the Brazilian id into a civilised ego (Castro, 2014).

Final Considerations

Aligning with public health trends in the early twentieth century, psychoanalysis became associated with mental hygiene in Brazil from around the same time, and was appropriated in Brazil as a supplementary tool intended to overcome the argument that miscegenation was a degeneration factor, and against the imposition of the description of the local population as inferior. With the help of psychoanalysis, psychiatrists began to affirm the universality of primitivism in all of humankind and within each individual during infancy, in keeping with the Kraepelian concept of the universality of mental illness and, at the same time, the Freudian *Totem and Taboo*.

Despite this, the psychodiagnosis of the nation was 'mediocrity.' For these psychiatrists, the lack of initiative, the lack of ideals to follow and, especially, the failure to constitute a Brazilian 'collective soul' and a 'collective superego' derived from this mediocrity (Porto-Carrero, 1933). The lack of sufficient investment in the areas of education and health had left families—which were themselves unable to control their impulses—with the role of educating children. As a result, education was often dominated by attitudes that contradicted the ideal advocated by the psychiatric 'elite,' impeding or paralysing intellectual and affective development, stagnating evolution and national adaptation to modernity.

Thus, the diagnosis was also a warning about the need to proceed with the scientific-sexual-sublimatory education project. Adapting psychoanalysis to local needs, the group combined sublimation with early intervention and prevention, functioning as an instrument of mental hygiene for sexual and scientific education capable of contributing individually and collectively so that the id—the 'Brazilian unconscious'—could become a stable ego, defending modernising ideals.

The break with racial degeneration did not prevent Brazil from continuing to be associated with barbaric, backward conditions, nor did it provide a new reading of its population, which continued to be characterised by excesses, wildness and uncontrolled instincts (Porto-Carrero, 1933). However, psychoanalysis appeared to offer these physicians a key to modify this interpretation, by removing hereditary determinism from the core of the problem, since all nations supposedly experienced the same 'infancy of humanity.' This was the approach taken by these psychiatrists in the early twentieth century for the short term, since it allowed them to intervene socially in support of the improvement of 'mentally healthy' Brazilians, to build 'civilised families,' attuned to the 'prevailing evolutionary stage' and with its continuity, creating a society balanced through its different forces, a 'strengthened country' and a 'regenerated national human species' (Porto-Carrero, 1928, pp. 97–101).

References

Atas da Sociedade Brasileira de Psychiatria, Neurologia e Medicina Legal. (1914). Archivos Brasileiros de Psychiatria. *Neurologia e Medicina Legal, 10*(3–4), 241–279.

Austregésilo, A. (1908). Novas concepções sobre a histeria. *Archivos Brasileiros De Psychiatria, Neurologia e Medicina Legal, 4*(1–2), 52–66.

Austregésilo, A. (1919). Sexualidade e Psico-Neuroses. *Archivos Brasileiros de Medicina 9*, 85–91

Austregésilo, A. (1922). Psicanálise nas doenças mentais e nervosas. *Arquivos Brasileiros De Neuriatria e Psiquiatria, 4*(1–2), 87–114.

Ayrosa, J. C. (1932). O comportamento e seus motivos psicológicos. *Arquivos Brasileiros De Medicina, 22*, 56–66.

Benchimol, J. L. (1992). *Pereira Passos: um Hausmann Tropical. A renovação urbana na cidade do Rio de Janeiro no início do século XX*. Secretaria Municipal de Cultura, Turismo e Esportes.

Castro, R. D. (2014). *A sublimação do 'id primitivo' em 'ego civilizado': o projeto dos psiquiatras-psicanalistas para civilizar o Brasil*. PhD Thesis, Casa de Oswaldo Cruz – Fiocruz.

Castro, R. D. (2015). Correspondência de Julio Porto-Carrero a Arthur Ramos: a Sociedade Brasileira de Psicanálise e a preocupação com a tradução dos termos psicanalíticos, décadas de 1920 e 1930. *História, Ciências, Saúde – Manguinhos 22*(4), 1451–1466. https://doi.org/10.1590/S0104-59702015000400014.

Castro, R. D. (2016). Associação Brasileira de Educação e a inserção da psicanálise no campo educacional: Julio Porto-Carrero, Pedro Deodato de Moraes e Renato Jardim (1927–1931). *Histedbr 16*(68), 89–108. https://doi.org/10.20396/rho.v16i68.8644071.

Cerqueira, E. C. B. (2014). *A Sociedade Brasileira de Neurologia, Psiquiatria e Medicina Legal: Debates sobre ciência e assistência psiquiátrica (1907–1933)*. Dissertation. Casa de Oswaldo Cruz, Fiocruz.

Engstrom, E. J. (2003). *Clinical psychiatry in Imperial Germany: A history of psychiatric practice.* Cornell University Press.
Facchinetti, C. (2018). História das Psicoterapias e da Psicanálise no Brasil: o caso do Rio de Janeiro. *Estudos e Pesquisas em Psicologia 18*(SPE), 1106–1117.
Facchinetti, C., & Castro, R. D. (2015). Die Psychoanalyse als psychiatrisches Werkzeug: Die Rolle Juliano Moreira (1900–1930). In C. Santos-Stubbe, P. Theiss-Abendroth, & H. Stubbe (Eds.), *Psychoanalyse in Brasilien – Historische und aktuelle* (pp. 85–112). Psychosozial-Verlag.
Facchinetti, C., Muñoz, P. F. N. (2013). Emil Kraepelin na ciência psiquiátrica do Rio de Janeiro, 1903–1933. *História, Ciências, Saúde – Manguinhos 20*(1), 239–262. https://doi.org/10.1590/S0104-59702013000100013.
Facchinetti, C., & Ponte, C. F. (2003). De barulhos e silêncios: Contribuições para a história da psicanálise no Brasil. *Psychê, 7*(11), 59–83.
Freud, S. (1908). Moral sexual civilizada e doença nervosa moderna. In S. Freud, *Edições Standard Brasileira, vol 9* (1986). Imago Editora.
Freud, S. (1913). Totem e Tabu. In S. Freud, *Edições Standard Brasileira, vol 13* (1986). Imago Editora.
Freud, S. (1916). A história do movimento psicanalítico, artigos sobre metapsicologia e outros trabalhos. In S. Freud, *Edições Standard Brasileira, vol 14* (1986). Imago Editora.
Freud, S. (1923). O Ego e o Id. In S. Freud, *Edições Standard Brasileira, vol 19* (1986). Imago Editora.
Marcondes, S. R. A. (2015). *'Nós, os charlatães': Gastão Pereira da Silva e a divulgação da psicanálise em O Malho (1936–1944).* Dissertation, Casa de Oswaldo Cruz / Fiocruz.
Moreira, J. (1920). O pan-sexualismo na doutrina de Freud, pelo Prof. Franco Da Rocha. *Brazil Medico, 34*(23), 365–366.
Muñoz, P. F. N. (2015). *À luz do biológico: psiquiatria, neurologia e eugenia nas relações Brasil-Alemanha (1900–1942).*PhD thesis, Casa de Oswaldo Cruz, Fiocruz.
Nina-Rodrigues, R. (2006). *As coletividades anormais,* 2nd ed. Senado Federal - Conselho Editorial.
Oda AMGR. (2003). *Alienação mental e raça: a psicopatologia comparada dos negros e mestiços brasileiros na obra de Raimundo Nina Rodrigues.* PhD Thesis, Universidade Estadual de Campinas.
Oda, A. M. G. R., & Dalgalarrondo, P. (2000). Juliano Moreira: Um psiquiatra negro frente ao racismo científico. *Revista Brasileira De Psiquiatria, 22*(4), 178–179.

Penafiel, C. (1913). O prof. Juliano Moreira. *Archivos Brasileiros de Psychiatria, Neurologia e Medicina Legal 9*(1–2), 122–136.

Pinto, G. A. S. (1914). *Da psicoanálise (a sexualidade das neuroses)*. Dissertation, Faculdade de Medicina do Rio de Janeiro.

Plotkin, M., & Ruperthuz, M. H. (2017). *Estimado Dr. Freud: una historia intelectual del psicoanálisis en América Latina*. Edhasa.

Ponte, C. F. (1999). *Médicos, psicanalistas e loucos: uma contribuição à história da psicanálise no Brasil*. Dissertation, Escola Nacional de Saúde Pública / Fiocruz.

Porto-Carrero, J. P. (1926). A psicanálise na Liga Brasileira de Higiene Mental. In: Porto-Carrero JP (1929) *Ensaios de Psicanálise*. Flores & Mano.

Porto-Carrero, J. P. (1927). O caráter do escolar – segundo a psicanálise. In J. P. Porto-Carrero, *Ensaios de psicanálise* (1929). Flores & Mano.

Porto-Carrero, J. P. (1928). Bases da educação moral do brasileiro. In J. P. Porto-Carrero, *Grandeza e Misérias do Sexo* (1934). Pongetti.

Porto-Carrero, J. P. (1929). A arte de perverter: applicação psychanalytica à formação moral da criança. In J. P. Porto-Carrero, *Ensaios de Psicanálise*. Flores & Mano.

Porto-Carrero, J. P. (1933). *Psicanálise de uma Civilização*. Guanabara.

Raj, K. (2007). Conexões, cruzamentos, circulações. A passagem da cartografia britânica pela Índia, séculos XVII-XIX. *Cultura - Revista De História e Teoria Das Ideias, 24*, 155–179.

Reis, J. R. (1994). *Higiene mental e eugenia: o projeto de 'regeneração nacional' da Liga Brasileira de Higiene Mental (1920–1930)*. Dissertation, Universidade Estadual de Campinas.

Roudinesco, E. (2000). *Por que a psicanálise?* Jorge Zahar.

Roxo, H. B. B. (1916). Nervosismo. *Archivos Brasileiros De Psychiatria, Neurologia e Medicina Legal, 12*(1–2), 73–106.

Roxo, H. B. B. (1919). Sexualidade e demência precoce. *Arquivos Brasileiros de Neuriatria e Psiquiatria 1*(1), 337–349.

Roxo, H. B. B. (1933). Psicanálise. In H. B. B. Roxo, Psicanálise e outros estudos. Conxson.

Roxo, H. B. B. (1938). Doutrina de Freud. In H. B. B. Roxo, *Manual de Psiquiatria*.

Russo, J. (2000). A psicanálise enquanto processo civilizador: um projeto para a nação brasileira. *Cadernos IPUB (UFRJ)16*(18), 10–20.

Schwarcz, L. M. (1994). Espetáculo da miscigenação. *Estudos Avançados, 8*(20), 137–152.

Skidmore, T. (1976). *Preto no branco: raça e nacionalidade no pensamento brasileiro*. Paz e Terra.

Stepan, N. (2004). Eugenia no Brasil: 1917–1940. In G. Hochman & D. Armus (Eds.), *Cuidar, controlar, curar: Ensaios históricos sobre saúde e doença na América Latina e Caribe* (pp. 331–391). Editora Fiocruz.

Venancio, A., & Facchinetti, C. (2005). Gentes provindas de outras terras - ciência psiquiátrica, imigração e nação brasileira. *Revista Latinoamericana De Psicopatologia Fundamental, 8*(2), 356–364.

9

Franco Da Rocha and the Psychiatric Discourse in São Paulo (1898–1914)

Raquel Saad de Avila Morales

In Brazil, the transition from Empire to Republic (1889) was marked by a government concern with lengthening the lifespan of its population, considered then to be the nation's wealth. From that point on, illness began to be seen as an obstacle to the country's progress. Within this context, physicians were given the task of regenerating health and national identity. The growth of cities produced the phenomenon of urban poverty, and medicine was one method that the government and the elites adopted to manage this phenomenon. The poverty and racial formation of the Brazilian population became a field of medical research, with public health intervention used to establish a civilised and modern nation (Mota, 2003).

From the end of the nineteenth century, Brazilian doctors began acting as social scientists and health was used as a means of political/medical control over the population, both individual and collective, within a

R. S. de Avila Morales (✉)
Universidade de São Paulo, São Paulo, Brazil

B. Mandelbaum et al. (eds.), *Brazilian Psychosocial Histories of Psychoanalysis*, Studies in the Psychosocial,
https://doi.org/10.1007/978-3-030-78509-3_9

preventive mindset (Machado et al., 1978). Medicine sought to standardise the habits and customs of society in the name of health and of the civility of republican society. The control over bodies was intended to establish a morally standardised, economically productive and potentially harmless model citizen, intended to contribute to the structuring of the rising capitalist system. Women, in turn, would be the moral example of the family and honour their roles as mothers, wives and caregivers, since the nation would be a larger family (Barbosa, 1903).

At that time, those individuals who did not adapt to a certain standard of behaviour—both productive and moral—could be considered insane and, under this justification, admitted to mental-health facilities, to learn to reproduce the type of behaviour promoted by the dominant classes. In the process of consolidating the Brazilian national state, psychiatry captured insanity as a scientific object of interest, investigation and medical intervention. The psychiatric discourse affirmed the dangers of the 'insane,' who would not only be a threat to themselves, but may harm others too. They should thus be isolated in psychiatric facilities in the name of urban safety, of republican order, and of national economic growth.

Brazilian psychiatrists, following the Philippe Pinel tradition, argued that, by being removed from the environment that would have driven them insane and undergoing appropriate treatment, those people could be rehabilitated for social participation.

> [This was] based on the conception that the origin of mental disorders resided in the 'evils of civilization', that is, the dynamics of work, family, economic, social, and religious concerns, as well as the use of alcoholic beverages, hallucinogenic substances and extramarital affairs. Precisely for this reason, removing the mentally ill from this context and placing them in a 'hygienic' and 'healthy' environment would be the first step towards the elimination of madness. (Cunha, 1986, p. 68)

In the city of São Paulo, the first record of an asylum for the 'alienated' dates back to 1829, located on Rua das Flores. Later, the Hospício de Alienados de São Paulo [Hospice for the Alienated of São Paulo] was built, which, under the care of Santa Casa de Misericórdia [Holy

House of Mercy], had two locations: first on Rua São João in 1852 and then in 1864, following the expansion of the city, on a farm on Ladeira Tabatinguera. In 1892, the São Paulo government decided to organise assistance to the insane under medical administration and the psychiatrist Franco da Rocha was invited to design this new institution, which was named Hospício de Alienados do Juquery [Hospice for the Alienated of Juquery].

Franco de Rocha was consequently a prominent figure in São Paulo's psychiatric establishment of the time. From the analysis of some of his publications in an important medical journal, the *Revista Médica de São Paulo: Jornal Prático de Medicina, Cirurgia e Higiene* [*São Paulo's Medical Journal: Practical Journal of Medicine, Surgery and Hygiene*], I intend to contextualise the field that psychoanalysis found when it began to circulate in São Paulo. Franco da Rocha's writings reveal a web of biologistic and racist ideas that were evident in psychiatric practices at the time, with which psychoanalysis had to contend and which it might have had to adapt when it was introduced into Brazil.

Franco Da Rocha (1864–1933)

Francisco Franco da Rocha was one of the main people responsible for structuring psychiatric knowledge in the city of São Paulo, which he did through education and clinical practice in the mental-health facility in addition to the scientific dissemination of his works and critiques. He was born in Amparo, São Paulo, on 23 August 1864. He studied at Faculdade Nacional de Medicina [National Faculty of Medicine] in Rio de Janeiro (1885–1890) and specialised at Hospício D. Pedro II [Hospice Don Pedro II], under the guidance of Teixeira Brandão, in addition to interning at Casa de Saúde Dr. Eiras. He returned to São Paulo in 1892, with the mission of reorganising assistance to the capital's alienated citizens. The Hospício de Alienados do Juquery began operating in 1898, with its first agricultural colony. The official date of its inauguration, however, was 6 May 1901 (Rocha, 02/28/1902). In 1903, the last group of patients was sent there (the women's pavilion), and the Hospício de

Alienados de São Paulo was closed down that same year. Franco da Rocha spent much of his life living in Juquery with his wife and six children.

Franco da Rocha wrote scientific journal articles for national and international publication. In 1892, when he arrived in São Paulo, he began to write for the daily newspapers *Correio Paulistano* and *O Estado de São Paulo*. In 1898, he became the main name in psychiatry to contribute to the medical journal *Revista Médica de São Paulo: Jornal Prático de Medicina, Cirurgia e Higiene.*

Franco da Rocha became interested in psychoanalysis in 1914, when psychoanalytic ideas began circulating more systematically in Brazil(Oliveira, 2002), but his references to psychoanalysis were sparse. He quoted Bleuler in his article 'Paranoia e Síndrome Paranoide' [Paranoia and Paranoid Syndrome] (1914), published 'Do delírio em geral' [Of Delusion in General] in *O Estado de São Paulo* (1919) and wrote the well-known book 'O Pansexualismo da Doutrina de Freud' [The Pansexualism of Freud's Doctrine] (1920). In 1918, he was invited to be the first professor of neuropsychiatry at the Faculdade de Medicina de São Paulo [Faculty of Medicine of São Paulo]. In 1927, Franco da Rocha and Durval Marcondes founded the Brazilian Society of Psychoanalysis of São Paulo (SBPSP), the first psychoanalytic society in Latin America, and he became the first president; however, he never claimed to be a psychoanalyst. As Mandelbaum and Frosh state (2020): 'despite being a curious enthusiast, he felt it was too late to cast himself into this new professional activity' (p. 89). He passed away on 8 November 1933, a few years after founding SBPSP.

Revista Médica De São Paulo (1898–1914)

In the city of São Paulo, the medical press only began at the end of the nineteenth century. It aimed to organise the medical profession and to expand knowledge through experimental research, in search of a consensus on the aetiology of illnesses and their treatments as well as a universalised language that was supposedly both neutral and objective.

The *Revista Médica de São Paulo: Jornal Prático de Medicina, Cirurgia e Higiene* was founded in 1898 by the physicians Victor Godinho and

Arthur Mendonça (inspectors of the Public Health Service). It was the second medical journal published by health professionals in the city and survived almost 17 years.[1] The *Revista* aimed to focus mainly on applied practice in the areas of medicine, surgery and hygiene (Teixeira, 2001). In its early years, it was published monthly (1898–1900), then fortnightly (1901–1914), and was dependent upon subscriptions to survive. It was a journal produced by doctors, read by doctors and financed independently by its subscribers. It intermittently published the bulletins of the Sociedade de Medicina e Cirurgia de São Paulo [Society of Medicine and Surgery of São Paulo] and stopped circulating shortly after the foundation of the Faculdade de Medicina de São Paulo [Faculty of Medicine of São Paulo] (1912), where most of the doctors who published in the *Revista* became professors.

Contributing to the areas of psychiatry, neurology and forensic medicine of the *Revista* were, in addition to Francisco Franco da Rocha (São Paulo), physicians such as Ponciano Cabral (Campinas), Enjorlas Vampré (São Paulo), Henrique Britto de Belford Roxo (Rio de Janeiro),[2] Antônio Austregésilo Rodrigues de Lima (Rio de Janeiro), Raimundo Nina Rodrigues (Bahia), Homem Claro de Mello (São Paulo) and Juliano Moreira (Rio de Janeiro). The journal included diagnosis classifications and debates about the different forms of insanity, analysis of clinical cases, applied therapies and their results and praise and critiques of published dissertations in those areas, in addition to notes and news about physicians and their work. The publications included scientific articles, reviews of scientific papers, copies of papers published in other media (nationally and internationally) and brief notes on matters related to the topic.

Franco da Rocha was the most published psychiatrist in the *Revista*, with 44 articles credited throughout its editions. Most of his publications were reviews, but also included statistics, observations and projects for the mental-health facilities in São Paulo and Juquery. He wrote on

[1] The first medical journal in the city of São Paulo was titled *Revista Médica de São Paulo*. It was inaugurated in 1889 but stopped circulating the following year due to financial difficulties (Silva, 2014).

[2] A reference to Freud was found in a publication of this *Revista*, written by Henrique Roxo, on 31 August 1908, titled 'Dos Estados Mentais nas GrandesNevroses.'

a variety of themes, including the history and organisation of Juquery; diagnostic and treatment hypotheses, based on clinical observations in mental-health facilities; analysis of cases of hysteria, paranoia and racial degeneration; discussions about alienated offenders, legal medicine and the Brazilian penal and civil codes. He was also the main contributor responsible for the publications related to psychiatry in the 'Bibliography' column of the *Revista*, which gathered the works of European authors on different medical topics. Franco da Rocha also wrote about other areas of medicine, such as dentition, leprosy, syringomyelia, ainhum, beriberi and yellow fever. This is not surprising, as medical specialisation was still developing and 'the task of psychiatry was to define its specificity in the field of medicine and make its science recognized among other medical practices.' (Foucault, 2014, p. 8).

Franco Da Rocha's Discourse in the *Revista*

The publications in the *Revista* clearly reveal the difficult task psychiatrists had in establishing themselves as scientific among medical peers. With regard to insanity, the psychiatrists who published in the journal sought to establish a consensus in the identification of its aetiology and symptoms, as well as in the classification of psychopathological conditions and in the most appropriate treatment for so-called mental illnesses. Often times, information on patients was lacking, or the information collected was scarce. In the publication 'Hospício de Alienados' [Hospice for the Alienated] (03/15/1898), Franco da Rocha stated that the information on patients at the Hospício was incomplete, even omitting references to age and marital status in their medical records. In his article 'Causas de alienação mental no Brasil' [Causes of Mental Alienation in Brazil] (05/15/1901), he described psychiatry in Brazil as 'a very delayed field, so the publication of this information is always another brick in the foundation of a future building. Those who come later will not fail to appreciate the service of the first workers' (p. 155).

Franco da Rocha (15 March 1898) reported that, on 1 January 1898, there were 337 patients in mental-health facilities and that 246 more were admitted throughout the year. However, not all of the 'sick' were classified: 'some because they had arrived recently, others because they were not insane and left after a few weeks of observation' (p. 33). He attributed the imprecision in the diagnosis of insanity to 'difficulties arising from the lack of good classification and, in addition, from the lack of information with which we struggle in the *Hospício*' (15 March 1901, p. 74). His contribution, in this sense, was to share annual statistics on the mental-health facilities in São Paulo based upon their classification in the statistical study *Ensaio de Estatística - 1896*, proposing slight changes over the years that they were published.

In Franco da Rocha's classification, his search for an anatomical-physiological justification for the possible causes of the onset or development of mental illnesses is evident. For the psychiatrists and neurologists who published in the *Revista,* the brain and the nervous system would be a fundamental part of the investigation into the causes of insanity, although studies involving nerve centres were still very controversial, as stated by Franco da Rocha (15 November 1898) in a review of Miguel Couto's dissertation, titled 'Dos espasmos nas afecções nervosas' [Spasms in Nervous Disorders].

In a review of Costa Pinto's dissertation, 'A grafologia em Medicina Legal' [Graphology in Forensic Medicine], Franco da Rocha (15 February 1901) reiterated the importance of finding objective signs to determine the character and temperament of both alienated and criminal individuals. He brought as an example Lombroso's contribution on the criminal's physical or somatic stigmas. Costa Pinto, in turn, proposed that graphology may be used in this same way, since it could reveal the individual's character, being less subject to disguise than physiognomic expressions. Franco da Rocha suggested that graphology should be studied and made an essential part in the schooling of physicians and lawyers.

Another dissertation analysed by Franco da Rocha (31 March 1901) was that of Henrique Roxo, titled 'Duração dos atos psíquicos elementares nos alienados' [Duration of Elementary Psychic Acts in the Alienated]. Roxo defended the use of reaction time studies in the description of the forms of insanity, which could contribute to diagnosis, being the physician's duty 'to identify as many symptoms as possible to establish a correct diagnosis' (p. 104). Franco da Rocha believed that 'the progress of laboratory studies will bring, sooner or later, an improvement in the techniques and ease in the application of such studies' (p. 105). The Pathological Anatomy Laboratory at Hospício do Juquery, however, only started to function in 1921: it was organised and directed by Antônio Pacheco e Silva. Before that, the psychiatrists who worked there sought to understand the causes of insanity by observing and describing the behaviour of hospitalised people, by looking at the results of tested therapies and by reading works on insanity produced internationally, especially in Germany, France, England, the United States and Argentina.

All psychiatrists agreed that heredity was the main cause of insanity. In the article 'Apontamentos e estatísticas: causas da loucura; alienados perigosos' [Notes and Statistics: Causes of Madness; Dangerous Cases] (15 March 1901), Franco da Rocha wrote that:

> In rare cases, the doctor may attribute insanity to a single cause, one that is enough to trigger this disorder. There are always merging factors. Among these, it is possible, in most cases, to distinguish what is essential from what is occasional. (p. 73)

In that same publication, Franco da Rocha maintained that, in addition to the 'genetic load,' social factors would also play a role in the development of insanity. He stated that the character and customs of parents could have an effect by 'conditioning the evolution of the central nervous system starting on the first day of pregnancy until the end of development' (p. 76), even without evidence of neuropathy in the family.

> A drunkenness... *familiar*, very intimate, can thus be the source of future sorrows, apparently without a more sensitive, more palpable explanation: excess mental work, a terrible heartbreak; an interruption of menstruation; a very strong fever, an endless number of causes, in short, which usually bring about nervous breakdowns and circulatory disorders. (p. 76)

The level of 'civility' of an individual and the society in which they are raised would also influence the development of insanity. General paralysis, for example, would be more frequent in more civilised countries, in which 'the struggle for existence is more fierce,' which would explain why, on the one hand, black people and women in Brazil do not present 'this form of insanity here among us' and, on the other hand, insanity is more frequent in black Americans than Brazilians, since 'they are much more civilised than us and fight more with the brain' (p. 77).

Regarding race, Franco da Rocha, who was influenced by the theory of degeneration, defended the superiority of the white race over the black, which, except for individual exceptions, possessed a 'rudimentary state of mentality.' In the article 'Contribution à l'étude de la folie dans la race noire' [Contribution to the Study of Madness in the Black Race] (30 December 1911), he claims:

> Obviously, limited aspirations, a consequence of psychic inferiority and lack of culture, are manifested to some extent in mental illness. These aspirations, which are still maintained at a very low social level among blacks, do not push them towards fighting for life in a very intense manner; and when that does happen, the obstacles encountered in that struggle are rarely the direct cause of mental failure. When this happens, the insanity observed in them can present certain peculiarities that originate from them. This is what we think we have found about paralytic dementia, which is very rare in black people, although alcoholism and syphilis are not. Krafft-Ebing would say: 'There is syphilisation among them, but civilisation is lacking.' (p. 459)

Alcoholism was common among black men after slavery was abolished and syphilis among black women, due to the social conditions they were subjected to: they were abandoned to their own fate and excluded from the productive chain in São Paulo as an attempt to whiten the population through immigration. Given the situation in which they found themselves, many of the men were drunks, while many of these women sought to survive through prostitution, which was the main cause of the spread of syphilis. Despite the evident social cause for the higher incidence of alcoholism and syphilis in the black population, Franco da Rocha, like many doctors, argued that these were ailments to which these people's bodies were more susceptible.

Franco da Rocha was also an admirer of Nina Rodrigues: the physician from Bahia is mentioned several times in at least seven of his publications in the *Revista*. On 31 October 1903, Franco da Rocha wrote a note about Nina Rodrigues' visit to São Paulo, calling him 'one of the most outstanding individuals in Brazilian medicine' (31 October 1903, p. 445).

> A robust intelligence, of improved and fruitful cultivation. Nina Rodrigues is an indefatigable science worker. Understanding this sentence well - 'the Portuguese language is a prison' – introduced the results of his research to a wider idiomatic circle, showing the scientific world that in Brazil people work and science is cultivated with love. (p. 446)

The main follower of Lombroso's ideas[3] in Brazil, Nina Rodrigues was the founder of Brazilian criminal anthropology and focused on the study of race, especially within the area of forensic medicine. According to Franco da Rocha, Nina Rodrigues 'does not spare sacrifices in order to compete with his lights to improve our laws. His name brings pride to the medical profession' (p. 446).

In a review of Nina Rodrigues' work titled: 'Épidémie de folie religieuse au Brésil' [Epidemic of Religious Madness in Brazil] (15 August 1899), Franco da Rocha praises the 'superb article' by his peer from Bahia. Nina Rodrigues' article was a 22-page leaflet about Antônio Conselheiro, leader of a religious movement, which had gathered thousands of followers in the village of Canudos (1893–1897), a rural community that had developed a self-sustainable economy based on solidarity. Nina Rodrigues said that Antônio Conselheiro was insane, diagnosing him with 'chronic systematised psychosis.' His followers, on the other hand–poor farmers, newly freed natives and slaves, the homeless and the victims of drought–were people of non-white races, that is, supposedly of inferior mentality.

> [On] the one hand a madman – Antônio Conselheiro – with a coherent, logical-looking delusion, in the ambitious phase of *messianismo*, and on

[3] In an article from 15 November 1909, titled 'Professor Cesare Lombroso,' Franco da Rocha pays tribute to him on the occasion of his death: 'An entire life devoted to science, to the fight for truth, filled his memory with the common law of death – oblivion. Lombroso's work is imperishable. Modified, retouched, corrected and increasingly grounded in the fight with opposing ideas, his doctrine is now true in the scientific world. The modification that criminal law underwent in the light of Lombroso's genius is enough to make him immortal' (p. 434).

> the other hand the ethical and social terrain in which the madman opened the foundations of his castle – the *jagunço*, fetishist in religion and monarchist in politics. The *jagunço*, a mestizo from the backlands, different from a coastal mestizo, preserves the indomitable character of the savage, the taste for wandering and a nomadic life, a resistance to psychic suffering, hunger, thirst, and bad weather; he is always resolute and ready for armed depredations and to serve the interests of those who know how to direct him, he is a lesser-minded creature, still late to understand both a more abstract religion and form of government; he is a monarchist because he needs a king to make government concrete for him; he is a fetishist because he needs images of saints, missionaries, and direct messengers from God. The reasoning of the *jagunço* does not go beyond this: in the monarchy life was easy, in the Republic it is expensive ...*post hoc, ergo propter hoc*, nothing more. (p. 238)

Like Antônio Conselheiro, those who opposed the ruling powers were often considered enemies of the Republic and diagnosed as insane: a good example of this was the category of the so-called 'morally insane.' In a review of Álvaro Fernandes' dissertation entitled 'Moral insanity,' published on 15 July 1899, Franco da Rocha classified some artists–Bacon, Bocage, Benvenuto Cellini–as 'morally insane' and asks: 'But… how does one clearly limit moral insanity? Where does the selfish, neglected and pernicious politician end and the insane begin?' (p. 206). Despite being able to differentiate something from its opposite, the insane would lack 'the emotional tone that usually accompanies these ideas,' due to a 'vicious brain development,' with a vast diversity of types of 'degenerates' that is difficult to define.

> This is the heart of the matter. They include journalists, lawyers, doctors, scholars; in all these professions there is a huge group of disqualified, recently mentioned by Le Bon, in *Psychologie du Socialisme* [Psychology of Socialism], as the proper ground for the germination of socialist ideas. (p. 206)

Franco da Rocha argued that the criterion for hospitalisation in these cases must be 'the harm that the individual is causing to society: his freedom should be limited by the well-being of others' (p. 206).

Another psychiatric category that made evident the social aspect of the psychopathological diagnosis was the so-called 'declassified':

> They are the igniters of emotional fires; they are the first to explode, sometimes for good, often for bad. The thermometer of their enthusiasm immediately rises to 100 degrees and drops in the same way. They lack perseverance in everything they attempt; there is no ideal for these beings to serve as a beacon on the path of existence, that encourages them to persist in their work to achieve it. (03/15/1901, p. 75)

The 'disqualified' would be those who do not fit in society or in the psychiatric facility: 'in society they are crazy, in the *Hospício* they are not (…). They are a torment to their acquaintances and live in a constant struggle with the police' (p. 75). Through abstinence and the everyday routine at the facility, the individual would return to their 'normal' state.

In that same article, Franco da Rocha questioned what the state's role would be in assisting the alienated. He believed that governmental inspection of alcohol is ineffective ('like in Russia') and that it is absurd to ban the marriage of degenerates. Neither did it seem 'promising' to sterilise the alienated ('like in the United States'), due to the resistance that such a procedure would generate in the population. Despite this, he was in favour of sterilising the 'degenerate' and defended the state regulation of prostitution, thus opposing physicians who were in favour of abolishing this.

In addition to the diagnosis and prophylaxis of insanity, another controversial point debated by Brazilian psychiatrists at the time was the notion of cure: the *Revista* showed that this was often relative. This can be seen in Franco da Rocha's comments on cases that he was able to monitor in the *Hospício*, such as the one presented in the article 'O 'Salvarsan' na Paralisia Geral' ['Salvarsan' in General Paralysis] (31 December 1912):

> He currently works in the establishment's pharmacy, without anyone noticing the symptoms described above. Upon closer examination, there is no doubt a mental deficit, which would be enormous if this poor man belonged to a high social class; for his social condition, however, he is doing well, just like the other, who currently works in tailoring. (p. 22)

What draws the most attention in the transcribed passage is the relativisation of the notion of cure, depending upon the social class to which the person belonged: a 'mental deficit' can be a problem for a person of 'high social class,' but it is not for a poor man who manages to work in tailoring at the mental-health facility. Having a work routine and providing for their own subsistence seems to be central points in the psychiatric evaluation, as this ensured that the individual would no longer be a burden for his family. It is also important to note that there were many reports about patients who, even after being discharged, remained in the psychiatric facility as employees.

In the statistics published about the mental-health facilities in São Paulo, Franco da Rocha divided the patients into cured and recovered, without explaining what the basis for this differentiation was. It also appears that unrecovered people left the facility, which is evident from the statistics published in 'Hospício de Alienados de S. Paulo: Seção de Juquery, Colônia agrícola e Hospício da cidade' [Hospice for the Alienated of São Paulo: Juquery Section, Colony and City Hospice] (28 February 1902).

> In 1901, 186 new patients were taken to the different units, 81 women and 105 men.
>
> Forty-five were cured, 15 recovered, 9 were not cured and 53 died.
>
> The total number of patients undergoing treatment during the year was 818.
>
> Mortality was 6.5%. (p. 75)

In the publication 'Hospício de S. Paulo. Estatísticas e apontamentos' [Hospice of São Paulo. Statistics and Notes] (15 November 1903), Franco da Rocha asserted that the patient's healing prognosis was a matter to be answered by psychiatry: 'It can be guaranteed that in this area, more than in any other, the prognosis is doubtful, lacking a strong foundation, and therefore, very risky' (p. 465). The only case presented in the *Revista* that gives us a clue as to what would be considered a patient's improvement appeared in this publication, when Franco da Rocha discussed a 'paranoid with an ambitious delirium' who spent 14 years at Hospício do Juquery. He considered himself immortal and had constant tantrums, which 'made him incompatible with the social environment he lived in' (p. 465). At the *Hospício*, his delusional ideas were tempered.

> (...) today this patient is not angry with those who do not accept his ideas. He smiles and moves on to another subject without any affective alteration. He has been living with his family for a year, very happy, working, without colliding with his social environment.
>
> He is one less burden for the state.
>
> He was not cured, it is true, but improved and disciplined so that he could be useful to his own. (pp. 465–466)

The main treatment for insanity used at Hospício do Juquery was work therapy on agricultural colonies. In the publication 'Apontamentos e estatísticas' [Notes and Statistics] (15 May 1900), Franco da Rocha recommended agricultural work for the insane 'because it requires less intellectual effort' (p. 93). He wrote that there are countless successful experiences in Germany, Belgium and France and that he was driven to make use of this 'granite wall'–the international references–to defend his point of view: 'If everything mentioned above had not been said in Europe, our own resources would be useless' (p. 92). One of the theorists he cited in support of work therapy, was Hack Tuke:

> If idleness is a disgrace for the healthy spirit, it is also a cause of unhappiness and boredom for the insane and especially for the teenager. (...)
>
> Occupation, the universal law of nature for a healthy body and soul is especially beneficial for the insane, since it replaces morbid ideas with new and wholesome thoughts, revives the familiar habit of daily activity, restores the esteem of one's own personality, showing the patient that he is useful, while promoting general health. (p. 89)

Franco da Rocha believed that physical work was fundamental in the treatment of 'nervous and mental illnesses': 'First, from a physiological point of view, like all movement; second, under a hygienic point of view, as a means of development; third, as a moralising means; fourth, as a pedagogical means; and fifth, as a means of balancing brain functions.'

(p. 91). If occupation is a 'universal law of nature for health,' idleness would also be an important element in the 'formation of a criminal,' as stated in a review of Ribeiro Gonçalves' dissertation, entitled 'Menores delinquentes' [Delinquent Minors] (28 February 1903).

> An individual with a poorly conformed brain, unbalanced by neuropathic inheritance may, under certain conditions – a good education and good financial conditions – not come to crime frankly, but simply skip the penal code, using the fear of prison and the police as a balance beam. There is no denying, there are individuals of this nature occupying a normal position in society. If they did not have a fortune (sometimes acquired with little fairness) they would be murderers of the worst kind. (p. 78)

In this sense, he affirms the importance of correctional facilities for 'wandering boys,' to save those who would otherwise lose themselves in vagrancy and misery.

The aetiology of crime, according to Franco da Rocha, arose from two sources: inheritance and environment (social or domestic). Education would thus play a fundamental role in the control of crime, being able to 'regenerate customs,' 'virilize the character,' 'form the heart' so that the new generation could 'fulfil their mission on earth of good and of duty' (p. 78).

> All passion, cruelty and lies are found in children. A brutal selfishness dominates which goes unseen only by the loving parent. These tendencies in the normal child, however, are undermined by education, which becomes all the easier the better the family history in each particular case. The heritage of good tendencies smooths the path to education.
>
> Selfishness starts giving way, but at the expense of the development of intelligence and reason, which come to show that this concession is for the benefit of selfishness itself.
>
> That the origin of altruistic tendencies is still selfishness cannot be denied without the subterfuge of dialectics. (p. 78)

Another concern regarding the crime was the so-called alienated delinquent. In many publications of the *Revista,* there were repeated concerns expressed by the psychiatric class to propose what should be done with this type of 'madness.' Despite heated discussions, the physicians agreed that 'the alienated person who committed a crime should be considered a dangerous patient and not guilty' (p. 20), as stated by Franco da Rocha in a comment on the work by José Igenieros, titled 'Dos Páginas de Psiquiatria Criminal' [Two Pages of Criminal Psychiatry] (15 January 1901). In that piece, Franco da Rocha argued that the construction of institutions for insane delinquents was not yet necessary in Brazil, 'where the number of insane people does not yet justify the enormous expense of an independent, special asylum' (p. 20). Two years later, however, he claimed (15 April 1903) to have sent a letter to the government of the state of São Paulo, requesting that an action be taken regarding the 'promiscuity of *certain* delinquents,' whom he considered 'unbearable.'

> Four calm easy-going criminals are found in Juquery, who seem to reason well, barely showing episodic alteration, having one or another idea of persecution that does not prevent them from providing services. It turns out, however, that they are addicts and masters of looking for ways to escape, something in which they display incredible shrewdness and an unshakable tenacity. Now, the *Hospício* is not a prison; the bars are fragile, and the escapes are many, leaving us constantly startled, diverting our attention entirely from everything else to meet this constant fear. (...)
>
> 'We have other alienated criminals who in no way disturb the order of the *Hospício*. These can and must remain in the establishment; not the others, a measure is needed to get us out of our embarrassment.' (p. 135)

Franco da Rocha (15 April 1903) took advantage of the review of Francisco Pondé's dissertation– 'Assistência Pública aos alienados delinquentes no Brasil' [Public Assistance to Alienated Delinquents in Brazil]–to ask that an annex to the prison be built as a means of transitioning 'to a more complete and proper system' (p. 135), since he still did not see the need for an exclusive facility for alienated delinquents. The annex would serve provisionally until 'the increase in the number of patients of this sort made an independent creation necessary' (p. 135). He argued that an effort had been made to bring life in the facility closer to ordinary life in society, but that these 'disturbers' had made it difficult for this goal to be achieved. He denounced the disorder in which most mental-health facilities were found in Brazil, even for the common alienated: 'If even the others have no proper asylum (except in two or three states), how can we jump in and deal with the special cases that have been pointed out?' (p. 136).

In this publication too, Franco da Rocha criticised the fragility of Brazilian law in relation to the alienated delinquent who suffers from 'transient mental alienation.'

> An individual commits a murder in a state of transient mental alienation, goes to the jury and is acquitted due to the illness, because shortly after the crime he was taken to a facility and recognised as mad. He is cured of madness at the end of a month of treatment and is released. Is this fair? Who can guarantee that within a year he will not commit another murder? (p. 136)

Eight years later, in the publication 'Os alienados perigosos e o Código Penal' [The Dangerous Deranged and the Penal Code] (12/15/1911), Franco da Rocha resumed this discussion, denouncing the deficiency and anachronism of the Brazilian penal code: 'If the law is defective, what will the decision be? It must be defective. This is common sense' (p. 437). He then claimed that there is a 'social responsibility' for the alienated delinquent.

> We need a well-written law, discussed at length by men of value, as was done in England, in the House of Lords, in whose debates sometimes Lord Brougham's firmly sarcastic spirit shone with the mention of the terms 'fair, unfair, good, bad, correct and perverse'.
>
> What is happening in relation to the penal code is what is always observed in transition phases, be it in organic, individual or social evolution: confusion and disorder. It is, in this case, the cracking of the joints of old classic moulds by modern ideas, which impose themselves, but do not fit them. (p. 438)

At that historical moment, medicine was disputing power with law within the field of legal medicine. This dispute aimed to demarcate a field of professional activity, in search of the legitimation of the medical discourse, which would allow medicine to increase its authority over the social body of the Brazilian Republican state. There were many dissensions among the doctors of the period, so it was essential to create a kind of fraternity among them, joining forces to legitimise their discourse before other authorities and thus consolidate themselves as authorised speakers, gaining the power to decide, plan and carry out measures that were both medical and political. The *Revista Médica de São Paulo: Jornal Prático de Medicina Cirurgia e Higiene* sought to fulfil this mission and make contributing authors the spokesmen for medicine in São Paulo.

Final Remarks

With the proclamation of the Republic, Brazilian medicine sought to legitimise its practice based on scientific discourse, institutional class organisation and partnerships with the government to guarantee its exclusive position in public health intervention in cities. In this context, psychiatry sought to capture insanity as a scientific object of investigation and medical intervention. Franco da Rocha's publications in the medical journal *Revista Médica de São Paulo* can be understood as an attempt to share the accumulated knowledge in the field, but also to legitimise psychiatry as a scientific field. The search for consensus among psychiatrists was also notable in order to strengthen themselves as a class in the face of other medical areas, other fields of knowledge, as well as the state and society.

When psychoanalysis arrived in São Paulo, it found a medicine that positioned itself in defence of a civilising project for Brazil, based on scientific racism and concerned with infant health education for the prevention of delinquency. Although Franco da Rocha produced publications that dealt with cases of hysteria and paranoia, topics that could interest the readers of this book, I chose to focus on the ideas that formed the field that psychoanalysis found upon arriving in the city of São Paulo, through the discourse of this famous representative of psychiatry there.

References

Barbosa, R. (1903). *Speech at Colégio Anchieta* [online]. http://www.casaruibarbosa.gov.br/dados/DOC/artigos/rui_barbosa/FCRB_RuiBarbosa_Discurso_no_Colegio_Anchieta.pdf (Accessed on September 01, 2020).

Cunha, M. C. P. (1986). *O Espelho do Mundo: Juquery, A História de um Asilo.* Paz e Terra.

Foucault, M. (2014). 'A Evolução da Noção de Indivíduo Perigoso na Psiquiatria Legal do Século XIX' in Motta, MB (Org.) *Ditos e escritos, volume V: ética, sexualidade, política,* 3rd ed. Forense Universitária.

Machado, R., Loureiro, A., Luz, R., & Muricy, K. (1978). *Danação da norma: Medicina social e constituição da psiquiatria no Brasil.* Graal.

Mandelbaum, B. P., & Frosh, S. (2020). Durval Marcondes, a Psicanálise e a modernização conservadora no Brasil. *Revista USP, 126*, 85–98.

Mota, A. (2003). *Quem é bom já nasce feito: Sanitarismo e eugenia no Brasil.* DP&A Editora.

Oliveira, C. L. M. V. (2002). Os primeiros tempos da psicanálise no Brasil e as teses pansexualistas na educação. *Ágora: Estudos em Teoria Psicanalítica, 5*(1), 133–154.

Rocha, F. F. (1898, March 15). Hospício de Alienados. *Revista Médica de São Paulo, 1*(2), 32–34.

Rocha, F. F. (1898, November 15). Dos espasmos nas afecções nervosas (Tese de concurso de Dr. Miguel do Couto). *Revista Médica de São Paulo, 1*(10), 193–195.

Rocha, F. F. (1899, July 15). Moral insanity (Dissertation by Dr. Álvaro Fernandes). *Revista Médica de São Paulo, 2*(7), 204–207.

Rocha, F. F. (1899, August 15). Épidémie de folie religieuse au Brésil par le Dr. Nina Rodrigues. *Revista Médica de São Paulo, 2*(8), 237–238.

Rocha, F. F. (1900, May 15). Apontamentos e estatísticas. *Revista Médica de São Paulo, 3*(5), 89–94.

Rocha, F. F. (1901, January 15). Dos Páginas de Psiquiatria Criminal (by José Ingenieros). *Revista Médica de São Paulo, 4*(1), 19–21.

Rocha, F. F. (1901, February 15). A grafologia em Medicina Legal (Inaugural dissertation by Dr. Costa Pinto, Bahia, 1900). *Revista Médica de São Paulo, 4*(3), 56–57.

Rocha, F. F. (1901, March 15). Apontamentos e estatísticas: causas da loucura; alienados perigosos. *Revista Médica de São Paulo, 4*(5), 73–80.

Rocha, F. F. (1901, March 31). Duração dos atos psíquicos elementares nos alienados (Dissertation by Dr. H. Belfort Roxo). *Revista Médica de São Paulo, 4*(9), 104–105.

Rocha, F. F. (1901, May 15). Causas de alienação mental no Brasil (by Dr. Henrique Roxo). *Revista Médica de São Paulo, 4*(9), 155–157.

Rocha, F. F. (1902, February 28). Hospício de Alienados de S. Paulo: Seção de Juquery, Colônia agrícola e Hospício da cidade. *Revista Médica de São Paulo, 5*(4), 75–76.

Rocha, F. F. (1903, February 28). Menores delinquentes (Inaugural dissertation by Dr. Ribeiro Gonçalves). *Revista Médica de São Paulo, 6*(4), 77–79.

Rocha, F. F. (1903, April 15). Assistência Pública aos alienados delinquentes no Brasil (Inaugural dissertation by Dr. Francisco Pondé, Bahia, 1902). *Revista Médica de São Paulo, 6*(7), 135–136.

Rocha, F. F. (1903, October 31). O professor Nina Rodrigues. *Revista Médica de São Paulo, 6*(20), 445–446.

Rocha, F. F. (1903, November 15). Hospício de S. Paulo. Estatísticas e apontamentos. *Revista Médica de São Paulo, 6*(21), 463–466.

Rocha, F. F. (1909, November 15). Professor Cesare Lombroso. *Revista Médica de São Paulo, 12*(21), 434.

Rocha, F. F. (1911, December 15). Os alienados perigosos e o código penal. *Revista Médica de São Paulo, 14*(23), 437–440.

Rocha, F. F. (1911, December 30). Contribution à l'étude de la folie dans la race noire. *Revista Médica de São Paulo, 14*(24), 458–462.

Rocha, F. F. (1912, December 31). O Salvarsan na Paralisia Geral. *Revista Médica de São Paulo, 15*(2), 21–23.

Roxo, H. B. B. (1908, August 31). Dos Estados Mentais nas Grandes Nevroses. *Revista Médica de São Paulo*, 11(16), 327–332.

Silva, M. R. B. (2014). *O Laboratório e a República: Saúde pública, ensino médico e produção de conhecimento em São Paulo (1891–1933).* Fiocruz.

Teixeira, L. A. (2001). *A Sociedade de Medicina e Cirurgia de São Paulo (1895–1913).* PhD thesis, University of São Paulo.

10

For a Conservative Modernisation: The Introduction of Social Psychology in Brazil Through Psychoanalysis

Thiago Bloss de Araújo

This chapter aims to discuss some theoretical and political contributions of psychoanalysis to the introduction of social psychology in Brazil. This can be understood in terms of the impact of an important historical movement present in the 1930s at the national and international level. Specifically, at a national level, social psychology was pioneered by the physician Raul Carlos Briquet, who published the first Brazilian book in this discipline in 1935, and was part of the intellectual elites who spearheaded a conservative modernisation project throughout the country. As will be seen, psychoanalysis has had a strong presence in the development of social psychology, which was characterised by profound contradictions and attempts at ideological conciliation, guided by authoritarianism at both the theoretical and political level.

Psychoanalysis and psychology, as autonomous disciplines, have at least two points in common in the way they were constituted in Brazil:

T. B. de Araújo (✉)
Federal University of São Paulo, São Paulo, Brazil

B. Mandelbaum et al. (eds.), *Brazilian Psychosocial Histories of Psychoanalysis*, Studies in the Psychosocial,
https://doi.org/10.1007/978-3-030-78509-3_10

they were born into the hands of doctors and responded to the collective demands of their time, either to affirm them or to deny them.

Brazilian psychology has its birth in the doctoral theses defended by Raul Briquet (1887–1930) and Arthur Ramos (1903–1949) in the Faculties of Medicine of Rio de Janeiro and Bahia. Despite their distinct intellectual influences, they shared the merit of having collaborated in the consolidation of psychoanalysis in Brazil. Through them, the development of a Brazilian social psychology took place, together with the constitution and institutionalisation of psychoanalysis.

Raul Carlos Briquet was a recognised obstetrician and an important figure of the São Paulo elite during the first half of the twentieth century, being part of the same intellectual circle as Mário de Andrade, Fernando de Azevedo, and Antônio Carlos Pacheco e Silva. Consequently, he was present at the foundation of significant higher education and training institutions in the city of São Paulo. In 1927, Briquet participated in the creation of the Brazilian Society of Psychoanalysis alongside Franco da Rocha, Durval Marcondes, and Lourenço Filho, assuming the vice-presidency of that institution. In 1934, he was among the intellectuals responsible for founding the University of São Paulo, becoming a professor at the Faculty of Medicine. He was also a signatory to the *Manifesto dos Pioneiros da Educação Nova* (Manifesto of New Education Pioneers), which constituted the movement against authoritarian education named 'escolanovismo' (Progressive Education).

Briquet's presence at the inauguration of the Free School of Sociology and Politics of São Paulo in 1933 was essential for the introduction of social psychology into Brazil. At the Free School, Briquet was responsible for teaching the first social psychology course in the country, which later resulted in the first Brazilian book of this discipline, named *Social Psychology* (1935), which took the form of a handbook, similar to Handbooks of Social Psychology that were popular at that time in Latin America.

One Step Back: The Ancestors of Social Psychology in Brazil

There is no way to understand the introduction and consolidation of a given scientific field without referring to its prehistory. Just as Robert Farr (1998) places the ancestors of modern social psychology in the works of European theorists such as Wilhelm Wundt and Gustave Le Bon–who investigated a kind of collective psychology of peoples–it is possible to make the same reflexive movement in the case of Brazil. Specifically, the intellectuals of the 'Brazilian Social Thought' of the nineteenth century were responsible for the first formulations of a 'psychology of the Brazilian people,' as reflections on the impact of miscegenation on the formation of the Brazilian national character. Among its main representatives are Sylvio Romero (1851–1914), Raimundo Nina Rodrigues (1862–1906), and Manoel Bomfim (1868–1932), who sought intellectual coordinates for understanding the Brazilian nation in racist theories that had been imported from Europe. The idea of a 'national character' was considered essential and was typical of the nineteenth century, a period that was marked worldwide by the unification of European countries and, consequently, by strong theories of national identity.

In tracing the ethnic differences between 'us' and 'others,' nationalism developed from conservative and racist thinking, scientifically justified by the nascent human sciences of the time (including psychology), which focused on the classification of human races between upper and lower, civilized and wild. In this way, concepts such as race and nation were forged under the guidance of the supposedly scientific thinking of social Darwinism (Hobsbawm, 2013). It was not by chance that one of the main European authors present in the libraries of the Brazilian intellectual elite of the nineteenth century was Herbert Spencer.

These intellectuals defended, to a greater or lesser degree, the hypothesis that miscegenation would lead the Brazilian people to racial degeneration, requiring the 'Aryanisation' of the races in order to civilise the nation. Certainly, the first work to address this issue was Sylvio Romero's *História da Literatura Brasileira* (1888), which sought to establish the racial roots of the Brazilian people and, consequently, of their 'national psychology.'

Romero reproduced a very widespread thesis that was, and remains, popular among Brazilian intellectuals, and was elaborated upon by the Bavarian naturalist Karl von Martius (1794–1868). He postulated the formation of the Brazilian people through the metaphor of three rivers, with each river representing a specific race, either white, black or indigenous. As Schwarcz (2019) points out, this metaphor assumed that the main river, represented by the white race, would be responsible for absorbing the other smaller rivers, represented by blacks and indigenous people. In this way, the solution for the formation of a civilised nation would be in the 'Aryanization' of the lower races at the base of the Brazilian formation.

Sylvio Romero's thought was contradictory, because while defending miscegenation as something beneficial for the evolution of the people, he also believed that the whitening of blacks and indigenous people would take the Brazilian people to a higher stage of evolution. His concern with the Brazilian racial future did not come from nowhere; after all, his book was published in the same year as the abolition of slavery in Brazil.

> The future generations of Brazil, if German colonization is used, will constitute a mixed people of Brazilians, Portuguese and German. The descendants of the new mixed people will be superior to their predecessors, Portuguese and German, as an element of colonization. Let us move, in spirit, to the future of Brazil: there we will see a mixed people, more apt and capable than their parents for the culture of the lands; because they will be accustomed from birth to the country's climate and life. (Romero, 1888/1902, pp. 55–56)

It is not the intention of this text to delve into the questions posed by these studies of the psychology and character of the Brazilian people. However, it is noteworthy that they directly influenced later works of the two intellectuals representing the phase of the introduction of social psychology in Brazil: Raul Briquet and Arthur Ramos. Likewise, the limits and contradictions presented in the reflections of the intellectuals of 'Brazilian Social Thought' were also inherited by their successors, mainly because they started from theoretical references that had been imported from Europe; that is, because they thought the Brazilian reality from 'ideas out of place' (Schwarz, 2007). As we shall see, the appropriation of psychoanalysis was instrumental in setting up the ideas of Briquet and likewise reinforced the contradictions of his thought, on the one hand strengthening hereditary and instinctive aspects of the individual, on the other, seeking to mediate between the individual and society.

Social Psychology and Conservative Modernisation

If we asked ourselves what would be the historical need for social psychology in Brazil, we would certainly find a clue through Briquet's 1930 translation of Ernest Jones's important work *Psychoanalysis*. In a brief introduction to his study, the Brazilian doctor states that his intention was to allow 'the reader to get a grip on psychoanalytic knowledge, which would allow him to harmonise psychic life with the social environment' (Bomfim, 2002). The premises of 'harmony' and 'adaptation,' enhanced by the natural sciences, are present in both the constitution of the rationality of modern psychology (Picheler-Harrous, 2018), as well as in the ideological apology of elites during a historic moment of polarisation and social, political and economic conflict.

The interwar period, when social psychology was introduced in Brazil, comprises part of what Hobsbawm (2004) considers the 'Age of Catastrophe,' which began with the First World War and ended with the end of the Second World War. During these years, the world saw a deep economic recession due to the costs of war and the impact of the stock market crash of 1929. In this political and financial context, most representative democracies were shaken and the rise of authoritarian regimes was enabled. The *Age of Catastrophes* called into question the very viability of liberalism as a system of political, economic and social values.

The two great wars represented the extreme result of the development of rampant and impersonal capitalism. The association between imperialism, expansionism and nationalism resulted in a level of mass destruction never before thought possible. Supported, above all, by technological development, genocide became impersonalised through the use of scientific administration–which was initially associated with the industrial production of goods–for the death of millions of human beings.

> But the production also required organization and management – even if its object was the rationalized destruction of human life in the most efficient manner, as in the German extermination camps. Speaking in the most general terms, total war was the largest enterprise hitherto known to man, which had to be consciously organized and managed. (Hobsbawm, 2004, p. 54)

The great economic depression that hit the world in 1929 is considered, by modern historiography, to be the necessary condition that led to the rise of authoritarian regimes, such as Italian fascism and German nazism. According to Hobsbawm (2004), only ten countries in the world kept their constitutional democracies intact during this period. In Latin American countries such as Argentina (Juan Domingo Perón) and Brazil (Getúlio Vargas), there was the emergence of regimes marked by nationalist populism, which were politically oriented towards the conciliation of antagonistic classes, above all, in a period of extreme insurgency and political radicalisation.

In Brazil, Getúlio Vargas instituted a coup that ended a four-decade oligarchic republic, and put the country into political turmoil by centralising power among the agrarian elites of São Paulo and Minas Gerais. Fausto (2013) has pointed out that the rise of Getulio Vargas to power brought three major political and economic changes in Brazil:

> A new type of state was born after 1930, distinguishing itself from the oligarchic state not only by its centralization and a greater degree of autonomy but also by other elements. We must emphasize at least three of them: 1. economic performance, gradually focused on the objectives of promoting industrialization, 2. social action, tending to give some type of protection to urban workers, incorporating them, next, into a class alliance promoted by state power; 3. the central role attributed to the Armed Forces – especially the Army – as support for the creation of a base industry and above all as a guarantee of the internal order. (Fausto, 2013, p. 208)

The conciliation policy and authoritarianism were present in Varguismo. The industrial and financial bourgeoisie, the urban middle class, and a part of the agro-export elite were among the classes that made up its base. Its opponents were part of the progressive military, the revolutionary left, and the Liberal Democrats, who were either eliminated or co-opted by the regime.

The counter-offensive to the coup came in 1932 from the São Paulo elites through a constitutionalist movement represented by the Frente Única Paulista (FUP), which was soon defeated by Vargas' 'Getulist' forces.

> The 1932 movement brought together different social sectors, from coffee farming to the middle class, to industrialists. Only the organized working class, which launched some major strikes in the first half of 1932, was left out of the picture. The struggle for the constitutionalisation of the country, the themes of São Paulo's autonomy and superiority vis-à-vis other states had electrified a good part of the population of São Paulo. A very effective image, at the time, associated São Paulo with a locomotive that pulled twenty empty wagons – the other twenty states of the Federation. (Fausto, 2013, p. 296)

Despite the defeat, these rebellious forces were soon integrated into the government, which was in charge of reconciling within limits liberal guidelines, the demands of the working class and interests of the agrarian elite, all under a strong nationalist populism with an authoritarian element.

However, it is worth mentioning that the defeat of 1932 was the main motivation that led the elite of São Paulo to inaugurate *Escola Livre de Sociologia e Política* (the Free School of Sociology and Politics) in 1933, in which Raul Briquet taught his first course in social psychology. Headed by Roberto Simonsen–who was one of the main representatives of the industrial and supposedly liberal elite of São Paulo–this institution had been created as an intellectual elite which would participate in the management of the state and public life 'to form personalities capable of collaborating effectively and consciously in the direction of social life' (Kantor et al., 2009, p. 238).

It was typical of scientific and positivist thinking at that time to try to bring 'men of science' closer to 'men of action,' that is, to form intellectual elites who would occupy public positions with the aim of creating a scientific management of society. The School's opening manifesto makes explicit the problem which they intended to solve:

> … it stands out naturally for its basic character, the lack of a large organised elite, instructed under scientific methods, alongside the institutions and conquests of the civilised world capable of understanding, before acting, the social environment in which we live. (Kantor et al., 2009, pp. 237–238)

The Brazilian elites were responsible for a mission typical of that decade, wherein the 'intellectual is elected the interpreter of social life because he is capable of transmitting the multiple social manifestations, bringing them to the heart of the State, which will discipline them and coordinate them' (Velloso, 2013, p. 155). In this sense, the São Paulo intellectuals presented themselves as the locomotive for the development and modernisation of the country. They were responsible for the insignia present on the flag of the city of São Paulo, which contains the Latin phrase *NON DVCOR DVCO*, that is, 'I am not being led, I lead.' This claim to a popular and avant-garde position appeared explicitly in the School's opening manifesto, and was an expression of their indignation at the defeat of the counteroffensive to the Getúlio Vargas coup.

> Not long ago, in the civil war unleashed in our state, and now, in the struggle to recover from the effects of that war and the afflictions that preceded it, the people feel more or less dizzy and vacillating. He wants to act, he wants to promote something useful, he considers a beneficial renovation, but he does not find the central spring of a harmonious elite, that inspires confidence, that teaches him steps, firm and safe. (Kantor et al., 2009, p. 238)

If the populist and scientistic plans of the *Escola Livre de Sociologia e Política de São Paulo* (*Free School of Sociology and Politics of São Paulo*) were explicit, so was its influence through social and racial evolutionism. In this sense, the main mentor of this institution, Roberto Simonsen, maintained the desire of the intellectual representatives of Brazilian Social Thought in the nineteenth century to improve the Brazilian race:

> Now, a school like the one imagined here aims to promote and systematize in Brazil the study of national sociology in harmony with research that guides the political, legal and economic institutions best suited to our environment and our race. The action of specialized technicians from our schools is already insufficient today if it is not inspired by safe and caring guidance for a healthy social evolution. (Simonsen, 1973, p. 464)

Through liberal and scientific consideration, the Brazilian intellectuals reproduced veiled racism, often justified by a culturalist or meritocratic argument. It was, therefore, the reproduction of what they precisely aimed to combat: authoritarianism. Velloso (2013) summarises this perspective in the following passage:

> Here we find one of the central tenets of authoritarian political thought, which is to understand society as being immature, indecisive and therefore in need of a capable guide to introduce standards of action and conduct. More than that: able to guess your wishes, to pinpoint them, in short, to provide solutions. Intellectuals appear as spokespersons for popular aspirations because they would be able to capture the 'collective subconscious' of nationality. This subconscious would contain the true reserves of 'Brazilian-ness' that the Estado Novo (New State) would recover, ensuring the continuity of the national conscience (...) Pointed out as the most lucid expressions of society, intellectuals are seen as the harbingers of the great historical changes and heralds of national renewal. (Velloso, 2013, pp. 156–157)

In this way, the conservative racial thinking of the nineteenth century is reproduced in a modern and liberal guise, a necessary condition for the establishment of the main driver of political, social and economic development in Brazil in the Vargas period: conservative modernisation.

As Maria Helena Souza Patto (2008) states, it was up to the elite of that period to reconcile racism and liberalism. It is within this paradox that social psychology was introduced in the country, constituting one of the disciplines of the social sciences responsible for the formation of future leading intellectual groups, who would be responsible for the scientific diagnosis of the 'evils of society.' For such a task, the social psychology proposed by Raul Briquet relied decisively on some European theories, among them psychoanalysis.

Social Psychology Through Psychoanalysis: Between Inheritance and the Environment

The attempt to establish social psychology on Brazilian soil has revealed a few insurmountable contradictions about the prevalent thought of the time. For Briquet, albeit important, social psychology could not be created as an autonomous science, because it did not have its own object of study. Indeed, the dimensions of human life which he intended to occupy were already the object of study in biology and sociology. In this way, social psychology would be situated between the methods of these two sciences.

Such premises supported Briquet's notion of the individual, which would be understood as the result 'to an equal extent' of the factors 'inheritance' and 'social environment.' For the author, genetics and evolutionism revealed the universal laws of the individual. Under strong organicist influence, Briquet (1935) appropriated concepts from biology, such as heredity and instinct, to explain such laws. Indeed, sexual and parental instincts would be responsible for the constitution of the family; private property, however, would be the result of the operation of nutritional instincts.

On the other hand, positivism had revealed the universal laws of society, mainly through the contributions of Auguste Comte and Émile Dürkheim. In this sense, society would be understood, in its 'normal' form, as the synthesis of order and progress, through the double condition of 'harmony of its constitutive parts' and 'progressive modification' through social consensus. *Harmony and consensus* would provide the basis for *order and progress* and, therefore, for the natural evolution of society and the improvement of the people. This way of thinking, also imported from Europe, was used in the Brazilian flag: 'order and progress.'

In both perspectives, either biological or sociological, we start from the theoretical-methodological reference of the natural sciences to think of the individual in society as subject to universal and natural laws. On the one hand, there would be the individual with instincts pre-shaped by race, which would provide the basis for social relations; on the other, the social environment that would be guided according to the rules of social evolution.

In this way, social psychology, whose function for Raul Briquet (1935) was to understand 'the psychic causes of social facts,' needed to be situated in some way in the limbo 'between' the dimensions of inheritance and the social environment, which were then understood as 'extrinsic' to the individual and guided by immutable natural laws. For this mission, psychoanalysis played a fundamental role, both by trying to offer an understanding of 'between,' and by providing the basis for the introduction of a modern social psychology in Brazil.

Indeed, to understand the movement of introducing social psychology in Brazil, it is necessary, first, to understand the entry of psychoanalysis in the construction of Brazilian psychosocial thinking. As already mentioned, the two pioneers of social psychology in Brazil, Raul Briquet and Arthur Ramos, were strongly influenced by psychoanalysis.[1] Specifically, Raul Briquet emphasises in his book the importance of psychoanalysis in the constitution of psychology itself: 'Until recently, scholastic psychology dismembered the whole of the Self, describing the elements or faculties of the soul in isolation: memory, perception, etc. But psychology can only deserve the name of science of the soul after Freud's discoveries' (Briquet, 1935, p. 185).

Throughout his handbook, Briquet (1935) applied contributions from psychoanalytic thinking to bear on social psychological themes. When discussing, for example, one of the most important factors of social identity, *suggestion*, Briquet uses works (usually in their French versions) such as *Traité Théorique et Pratique de Psychanalyse* by Ernest Jones, *Sex in Psycho-Analysis* by Sandór Ferenczi and *Psychologie Colletive et Analyse du Moi* (*Group Psychology and the Analysis of the Ego*) by Sigmund Freud. In his argument, Briquet assumes that *'le désir est pére de la pensée.'*

[1] See Chapter 11 of this volume for a discussion of Arthur Ramos' work.

Similarly, in the chapter dedicated to the study of social adaptation, he references Alfred Adler's *Le Tempérament Nerveux*, stating that the *compensation* mechanism is fundamental for 'psychosocial readjustment.' Briquet exemplifies *compensation* through the process of re-adjusting immigrant peoples, many of them fleeing the war, who tragically were common figures in that interwar period.

In the chapter dedicated to the theme of *leadership*, Briquet describes the psychodynamics of the leader and the masses through the work of *Modern Education* by Otto Rank. However, the chapter with the greatest reference to psychoanalysis is the one dedicated to the crowd, in which the works *Totem and Taboo* and *Group Psychology and the Analysis of the Ego* by Freud are referenced (in French), in addition to two Brazilian works: *Psicanálise da Alma* of Inaldo de Lyra Neves-Manta and *Psicanálise de uma Civilização* by Júlio Pires Porto-Carrero.

The theme of the crowd is central to the development of social psychology in the early twentieth century and there is no doubt about the importance of psychoanalysis in this. In the first paragraph of *Group Psychology and the Analysis of the Ego*, Freud stated:

> The contrast between individual psychology and social or group psychology, which at a first glance may seem to be full of significance, loses a great deal of its sharpness when it is examined more closely. It is true that individual psychology is concerned with the individual man and explores the paths by which he seeks to find satisfaction for his instinctual impulses, but only rarely and under certain exceptional conditions is individual psychology in a position to disregard the relations of this individual to others. In the individual's mental life someone else is invariably involved, as a model, as an object, as a helper, as an opponent; and so from the very first individual psychology, in this extended but entirely justifiable sense of the words, is at the same time social psychology as well. (Freud, 2011, p. 13)

In this way, the birth of modern social psychology took place through psychoanalysis, which offered a first model of synthesis between individual and culture. However, the field opened by Freud at that time was inhabited more by clinicians than by social scientists:

> The psychoanalytic contribution to the social sciences is in danger of being neglected, especially in the history of social psychology. It appears in the 1954 *Handbook of Social Psychology*, edited by Lindzey, as well as in the 1968-69 edition, edited by Lindzey and Aronson, but not in subsequent editions. The psychoanalytic heritage of psychology, more generally, is found primarily in the hands of clinicians and not social psychologists. Therefore, it has a bias in favor of the individual instead of in favor of culture, as the focus of its interest. (Faar, 1998, p. 72)

It is worth examining how Briquet appropriated psychoanalytical concepts in his attempt to explain the psychosocial phenomena resulting from the encounter between the individual's biological heritage and the social environment. To this end, the discussions in the chapters on *instinct* and *aggressive instinct* will be addressed here, understood, along with the phenomenon of *habit*, as 'psychic factors that motivate social behavior' (Briquet, 1935, preface).

In the chapter dedicated to *instinct*, Briquet offers a perspective present in practically the entire book: the need to harmonise the biological and social dimensions. Given this opposition between 'inheritance' and 'environment,' the author states that:

> It is necessary to combine them and not to exalt one to the detriment of the other. Excluding from the study of nature what is most spontaneous and innate, such as automatic responses to stimuli in the environment, any work of *reconstruction or social improvement*, which, if it is not an instinct or habit, must be artificial, outlined in apriorism and, therefore, destined for setbacks in practical results. (Briquet, 1935, p. 97)

This attempt at conciliation aiming at social improvement was also expressed in the parallels that Briquet drew between psychoanalysis and Auguste Comte's positivism. From Freud's *Au dela du Principe Du Plaisir* (*Beyond the Pleasure Principle*) and *Psychoanalysis* by the Italian psychoanalyst Edoardo Weiss, Briquet states (using the first Portuguese translation of 'trieb') that 'instinct is the tendency of every living organism to reproduce and restore the previous state which it had to renounce under the influence of external disturbing forces' (Briquet, 1935, p. 104). In this sense, he affirmed that the need for social sublimation of instincts in favour of the advance of civilisation is also present in Comtian work. Briquet then approaches Comte's positivist thinking by stating that the 'personal instincts' overlap with the social inclinations, which are characterised by the dominance of the intellect. In this way, the individual would represent the starting point of the psychosocial phenomenon through the 'affective-instinctual' emergence, with society as its counterpoint, representing the 'intellectual-rational' sphere.

In this kind of 'Freudo-Comtian' perspective, the possibility of human progress and improvement would reside in the sublimation of personal instincts:

> We must insist: the social order must rest on instincts, naturally sublimated, and controlled. Without a doubt, human perfectibility is in the acquisition of the method and the precepts that allow reaching the truth. Education does not attribute to individuals faculties that do not have or cannot develop, for reasons of inheritance or means, but shows each citizen, through early and systematic action, the vulnerable aspects of their psychic structure, and the most adequate resources to repress and ennoble them. (Briquet, 1935, p. 106)

It should be noted that, together with the defence of a supposed immutability of instincts and subjectivity, Briquet points to a need for psychosocial intervention based on psychoanalytic knowledge, through an 'early and systematic action' on what is fragile in the psyche of the individual. This was, therefore, precisely the assumption of hygienist thinking at the beginning of the twentieth century in Brazil, which had the support of psychoanalysis in the search to identify any evidence of abnormality in school-age children. In this period, the association of mental hygiene and orthophrenic clinics with school institutions was not an accident.

The same assumptions were also present in the chapter on aggressive instinct, in which Briquet starts from the works *La Déception de la Guerre* by Freud and *War, Sadism and Pacifism* by the English psychoanalyst Edward Glover, in order to reflect on the psychological factors that lead human beings to war, which, in his opinion, would be more important than the political and economic ones. In this sense, *sadism*, when not properly repressed, would constitute one of the main 'etiological factors of war.' According to Briquet (1935):

> Poor repression, in addition to disorienting primitive sadism, provokes the unreasonable hatred of neurotics. And what a sum of anguish he did not spend before the morbid symptom appeared! (...) The frustration of the impulses caused the anguish opposite to peace of mind. It is understood that, when the threshold is reached, the child proceeds as a harassed animal, and only sees a way out in aggression and attack. (Briquet, 1935, p. 110)

However, just as Briquet approached positivism, he now approached social evolutionism by understanding war as a biological adaptation. Thus, he states: 'about being an economic imposition, war is a derivative, an outlet for instincts that, dissatisfied, represent a strong potential for the disintegration of the family or the tribe. It is, therefore, a biological adaptation modality' (Briquet, 1935, p. 111). In effect, he believed that it reinforced evolutionary thinking by comparing the aggressiveness of children, guided by the projection mechanism, to that of the so-called 'primitive' peoples.

Further on, he quotes Glover to justify, once again, a form of preventive intervention with a strong hygienist tendency, especially in starting from an etiological perspective on an essentially social phenomenon:

> Pacifists, who see nationalism as the main cause of war, should not neglect such sexual factors, basic to nationalist sentiment. True nationalism promotes the cooperation of the motherland in the universal harmony of the peoples.
>
> Many protest the war. Indeed, the feeling that moves them is very noble, but it does not aim at the respective etiology. Men will only extinguish war by socializing and sublimating selfish instincts: such a great goal, which will only be achieved in pacifist education, especially for children. (Briquet, 1935, p. 112)

In this way, Briquet resumed his attempt to reconcile sexual and aggressive instincts with the impositions imposed by civilisation, or, in other words, between the spheres of the innate and the acquired. In this sense, he affirmed that 'the difference between the imposed conduct and the person's instinctual dispositions increases with the progressive repression that they must suffer, manifesting the resulting tension by the most extravagant phenomena of reaction and compensation' (Briquet, 1935, p. 113). In effect, adaptation to social life would occur through what the author calls 'libido-social transformation,' that is, a kind of interdependence, or middle ground, between the biological and social dimensions.

In both chapters, Briquet presents a perspective aimed at conciliation, adaptation and with an intervention proposal that, although well-intentioned through education and psycho-hygiene, did not hide its authoritarian dimension. It is also noticeable that his reference to social psychology through psychoanalysis starts with the individual and not society; in this sense, the insistence on thinking about the particular, despite the totality, reveals an essentially ideological perspective for considering any type of perspective of social transformation other than from the individual himself.

Even with the contribution of psychoanalytic theory, which would allow a more in-depth understanding of the 'between,' the social psychology proposed by Raul Briquet, found itself hostage to the contradictions of a philosophy that sought to reconcile such distinct theoretical and methodological perspectives as those of biology and sociology. Ultimately, social psychology, which should be a discipline responsible for thinking about the formation of the social being, relied on the erasure of the historical subject and the annulment of the individual by forces foreign to him, such as 'inheritance' and 'environment.'

The impossibility of thinking about mediation between individual and society would lead to an authoritarian perspective, on which psychoanalytic thinking had a strong influence. Specifically, psychoanalysis contributed both to the founding of authoritarianism present in hygienist practices of psychosocial intervention, and to a type of authoritarianism at the theoretical level, in its attempt to reconcile radically contradictory and irreconcilable instances. As mentioned earlier, these contradictions are present in the ancestors of social psychology in Brazil and were inherited by Briquet and other intellectuals during the 1930s, however, it is essential to understand that this is a contradictory process, and far from being merely intellectual and theoretical, is real and concrete.

Concrete Authoritarianism, Theoretical Authoritarianism: A Dialectical Conclusion

If there is one thing that historical and dialectical materialism carries as a precise axiom, it is that there is no contradiction in thought that does not reveal a real contradiction, present in its entirety. As Lukács (2003) states:

> …in the case of social reality, these contradictions [in thought] are not a sign of the imperfect understanding of society; on the contrary, they belong to the nature of reality itself and to the nature of capitalism. When the totality is known they will not be transcended and cease to be contradictions. Quite the reverse, they will be seen to be necessary contradictions arising out of the antagonisms of this system of production. (Lukács, 2003, pp. 79–80)

In this sense, theoretical production in capitalist society expresses itself subjectively as a *fetishistic form of objectivity*, that is, as an apparent autonomous manifestation of thought. However, this appearance is determined by the antagonistic and reified social totality of capital. The abstraction of thought, which divides human phenomena into universal laws and cause and effect relationships, reveals itself as the result of concrete, real abstraction, which underlies the production of our conditions of existence:

> The fetishistic character of economic forms, the reification of all human relations, the constant expansion and extension of the division of labour which subjects the process of production to an abstract, rational analysis, without regard to the human potentialities and abilities of the immediate producers, all these things transform the phenomena of society and with them the way in which they are perceived. In this way arise the 'isolated' facts, 'isolated' complexes of facts, separate, specialist disciplines (economics, law, etc.) whose very appearance seems to have done much to

> pave the way for such scientific methods. It thus appears extraordinarily 'scientific' to think out the tendencies implicit in the facts themselves and to promote this activity to the status of Science. (Lukács, 2003, p. 72)

Indeed, these *fetishist forms of objectivity* are expressed in the problem of the relationship between individual and society and, methodologically, in the contradiction between psychology and sociology. As Adorno (2017) points out, the contradiction between these two disciplines expresses both the division of social work that expands to other dimensions of life, and the alienated split between the individual and the totality:

> The separation of society and psyche is false consciousness; it perpetuates conceptually the split between the living subject and the objectivity that governs the subjects and yet derives from them. But the basis of this false consciousness cannot be removed by a mere methodological dictum. People are incapable of recognizing themselves in society and society in themselves because they are alienated from each other and the totality. Their reified social relations necessarily appear to them as an 'in itself'. What compartmentalized disciplines project on to reality merely reflects back what has taken place in reality. False consciousness is also true: inner and outer life are torn apart. (Adorno, 2017, pp. 74–75)

Briquet's attempt to conceive a social psychology through psychoanalysis is based on the radical split between individual and society; more precisely, on the conception of an individual who seeks his realisation 'between' forces extrinsic to him and over which he has no control. Inheritance and the social environment thus reveal themselves as alienated and ideological forces, which subject the individual to their laws. As Chauí (2012, p. 96) points out, ideology operates precisely in the justification of this alienation by 'making men believe that their lives are what they are as a result of the action of certain entities (Nature, the gods or God, Reason or Science, Society, the State), which exist in and by themselves and to which it is legitimate and legal to submit.'

Adorno (2017), points out that ideology, although false, reveals a truth: the alienation of the individual in relation to the production of his conditions of existence. This observation is particularly pertinent to the period when Briquet's social psychology manual was being prepared, specifically, between two wars characterised by mass destruction and impersonality. As already mentioned, the main characteristic of the 1930s was the radicalisation of the antagonism between social, political and economic forces in the world and the stubborn attempt to reconcile them in Brazil. The Getúlio Vargas government, which came to power through a coup, was guided mainly by the reconciliation of contradictory interests, of antagonistic forces, which was only possible through the use of authoritarianism. In Briquet, the elaboration of a social psychology in Brazil was also only possible through conciliation, with an authoritarian touch, of radically opposed and alienated dimensions such as inheritance and social environment.

In this manner, it is possible to understand two hegemonic forces in their conception of social psychology, which reveals the totality in which it was produced. On one hand, the conservative, traditional, oligarchic, landowning forces; and on the other hand, a liberal, bourgeois, industrialist force, which relied upon constitutionalist and republican principles as a means of scientifically 'guiding' politics. On one side, the exclusionary principle of race and heredity as the essence of a Brazilian national character; on the other, the principle of order and progress of society which, despite its limits, was aimed at the development of society and, therefore, a certain social transformation. Faced with this dead-end antinomy that operated on the individual and society, Briquet theoretically accomplished what Vargas operated in politics: a reconciliation through authoritarianism.This authoritarian theoretical reconciliation was made possible mainly by the contributions of psychoanalysis to social psychology, when trying to methodologically stitch together the concrete split between individual and society.

In conclusion, the introduction of social psychology in Brazil through the person of Raul Briquet was a singular expression of the movement of conservative modernisation that began in the country in the 1930s. This was done first, by situating social psychology as one of the subjects of the social sciences that would be responsible for the populist modernisations in the country, by men of science, as intended by the elites from São Paulo in that period. Secondly, by harmonising, in an authoritarian manner, radically distinct theoretical-methodological propositions, like those offered by biology supported by heredity and positivist sociology supported by the excuse of order and progress. From this, it is understood that the social psychology introduced on national soil was, without a doubt, the theoretical expression of a historical necessity determined by attacks, strong authoritarianism and denial of the individual, and, at the same time, by resistance, struggles for democracy and for the theoretical and concrete rescue of this individual. In this singular and contradictory movement of a conservative modernisation project made by 'men of science,' social psychology found its birth through the contributions and contradictions of nationally appropriated psychoanalysis.

References

Adorno, T. W. (2017). *Escritos de Psicologia Social e Psicanálise*. Editora Unesp.

Bomfim, E. M. (2002). *Raul Carlos Briquet. Coleção Pioneiros da Psicologia Brasileira*. Imago Ed., Brasília, DF: CFP, v. 7.

Briquet, R. (1935). *Psicologia Social*. F. Alves.

Chauí, M. (2012). *O que é ideologia*. Editora Brasiliense.

Farr, R. M. (1998). *As raízes da Psicologia Social Moderna*. Vozes.

Fausto, B. (2013). *História do Brasil*. Edusp.

Freud, S. (2011). *Psicologia das massas e análise do eu e outros textos (1920–1923)*. Companhia das Letras.

Hobsbawm, E. (2004). *A era dos extremos*. Paz e Terra.

Hobsbawm, E. (2013). *Nações e nacionalismo desde 1780: Programa, mito e realidade*. Paz e Terra.

Kantor, I., Maciel, A. D., & Simões, A. J. (2009). *A Escola Livre de Sociologia e Política: anos de formação (1933–1953)*. Ed. Sociologia e Política.

Lukács, G. (2003). *História e consciência de classe*. Martins Fontes.

Paicheler-Harrous, G. (2018) *A invenção da Psicologia Moderna*. Benjamin Editorial.

Patto, M. H. S. (2008). *A produção do fracasso escolar: histórias de submissão e rebeldia*. Casa do Psicólogo.

Romero, S. (1902). *História da literatura brasileira* (2nd ed.). H. Garnier.

Schwarz, R. (2007). *Ao vencedor as batatas: forma literária e processo social nos inícios do romance brasileiro*. Duas Cidades, Ed.34.

Schwarcz, L. M. (2019). *Sobre o autoritarismo brasileiro*. Cia das Letras.

Simonsen, R. (1973). *Evolução industrial do Brasil e outros estudos: seleção, notas e bibliografia de Edgard Carone*. Nacional, USP.

Velloso, M. P. (2013). Os intelectuais e a política cultural do Estado Novo. In J. Ferreira & L. A. N. Delgado (Eds.), *O Brasil republicano: O tempo do nacional-estatismo: Do início da década de 1930 ao apogeu do Estado Novo* (6th ed., pp. 145–179). Civilização Brasileira.

11

The Savage Rests in Every Soul: Social Misfits and the Primitive Unconscious in Arthur Ramos's Social Psychology

Fernando A. Figueira do Nascimento

Introduction

Brazil has the second highest number of deaths in the world caused by the new coronavirus. The pandemic, at its inception, was seen by the Brazilian government as a small flu that should not prevent people from working and should not stifle the economy. When Brazil reached 10,000 deaths, the president said he was not a gravedigger and defined his position with a smile and a resounding 'so what?' After twenty thousand deaths, the president encouraged his supporters to invade the campaign hospitals and to photograph the Intensive Care Centres to unmask the communist farce. At the time of writing, there have been more than 500,000 deaths and little care to establish preventive measures: the government has comforted us by saying that we must go on living—after all, we will all die one day.

F. A. F. do Nascimento (✉)
Universidade de São Paulo, São Paulo, Brazil

B. Mandelbaum et al. (eds.), *Brazilian Psychosocial Histories of Psychoanalysis*, Studies in the Psychosocial,
https://doi.org/10.1007/978-3-030-78509-3_11

It is under these circumstances that this text is written and these events that make us return to history. These episodes should be positioned as part of a movement that is anchored in scientific negativism, relativism and historical revisionism, which attacks the university, professors, students and artists and mobilises part of the population in a crusade against all critical thinking. This movement associates itself with, and finds its surface of emergence in, the political space preserved by Brazilian authoritarianism, tempered by religious fanaticism, neo-fascist discourse and neoliberal rationality, and marks much more than a possible theoretical–methodological insufficiency. The solidity of truth, once the basis for disciplinary societies, now seems fleeting, to the same extent that the society of control demands and produces other forms of organisation for the exercise of power.

The analysis of the history of psychological knowledge urges a reflection on the updating of the games of truth and the new relationships created between knowledge and power. In particular, for people working in the field of mental health, this implicates the notion of the subject that is produced in our field, raising questions about the political dimension of clinical practice. Beyond a common criticism of the supposed disciplinary and normative practice of psychology, it is important to ask ourselves where psychological discourses fit, in a time when neoliberal governance triumphs and offers its subjects both their method of enjoyment (*jouissance*) and their forms of subjection—a process for which the discipline no longer needs so many intermediaries (Dardot & Laval, 2016).

Foucault (2013) argued that if history has provided the bourgeoisie with the means to justify domination, naturalise processes of colonial violence and design methods of dominance until time immemorial, it is still through the roar of battles that its grimmest origins are shown. Thus, it is not a question of understanding that a theoretical–methodological error, or ideology, or even any misunderstanding, has diverted our knowledge and that a new elaboration of history makes it possible to correct these errors to finally reach an ideal state of pure science. It is about understanding who we are and, as Foucault (2005) has stated, revealing the devices that prevent us from having any other identity.

This chapter seeks to contribute to the critical analysis of the history of social psychology in Brazil. It is part of an ongoing research project on the genealogy of social psychology in the country, but will be limited here to presenting the propositions of Arthur Ramos (1903–1949). Ramos was a physician and anthropologist who wrote one of the first manuals on the new science in the country. In his *Introduction to Social Psychology* (1936), social psychology was not characterised as an autonomous scientific field, and its interfaces are not limited to psychological and sociological knowledge. Moreover, Ramos positions psychoanalysis as one of the fundamental tools for his historical-cultural analysis. He is considered a pioneer in psychoanalysis in the country, inspired largely by the works of Freud, Jung, Adler and Anna Freud among others.

A Historical Outline

Our approach to the historical constitution of psychological knowledge in Brazil, has as its fundamental axis the problem of social maladjustment. This enables us to examine the network of devices (institutions, discourses, laws, techniques and strategies of government, philosophical propositions and psychological practices) that have acted on individual bodies and the population as a whole.

Inspired by Oliveira (2005), Prado Filho (2014) and Ferreira (2007), for methodological purposes, we propose the following four fundamental periods for the study of social psychology in Brazil:

- 1850–1920: the period in which the studies of sociology prevailed, inspired by the positivism of Auguste Comte and the Social Evolutionism of Herbert Spencer;
- 1920–1945: the period of the first Brazilian social psychology manuals; it is also the period when the institutionalisation of social psychology began, with the first courses at the *Escola Livre de Sociologia e Política* (Free School of Sociology and Politics) in São Paulo and at the *Universidade do Distrito Federal* (University of the Federal District) of Rio de Janeiro;

- 1945–1979: the period of consolidation of social psychology, when the effects of its crisis were observed in the country, which in Latin America sparked efforts towards theoretical–methodological revision;
- 1980–to date: the founding period of the Brazilian Association of Social Psychology, which stimulated important discussions in the field. During this time, new possibilities for action and research opened up, with shared perspectives in notions of ethical–political commitment.

In this chapter, we will focus on the period from 1920 to 1945, and we will review the propositions of Arthur Ramos, a physician from Alagoas, who graduated from the Faculty of Medicine of Bahia and was one of those responsible for the dissemination of psychoanalysis in that state during the 1930s.[1]

Approaches

The first social psychology manuals written and published in Brazil, at the beginning of the twentieth century, made frequent references to psychoanalysis, American experimental social psychology, behaviourism, gestalt and a whole set of sociological and anthropological texts. These texts addressed the relationship between the individual and society, highlighting the specificity of social psychology as the science that studied the emerging psychic processes in the interactions among the individual, society, history and culture.

In Brazil during the 1930s, the social psychology that was beginning to be produced and institutionalised had presented American and European bibliographical references of the time and sought its validation in Brazil. However, with the arrival of psychological knowledge, Brazilian

[1] Menezes (2002) states that as early as the end of the nineteenth century, 1898, Afrânio Peixoto quoted Freud in his doctoral thesis Epilepsy and Crime. In 1919, Francisco Peixoto Magalhães Netto presented Freud's theories in his thesis on the etiopathogeny of Morel-Kraepelin disease. In 1924, José Júlio Calasans, still a medical student, presented a paper entitled *Freud's doctrine in neuroses and psychoses*, at the Alfredo de Brito Academy, and published in the Bahia Medical Gazette. In the following years, the Medical Society of Bahia witnessed several debates on psychoanalysis, although the comments did not indicate an adherence by doctors to Freudian theories. On psychoanalysis in Bahia between 1926 and 1937, see Menezes (2002).

authors could not distance themselves from the problems and contradictions that impacted on psychology itself since its emergence: to be characterised as a science of the norm in the interstices of the empirical sciences and, by pursuing the rigour of the natural sciences and their supposed objective precision, constructing a vision of the human being as no longer belonging to the order of nature (Foucault, 2007, 2011).

For those Brazilian authors who opposed the theories of racial inferiority and integrated anti-fascist intellectual movements and the renewal of teaching methods in the country, the normative and pedagogical function of psychology was not perceived as a contradiction, but rather as a break with the ancient authoritarian methods (Ramos, 1939/1949). Psychological discourses produced relations with psychiatry and education and presented themselves as rational foundations for medical and pedagogical practices dedicated to the problems that were gaining more and more political importance: school failure, the integration of the patient into society and the adjustment of individuals to work.

In this heterogeneous space of reception and invention of social psychology, Raul Carlos Briquet (1887–1953) and Arthur Ramos were two intellectuals recognised by historians as pioneers of psychoanalysis in the country (Morkejs, 1993; Perestrello, 1992; Russo, 2002, 2007). These authors believed that social psychology also presented an important approach to Freudian studies, as well as to its dissidents Carl Gustav Jung and Alfred Adler.

Although its oldest roots can be located in sociological studies mainly in the second half of the nineteenth century Teixeira (2009), social psychology found other paths in the first decades of the twentieth century, between Forensic Medicine and Criminal Anthropology, Mental Hygiene, Education and Psychiatry. These were fields in which it was possible to notice not only the presence of Comtean positivism and Spencer's social evolutionism, but also the ideal of the individual, which was based on the liberal values of the time, and contrasted with the increasingly authoritarian political atmosphere and the accentuation of the serious structural problems experienced in urban centres. These structural problems had resulted from population growth, precarious health and working conditions, low wages and housing shortages. It is in this context that we find the first texts dealing with, or at least alluding to, social psychology.

In the 1920s, the first manuscript to use the term social psychology in its title was by Oliveira Vianna (1883–1951). This was marked by the political events of his time including disenchantment with European knowledge after the first great war, the public demonstrations by urban workers, in which anarchists and communists[2] played an important role, and the organisation of workers and trade unions, which brought to life the threat of subversion. Moreover, in *Small Essays in Social Psychology* (*Pequenos Ensaios de Psicologia Social*, 1921), Vianna dealt with topics such as the mental roots of the Brazilian people, the repetition of scientific and cultural fashions from abroad, morality and problems related to modernisation which, according to him, caused the loss of traditional family values. Vianna believed that the loss of traditions and changes in political power were associated with the problems of identity and modernisation, which in his view would dismantle the social order.

Vianna highlighted notions such as 'subconscious of race' and 'instinct' to examine the difficulties of adapting individuals to new forms of organisation in society. When he classified every Brazilian man as a 'peasant,' he reiterated the problem of social maladjustment in its broadest sense, as a general crisis in the ways of existing:

> What is bestowing on our society this appearance of corruption and degeneration, on the one hand, and this impression of discouragement and selfishness, on the other, can be summed up in this synthetic formula: the tendency, of recent origin, of the country's upper classes and leaders to concentrate on capital cities; as a consequence, an intense and extensive crisis in their professional means of subsistence. (Vianna, 1921, p. 20)

The central question for Vianna (1921) seemed to rest on the notion of national identity, which had placed the population at the centre of medical and anthropological debates since the invention of the Republic.

---

[2] Vianna presents criticisms of communism, socialism and anarchism, classifying them as 'retrograde utopias,' anachronistic in the history of man because '(…) the type of man of the future, is the man liberated from every community, the individualist man, who seeks in himself the power of salvation and triumph' (Vianna, 1921, p. 92).

As a solution, he opined that the population should return to the spirit of early frontiersmen (bandeirantes) and accept the example of great men as the basis of healing. He believed that this was the best action for a sick nation that had little understanding of liberal morality, was mobilised by instinct and imitation, and consequently had little appreciation of the civic acts of republicanism (Vianna, 1921). The population, therefore, was presented as a problem for the government, and the formation of social identity and its maladjustment became a political and psychological category.

More than a decade later, the text by Raul Briquet, *Social Psychology* (1935), expressed significant discontinuities with the one published by Vianna and, in addition to an up-to-date bibliographical review for the time, presented the definitions of social psychology and its object according to different schools and traditions which highlighted the importance of scientific studies that supported his considerations.

Briquet positioned social psychology as a science at the interface between psychology and sociology. He also analysed, based on Tarde's writings, the processes related to identity formation, social adaptation, the movement of crowds and the mental processes of a revolution. To support his hypothesis about the fanatic spirit, the author applied the psychoanalytical notions of narcissism and the attempts of the Self to adjust to the outside life onto his analysis of religious feeling and the revolutionary spirit (Briquet, 1935). Briquet also considered that a primitive mental activity prevailed within crowds, that individuals would surrender their individuality to the group, letting go of their selves and embracing a new totality.

In the chapter devoted to social adaptation, Briquet used Alfred Adler's theories to locate the feeling of inferiority acquired in childhood experiences as the cause of deviations from social adaptation. 'The degree of psychic deviation depends on the non-adaptation to the impositions of the environment' (Briquet, 1935, p. 195). This perception offered the possibility for healing, as long as the patient was convinced and encouraged to engage in analysis.[3]

[3] See Chapter 10 of this volume for more detail on Raul Briquet.

At the point that Briquet's book was being printed, Arthur Ramos was lecturing in the Economics and Law courses of the *Universidade do Distrito Federal*. Whether at the *Escola Livre de Sociologia e Política*or at the *Universidade do Distrito Federal*, social psychology was directly linked to the problem of governance and the objective of forming a new set of intellectuals who would have the task of governing the country (Araújo, 2016; Teixeira, 2009).

Arthur Ramos (1933), believed that psychoanalysis opened up new possibilities for psychiatrists, through new methods of healing that recognised human values in individuals that normal science could not address. The dichotomy adjustment–maladjustment, added to the concepts of primitive or folkloric unconscious and social identity, was also important for the articulation between psychoanalysis and social psychology in a type of applied Mental Hygiene.

Arthur Ramos: Introductory Remarks

Arthur Ramos de Araújo Pereira was born in 1903 in the city of Pilar, in the State of Alagoas. After completing his primary education, he moved to Maceió, where he carried out preparatory studies for entering college with Faustino Magalhães da Silveira, the father of Nise da Silveira (1905–1999).[4]

In 1921, at the age of eighteen, he enrolled in the Faculty of Medicine of Bahia where, five years later, he received the title of Doctor of Medical-Surgical Sciences, defending a thesis entitled *Primitive and Madness* (*Primitivo e Loucura*), which in the same year was published by the Official State Press.

According to Gutman and Pereira (2007),

[4] Nise Magalhães da Silveira was a psychiatrist who fought against established psychiatric practices of electric shock, lobotomy and insulin therapy during the 1930s and 1940s. She pioneered a more humane approach in psychiatry, using art as a therapeutic resource. She was one of the first students of Carl Gustav Jung in Brazil and in 1952 she founded the Museum of Images of the Unconscious (Melo, 2001).

> the dissertation of Arthur Ramos, already at its beginning, takes up the position explained by Auguste Comte, according to whom 'the psychological portrait of "man" [must] be explained by humanity and not by that man' (p. 4). It is therefore a plan of work in which anthropology and ethnology are used to clarify questions arising from the field of psychology (p. 4).

In his inaugural text, Ramos presents his interest in social and collective psychology, and identifies the physician Raimundo Nina Rodrigues (1862–1906) as the precursor of studies on social psychopathologies and African peoples in Brazil. He also drew on Gustave Le Bon's theory on the irrational functioning and regressive processes of the masses, Gabriel Tarde's on the laws of imitation, as well as the Italian School of Criminal Anthropology, with Tanzi, Sighele and Rossi, on psychic atavism and the regressive character of pathological symptoms.

In relation to psychoanalysis, Ramos drew on at least three themes: its theories on child development, the study of psychopathology and research into the psychology of the masses and peoples. There are references to Sigmund Freud, Carl Gustav Jung and Alfred Adler, the latter for a teleological understanding of behaviour and maladjustment from the perspective of conflicts of inferiority. Ramos criticises Freud for his individualistic application of the concept of the unconscious, which, contrary to what Jung had contended, would not enable understanding of the collective and ancestral elements present in the psyche.

In the field of psychiatric studies, Ramos found in Juliano Moreira and Afrânio Peixoto (2005), in addition to reflections on the causes of delusion, a justification of the role of early childhood education as a device for the prevention and correction of mental illness, stating that these authors '(...) point out, as essential vices of the paranoid, a primitive and original autophilia, inadequacy between the individual and the environment, and consequent reactions of that against them: active, passive, or active-passive persecution' (Ramos, 1926, p. 34). Ramos argued that delirium is characterised as a process where the experiences bequeathed by previous generations reappear in the psyche, when 'the moderating functions die, or indirectly by extrinsic defect of the inhibiting functions, as in acute mental disorders and its chronic *reliquats*'[5] (Ramos, 1926, p. 33).

Ramos contributed to an important debate for the psychiatry of his time on the causes of mental illness and, although he partly agreed with Moreira and Peixoto's criticism of Tanzi's notion of psychic atavism, he stated that '(…) the essential fact is that these morbid pictures exist and their analogy to certain manifestations of the primitive cannot be denied' (Ramos, 1926, p. 40). He added to these considerations the influence of Jung's studies, and conceptualised the notion of the primitive or folkloric unconscious as a synthesis between the inter-psychic and ancestral unconscious. Thus, he defended the hypothesis that the construction of neurotic and psychotic symptoms had a trans-generational and phylogenetic basis, which was represented in cultural formations, language, dreams, the primitive mental functioning of children and uncultivated populations, and in universal psychopathological symptoms.

Following Freud's account, he generalised primitive mental functioning even to the adult individual considered sane and civilised. He believed that the savage that lurks in every soul reached the surface of the psyche under certain conditions, from oneiric activity to reverie and artistic creation, as well as in the behaviour of groups and crowds (Schreiner, 2005).

In 1927, Arthur Ramos was appointed medical assistant at St. John of God Hospital, a psychiatric asylum where he carried out his first psychopathological studies, which later (1928) helped him write his *habilitation* thesis *The Sordidness of the Alienated—An essay on a pathology of filth* (*A Sordice dos Alienados—ensaio de uma patologia da imundice*). In that text, Ramos reiterated the idea that the primitive aspects of development are represented in cultural formations such as folklore, and that pathological symptoms, such as the eschatological beliefs of the alienated, would correspond to points of fixation in psychosexual development that had caused their disturbance.

The analysis of the phases of development, with special emphasis on the anal phase and the enjoyment that excrement aroused in certain patients, led Ramos to affirm that there is the presence of an 'elemental

[5] Translated from French as remnants or remainders.

impulse' in the daily experience of the individual, discovered by psychoanalysis. From the psychotic symptom, Ramos reached out to other subjects, those who were deemed to be sane, and to the different dimensions of daily life: the use of money, the taste for perfumes, acquisitiveness, possessiveness, the creation of folkloric myths and the whole psychic game of attractive and repulsive activities (Ramos, 1928).

At the end of his text, drawing on the studies of Julio Pires Porto-Carreiro (1887–1937), Ramos presented characterological types among schoolchildren in which it is possible to identify the presence of the anal-erotic complex at the centre of failed adaptation to the environment: the complainants, the lovers of their self, the homosexuals, rebels constituted by self-centredness who were resistant to the recognition of their inferiority derived from the castration complex (Ramos, 1928).

In 1928 Arthur Ramos also became a medical examiner at the *Instituto Médico Legal da Bahia* (Medical Legal Institute of Bahia), which later became the Nina Rodrigues Institute and, under the influence of Professor Estácio de Lima, began his studies on black people, African religions and forensic psychopathology. In the 1930s, he continued to dedicate himself to these studies and was inspired by the work of Nina Rodrigues—to whom he became a disciple—and by his experiences as a medical examiner and clinician, which put him in contact with the black and mestizo populations (Ramos, 1942, 2001).

In his 1934 manuscript, *O Negro brasileiro: etnografia religiosa* (*The Brazilian Black People: Religious Ethnography*, 2001), Ramos stated that it was important for education to recognise the primitive psychic mechanisms that worked in any culture. He affirmed that pre-logical thinking acted in any ethnic group that was culturally backward, in the poor classes, in neuralgic adults, in art and in special conditions of psychic regression. The study of collective representations would provide routes for overcoming these elements by sublimation.

> (For) educational and cultural work, it is necessary to know these modalities of 'primitive' thinking, in order to correct it, raising it to more advanced stages, which will only be achieved by an educational revolution that acts in depth, a 'vertical' and 'interstitial' revolution that goes down

> the remote steps of the collective unconscious and loosens the pre-logical ties to which it is chained. (p. 32)

The primitive was defined by the author in purely psychological and social terms, as opposed to the racial element, which had been used to justify and naturalise the position of the black in society. In addition to the possibility of understanding the collective psyche of the Brazilian people, Ramos added a political element: the social inequalities in the country, as the cause of the prevalence of primitive thinking.

In his 1935 work, *O folclore negro do Brasil: demopsicologia e psicanálise* (*The Black Folklore of Brazil: Demopsychology and Psychoanalysis*), he dedicated himself to the study of African myths, stating that they could only be fully understood in the light of psychoanalytical theories, especially from the perspective of the family romance. With this, he analysed the ancestral element in the formation of the collective and individual psyche:

> When cultural interpenetration intervenes, underground psychological work of extraordinary importance begins to take place. It happens in the collective psyche the same as in the individual psyche. The old elements do not disappear. They are repressed and encrusted in the collective unconscious. They become private. And they entwine as survivors or superstitions. (Ramos, 2007, p. 25)

Ramos (2007) stated that it would be up to social psychology to present the ideological aspects, which were often unconscious, that determined the methods and results of research on black cultures in Brazil. Social psychology, besides its adaptive aspect, had a dimension of critique of scientific knowledge:

> It is social psychology, with the methodological position to which I allude [the historical-cultural and psychoanalytical method], that will come to 'psychologically' clarify the motives of these discussions and controversies, denouncing the often unconscious plots of their exclusivism, almost always at the service of certain philosophical beliefs and convictions and even of political-social ideologies. (Ramos, 2007, p. 7)

In addition to his studies on black people in the early 1930s, he published *Estudos de psicanálise* (*Studies in psychoanalysis*, 1931), *Freud, Adler and Jung* (1933), *Psiquiatria e psicanálise* (*Psychiatry and psychoanalysis*, 1933), *Educação e psicanálise* (*Education and psychoanalysis*, 1934), *Introdução à psicologia social* (*Introduction to social psychology*, 1936). After the launching of the *Introduction*, Ramos published, in 1937, *As culturas negras no novo mundo* (*Black cultures in the new world*), *Loucura e crime: questões de psiquiatria, medicina forense e psicologia social* (*Madness and crime: Questions of psychiatry, forensic medicine and social psychology*) and, two years later, *A criança problema* (*The problem child*, 1939).

In 1934, he went to Rio de Janeiro and accepted Anísio Teixeira's invitation to direct the Service of Orthophrenia and Mental Hygiene (SOHM), linked to the *Instituto de Pesquisas Educacionais do Distrito Federal* (Educational Research Institute of the Federal District). Between 1934 and 1939, he made two thousand observations of children, which resulted in the book *A Criança Problema* (*The problem child*), where he wrote:

> The 'class tail' children in schools, insubordinate, disobedient, unstable, liars, runaways... in their great majority are not the bearers of any 'moral anomaly' in the constitutional sense of the term. They have been 'ab-normalised' by their environment. Like primitive man whose 'savagery' was a creation of the civilised, also in the child, the concept of 'abnormal' was, above all, the adult point of view, the consequence of an enormous unconscious sadism of parents and educators. (Ramos, 1939, p. 18)

In this perspective, social maladjustment was a fundamental concept for the elaboration of the notion of the 'problem child,' as opposed to the 'abnormal child,' which meant a shift in the focus from heredity to social, family and institutional conditions as determinants for the study of personality. He established the correction of deviations as the central objective of child mental hygiene (Patto, 1999). Ramos broke with the idea of biological determinism and, in treating the health of the spirit as a historical and socio-cultural phenomenon, he revealed his anti-determinist approach (Maio, 2015).

In 1935, with the creation of the *Universidade do Distrito Federal* (University of the Federal District), Ramos was invited by Anísio Teixeira and Afrânio Peixoto to assume the chair of social psychology. Between July and December of the same year, he taught social psychology at the School of Economics and Law and, between February and May of the following year, he wrote his *Introdução à Psicologia Social* (*Introduction to Social Psychology*), which aimed to systematise the recent discipline within the framework of the social sciences (Ramos, 2003).[6]

In the preface of its first edition Ramos presented social psychology as having been central to his studies since his first works:

> I could not escape, however, some personal views on this or that point: the presentation of the subject and division of the book, criteria of methodological convergence, some applications of social psychology to Brazilian problems, child maladjustments at home and school, use of psychopathological and ethnographic material, and especially the whole third part, object of ancient studies, which, on affective logic, primitive thinking and the magical-schizophrenic mentality, I have been carrying out since 1926. (Ramos, 2003, p. 23)

His propositions regarding social maladjustment corresponded with the modernisation ideal of his time and with the process of extending psychiatric power beyond asylum walls as part of this same ideal. However, the historical-cultural approach also opened up the possibility of analysing subjectivity in individual terms (Sodré, 2015). For Ramos, maladjustment became the main object of the work of psycho-sociologists and combined collective, social and individual causes. Among these causes were hereditary aspects, fight conflicts (according to Allport), regression and the inferiority complex, the permanence in the psyche of ancestral images, psychic atavism and educational and affective factors (Ramos, 2003).

In this sense, in the *Introduction*, Ramos once again advocated a contrast to the theories on racial degeneration that had defined mestizaje

[6] The course of introduction to social psychology at the University of the Federal District took place between the years 1935 and 1938. In 1937, Ramos organised the course in general psychology, also in the School of Economics and Law (Schreiner, 2003).

and the black as the central cause of the various problems of Brazilian society. During the 1930s, psychoanalysis and social psychology, in his perspective, meant openness to the function of educating and improving what had been corrupted by social conditions (Tamano, 2013).

When the *Estado Novo* (New State)[7] closed the University of the Federal District, which employed social scientists who were gaining prominence at the time, such as Gilberto Freyre and Sergio Buarque de Holanda, Ramos became professor of anthropology and ethnography at the *Faculdade Nacional de Filosofia* (National Faculty of Philosophy, FNFi) of the University of Brazil, where he remained from 1939 until 1949 (Maio, 2015).

In 1949, he was invited by the UNESCO General Director to chair the Department of Social Sciences. In Oslo during the same year, he chaired the Conference of the International Association of Sociology on behalf of the General Director and, at the General Conference of UNESCO, he presented the programme of the Department of Social Sciences for the following years, which indicates the extent of his international influence. Arthur Ramos passed away in Paris on the evening of the 30th to the 31st of October 1949.[8]

Between Eras: The *Introduction to Social Psychology*

Introdução à Psicologia Social (*Introduction to Social Psychology*, 2003) was conceived during a period of transition in Arthur Ramos' research: the studies that he developed in the following years were close to anthropology and, although we find references to social psychology and psychoanalysis, his dedication to anthropological studies appeared to be

[7] With the closing of the National Congress in 1937, Getúlio Vargas established the dictatorship of the *Estado Novo* (New State, 1937–1945), under the claim of defending society against political disputes and the communist threat. Moreover, the period is marked by affinity and receptiveness to the fascist ideals coming from Europe.

[8] Arthur Ramos joined numerous medical and scientific institutions in Brazil, including the Bahia Society of Forensic Medicine, Criminology and Psychiatry, where he proposed the creation of a section dedicated to psychoanalytical studies; the Bahia Society of Medicine; the Brazilian League of Mental Hygiene; the Bahia Penitentiary Council; the Society of Neurology, Psychiatry and Forensic Medicine; the Brazilian Society of Psychology; and was one of the founders of the Brazilian Society of Anthropology and Ethnology.

increasing. Likewise, the work was written at a time of profound turbulence in the country, amidst the political upheavals, such as the military uprising of November 1935, which later resulted in the closure of the National Congress and the beginning of the *varguista* dictatorship of the *Estado Novo*.

Since the nineteenth century, controversies about human nature, as well as the breakdown of ancient customs and moral values, were perceived as a risk for Brazilian society. This intensified the perception of an entire population as potentially dangerous: freed slaves, *capoeiristas*,[9] thieves, gypsies, itinerant people, deserters, prostitutes, anarchists, madmen, etc. (Carvalho, 2015; Schwarcz, 2017). At the same time, debates between the 'civilised' and the 'savage' were reconfiguring themselves into the opposition between modernisation, which directly implied control of the masses, and the country's backwardness.

For the construction of a new power pact that would break with colonial traditions and simultaneously keep political power in the hands of the children of the Brazilian bourgeoisie, 'some solid normative element, innate in the soul of the people, or even implanted by tyranny, is necessary for social crystallisation' (Holanda, 2014, p. 221). The call towards this 'normative element' denounced the crisis of adaptation of individuals and the triumph of anti-family virtues that had lurked in the growing spirit of competition among citizens, resulting from modernisation. It also revealed the appeal of, and continuous flirtation with, authoritarianism that arose in Brazil after 1929 following disenchantment with liberalism, with the persistent presence of patriarchal colonialism and the heritage of slavery that had spread through daily social relations. Fears of the dismantling of society called for psychology, together with psychoanalysis and mental hygiene, as another important political element for the understanding, elaboration and application of the norm on the behaviour of individuals and groups.

[9] Capoeira is a fighting style, a martial art, which originated in the sixteenth century among black people kidnapped in Africa and brought to the Portuguese colony for plantations and sugar cane mills. During the colonial period, as it was considered a threat to the enslavers, it was the target of repression by the Imperial Police and then the Republican Militia. Until the 1930s, capoeira was forbidden in the country. Capoeirista is a practitioner of capoeira.

In this context, Ramos (2003) defined social psychology in three fundamental perspectives and highlighted the psychological bases of social behaviour: inter-psychology, the concept of personality and its quality of cultural psychology:

> First of all, social psychology studies the psychological bases of social behaviour and thereby approaches the psychology of the individual. Secondly, it studies the psychological inter-relationships of individuals in social life. It then becomes an inter-psychology, in the old sense of Tarde. Finally, social psychology has to consider the total influence of groups on the personality. It will then be a psychological sociology and a cultural psychology. (Ramos, 2003, p. 36)

Social psychology and cultural psychology were tools for understanding the unconscious elements that circulate in culture and are the expression of primitive mentality. In this sense, although the notion of personality, based on the elaborations of Kimball Young (1935), has importance in Ramos' bibliography, his social psychology seems to be based on three different devices: social identity, social maladjustment and the primitive unconscious.

In the laws of imitation of Gabriel Tarde, Ramos found the concepts of suggestion, imitation and sympathy as fundamental factors for the formation of social identity. He first looked at suggestion and, in analysing the perspectives of Ellwood (1917), McDougall (1908) and Tarde (1903), he defined it as the intellectual or cognitive dimension of the process of mental interaction. He then turned away from these authors in favour of psychoanalytical theories and devoted himself to analysing the psychic dynamism involved in hypnotism. In his subsequent consideration of the relationship between suggestion and hypnosis, he reflected on the transference aspect involved in each of these phenomena and, at the same time, the relationship of power and domination that they could mean.

Tanzi's studies (1890) had previously inspired his thesis and other works. Ramos reaffirmed the idea that a wild, irrational dimension lurked in the psyche of all civilised individuals and, if at first he considered neuroses and psychoses as the major terms of social maladjustment, he later stated that 'we all bring with us the germ of delirium, says the eminent psychiatrist, because we inherited it from our great-grandfathers, and because it does not leave the normal function of primitive man' (Andrew Lang, 1896, *quoted in* Ramos, 2003, p. 172).

Ramos sought to investigate the functioning of the primitive mental structures that would prevail in what he called an adult, normal and civilised mentality. In addition to the *individual* soul, he considered that investigating the *ethnic* soul, a popular spirit that survives in modern societies, was necessary: the most civilised man does not completely free himself from these primitive-undifferentiated structures:

> A social psychology that does not investigate these relationships between the overt forms of culture and their unconscious contents will be a descriptive, superficial, *ad usum delphini* social psychology. It has to go beyond: it has to descend into the analysis of the pre-logical categories of a cultural cycle, by researching the folkloric unconscious. (Ramos, 2003, p. 316)

The problem of social maladjustment was directly related to the social changes and the fear of the shattering of the social fabric that had been experienced in the first decades of the twentieth century. Articulated with the notion of a folkloric, or primitive, unconscious, it had mobilised the policies of prevention of mental illness, which meant the extension of psychiatric domains and power. Therefore, while psychological discourses encountered some vulgarisation and resistance, they also provided psychiatry with the possibility of expansion. It was not a question of establishing the confrontation of the alienated with his truth in the isolation of hospitals and colonies: it was a question of understanding the whole of civilisation as potentially ill, and as a fertile field for the emergence of the primitive functioning latent in the psyche, which resulted in the multiplication of social risk.

In short, we find in Ramos a theoretical elaboration that articulated social psychology, in addition to medicine and pedagogy, with the social sciences, history and psychoanalysis, positioning its studies in a historical-cultural perspective that in turn reconciled clinical observations with the study of culture, groups and collective memory. Until the 1940s, his studies of black people were largely inspired by the works of Freud and Jung. Furthermore, psychoanalysis was central to his research on the behaviour of schoolchildren, which became part of his social psychology approach. Therefore, psychoanalysis and social psychology were deeply interwoven in Ramos' studies.

Ramos' approach to social psychology, according to Sodré (2015), makes us reflect on the current paths of Critical Social Psychology, which affirms its interdisciplinary character, recognises its political dimension, and distances itself from an experimental, cognitivist and individualistic psychology. It opens new possibilities for understanding the discontinuities produced in these paths and what their ethical and political impacts may be.

References

Araújo, T. B. (2016). *Raul Briquet e a modernização conservadora: crítica ao primeiro manual sobre psicologia social no Brasil* (Dissertação de Mestrado). Universidade de São Paulo, São Paulo.

Briquet, R. (1935). *Psicologia Social*. Livraria Francisco Alves.

Dardot, P., & Laval, C. (2016). *A nova razão do mundo; ensaio sobre a sociedade neoliberal*. Boitempo.

de Carvalho, J. M. (2015). *Os bestializados: o Rio de Janeiro e a República que não foi*. Companhia das Letras.

de Holanda, S. B. (2014). *Raízes do Brasil*. Companhia das Letras.

Ellwood, C. A. (1917). *An introduction to social psychology*. Appleton and company.

Ferreira, A. (2007). O múltiplo surgimento da Psicologia. In A. Jacó-Vilela, A. Ferreira, & F. Portugal (Eds.), *História da Psicologia - Rumos e percursos*. Nau Editora.

Foucault, M. (2005). *Em defesa da sociedade*. Martins Fontes.

Foucault, M. (2007). *As palavras e as coisas*. Martins Fontes.

Foucault, M. (2011). A psicologia de 1850 a 1950. In M. Foucault (Ed.), *Ditos e Escritos - Volume I: Problematização do sujeito: psicologia, psiquiatria e psicanálise. Forense Universitária.*

Foucault, M. (2013). Nietzsche, a Genealogia, a História. In M. B. Motta (Org.), *Arqueologia das ciências e história dos sistemas de pensamento – Ditos e Escritos II* (pp. 273–295). Forense Universitária.

Gutman, G., & Pereira, M. E. C. (2007). Primitivo e loucura, ou o inconsciente e a psicopatologia segundo Arthur Ramos. *Revista Latinoamericana de Psicopatologia Fundamental, X*(3), 517–525.

Maio, M. C. (2015). Caminhos de Arthur Ramos: a busca do Brasil como projeto civilizatório. In G. Hochman & N. T. Lima (Org.), *Médicos intrérpretes do Brasil*. Editora Hucitec.

McDougall, W. (1908). *An introduction to social psychology*. Methuen.

Melo, W. (2001). Nise Magalhães da Silveira. In R. H. F. Campos, *Dicionário biográfico da Psicologia no Brasil – Pioneiros*. Imago Editora.

Menezes, M. O. (2002). *A Psicanálise na Bahia (1926–1937): os estudos de Arthur Ramos sobre a loucura, educação infantil e cultura.* Universidade Federal da Bahia, Universidade Estadual de Feira de Santana - Mestrado em Ensino, Filosofia e História das Ciências.

Morkejs, E. (1993). *A Psicanálise no Brasil. As origens do pensamento psicanalítico*. Editora Vozes.

Oliveira, C. L. M. V. (2005). *História da Psicanálise – São Paulo 1929–1969.* Editora Escuta.

Patto, M. H. S. (1999) *A produção do fracasso escolar – Histórias de submissão e rebeldia*. Casa do Psicólogo.

Moreira, J., & Peixoto, A. (2005). As doenças mentais nos climas tropicais. *Revista Latinoamericana de Psicopatologia Fundamental, VIII*(4), 794–811.

Perestrello, M. (1992). Histoire de la psychanalyse au Brésil des origines à 1937. *Frénésie, 10,* 283–302.

Prado Filho, K. (2014). Para uma genealogia da Psicologia. In N. Guareschi, S. M. Hüning, & M. A. Azambuja, *Foucault e a Psicologia na Produção do conhecimento.* EdiPUCRS.

Ramos, A. (1926). *Primitivo e loucura.* Official do Estado.

Ramos, A. (1928). *A sordice nos alienados: ensaio de uma psycho-patologia da immundice*. Livraria e Typ. do Commercio.

Ramos, A. (1933). *Psiquiatria e Psicanálise*. Editora Guanabara.

Ramos, A. (1937). *Loucura e crime*. Globo.

Ramos, A. (1939). *A Criança Problema*. Livraria Editora da Cada do Estudante do Brasil, 1949. 2o edição.

Ramos, A. (1942). *A aculturação negra no Brasil*. Companhia Editora Nacional.
Ramos, A. (2001). *O negro brasileiro*. Graphia.
Ramos, A. (2003). *Introdução à Psicologia Social*. Casa do Psicólogo. Conselho Federal de Psicologia, Brasília.
Ramos, A. (2007). *O folclore negro no Brasil: demopsicologia e psicanálise*. Marftins Fontes.
Russo, J. (2002). *O mundo Psi no Brasil*. Jorge Zahar.
Russo, J. (2007). Psychoanalisis in Brazil – institutionalization and dissemination among the Lay Public. *Estudios Interdisciplinarios De América Latina Y El Caribe, 18*(1). http://cial.tau.ac.il/index.php/eial/article/view/431.
Schreiner, A. (2003). Preface to the fourth edition of Introdução à Psicologia Social. In A. Ramos, *Introdução à Psicologia Social*. Casa do Psicólogo. Conselho Federal de Psicologia, Brasília.
Schreiner, A. (2005). Uma aventura para o amanhã. Arthur Ramos e a neurohigiene infantil na década de 1930. In A. T. Venancio, L. F. D. Duarte, & J. Russo (Orgs.), *Psicologização no Brasil: atores e autores*. Contra Capa Livraria.
Schwarcz, L. M. (2017). *Retrato em branco e negro: jornais, escravos e cidadãos em São Paulo no final do século XIX*. Companhia das Letras.
Sodré, O. (2015). A dimensão histórica da psicologia social de Arthur Ramos. In L. O. C. Barros, *Arthur Ramos*. Fundação Miguel Cervantes.
Tamano, L. T. O. (2013). *Arthur Ramos e A mestiçagem no Brasil*. EdUFAL.
Tanzi, E. (1890). *Il Folk-lore nella patologia mentale*. Rivista di Filosofia.
Tarde, G. (1903). *The laws of imitation*. Henry Colt and Company.
Teixeira, A. (2009). Discurso de Anísio Teixeira por ocasião da instalação dos cursos da UDF (31/07/1935). In M. L. A. Fávero & A. C. Lopes, *A Universidade do Distrito Federal (1935–1939): um projeto além de seu tempo*. Liber Livros.
Vianna, F. O. (1921). *Pequenos estudos de Psicologia Social*. Revista do Brasil.
Young, K. (1935). *Social psychology*. F.S. Crofts & Company, Inc.

12

The "Fearless Bandeirante": Durval Marcondes, Psychoanalysis and Conservative Modernisation in Brazil

Belinda Mandelbaum and Stephen Frosh

Introduction

In a classroom of the Brazilian Society of Psychoanalysis of São Paulo (SBPSP), a small black-and-white portrait on the blank rest wall shows Durval Marcondes, the founder of the institution, posing in front, riding a horse. Born in 1899 in the city of São Paulo, Durval lived through in his youth the transformations of a traditional patriarchal society, based on the coffee economy, with its elites of landowners and only recently

B. Mandelbaum (✉)
Department of Social and Work Psychology, University of São Paulo, São Paulo, Brazil
e-mail: belmande@usp.br

S. Frosh
Department of Psychosocial Studies, Birkbeck, University of London, London, UK
e-mail: s.frosh@bbk.ac.uk

B. Mandelbaum et al. (eds.), *Brazilian Psychosocial Histories of Psychoanalysis*, Studies in the Psychosocial,
https://doi.org/10.1007/978-3-030-78509-3_12

abolished slavery, to a society in the process of industrialisation, urbanisation and modernisation. The trajectory of Durval Marcondes in the psychoanalytic field in São Paulo is an expression of these modernising processes, which in his case were made in the form of the struggle for the introduction of psychoanalysis as a psychotherapeutic method alternative to hegemonic psychiatric practices in the period. However, although recognising his pioneering role in the struggle for the establishment of the new science of psychoanalysis in the territory of São Paulo, we will try to show how this took place within a socially and culturally conservative framework, to which the psychoanalysis that arrived here could adapt and serve. We hope to show how it was within this conservative framework that Durval Marcondes carried out his entire clinical and academic career, including as a teacher at the University of São Paulo during the 1960s, in the period of the civil-military dictatorial government.

In a previous article, which dealt with the conservative bias present in Brazilian Psychoanalysis throughout its history (Frosh & Mandelbaum, 2017), we present evidence of how psychoanalysis, so often characterised by its transforming and liberating power, has been absorbed in Brazil since its beginnings, in clinical and institutional practices that operated in the service of maintaining the *status quo* in an elitist and deeply unequal society. In Durval Marcondes' case, the coexistence of these seemingly contradictory aspects—on the one hand, his pioneering in the implantation of the new science in the lands of São Paulo and, on the other, his conservatism in the cultural, social and political spheres—marked the psychoanalytic institution in São Paulo, with deep reverberations in the institutional functioning and in its clinical practices until today. It is important to remember that these conservative-originary—or even reactionary—practices, conniving with periods of rupture of the democratic rule of law, as various researchers have shown (Besserman Vianna, 1994; Frosh & Mandelbaum, 2017; Russo, 2012), are part of the history of the modes of functioning of most psychoanalytic societies in Brazil. More broadly, scholars of Brazilian social life in the first decades of the twentieth century (Fernandes, 1975; Werneck Vianna, 1996) have detected, in the adoption of new ideas and practices within the modernisation movements themselves, the preservation of traditional social and cultural structures. Such movements have been encompassed under the term of *conservative modernisation*, to name an arrangement between landowners and the emerging bourgeoisie that allowed the integration, in social and cultural terms, of new ideas and practices originating in "First World" countries—particularly Europe and the United States of America—without being accompanied by structural social transformations. This means that the old forms of production and distribution of wealth, the traditional forms of exploitation in the relations between capital and labour, and the hegemonic morality of a patriarchal society marked by inequalities of class, race, sex and gender, were preserved in coexistence with industrial and urban modernisation processes. New ideas and practices such as psychoanalysis have often served to give new clothes and justifications for old ways of living (Russo, 2012), while preserving them untouched.

The trajectory of Durval Marcondes, like that of others, mostly doctors, who introduced psychoanalysis in several Brazilian cities in the first half of the twentieth century, is expressive of this paradoxical, modernising and conservative pattern. This can be observed in the way they sought to reproduce on Brazilian soil a psychoanalytic institution that would follow in an integral and unquestioned way the dictates of the International Psychoanalytic Association,[1] as in private clinical practices directed to the rural and bourgeois elites of the main Brazilian cities, or even in its insertion in the field of public health, in which psychoanalysis was proposed as a tool to aid the social adjustment of poor children (Lima, 2012). It is in this sense that Durval Marcondes can serve as an *analyser*—the term is inspired by the work of Cecilia Coimbra (1995)—of the ways psychoanalysis has contributed and developed in Brazil, in its relations with the wider society. His articles and books (see, for example, *Medicina e Psicologia* [*Medicine and Psychology*], 1952) reveal the reproduction in his clinical work of Freudian theoretical and technical conceptions, with special emphasis in the field of Psychosomatic Medicine, where he makes use of studies of Freud on hysterics to deal with the psychogenic origin of the physical symptom, as well as

[1] The daily São Paulo newspaper *A Gazeta* published, on February 5, 1935: "What we do need—Dr. Durval declared—is a psychoanalytic institute like the ones existing abroad. I have here some leaflets where you can see what these establishments in Berlin, London, Vienna, Budapest, New York, Chicago and other big cities already have in excellent conditions."

drawing on the work of Franz Alexander (1943, quoted in Marcondes, 1952) on psychogenesis and conversion as fundamental concepts of psychosomatic research. Armed with these readings and his clinical experience as a psychoanalyst, Marcondes challenged the local medicine of his time which, as he discusses in his book, privileged an organicist perspective, thus denying psychological factors in the production of the disease. Marcondes also confronted the hegemonic psychiatry in São Paulo, which sought the causes of mental disorders in the physiology of organisms. He claimed for himself the introduction of psychology into medical training, always operating within the psychoanalytic theories and practices consecrated internationally by the psychoanalysis of his time, to which he adhered unconditionally. In his work for children, which was at the centre of the Brazilian developmentalist project during the dictatorial period of the *Estado Novo*[2]—as the focus of a civilising investment aimed at eliminating traits of social primitivism—Freudian psychoanalysis, as read and applied by Marcondes at the School Mental Hygiene Service, where he worked from the 1920s onwards, proved to be an effective theoretical and practical tool to achieve social adjustment.

Our concerns with these apparent contradictions present in the history of the Brazilian psychoanalytic field—on the one hand psychoanalysis in its transforming power and on the other hand its uncritical and adaptive use—are expressed in the words of Elisabeth Roudinesco, at a conference in São Paulo in the cycle Fronteiras do pensamento [Frontiers of thought], in 2017, when she stated that

> Psychoanalysis has never been able to establish itself in countries where there is no democracy and the rule of law. In other words, in order to have access to the unconscious, so that someone can have the freedom to explore his/her unconscious, you need a state of law and democracy. The rule of law, that is, a state in which subjective freedom is guaranteed. It is necessary to have political freedom in order to have access to the determinations of the unconscious.[3]

---

[2] Estado Novo was the Brazilian political regime established by Getulio Vargas on November 10, 1937, which was in force until January 31, 1946. It was characterised by the centralisation of power, nationalism, anti-communism and authoritarianism.

[3] https://www.fronteiras.com/videos/o-principal-fator-para-o-desenvolvimento-da-psicanalise.

If this is true, how was it possible for psychoanalysis to contribute and develop in Brazil throughout the twentieth century, with marks of its flowering during the two dictatorial periods—the Vargas era in the 1930s and the civil-military dictatorship of the years 1960–1980—marked by the curtailment of freedom of expression? Or perhaps, by making the question more precise: What psychoanalysis has developed here, with what characteristics, in such a way to accommodate and even serve as a tool for ongoing social policies? Let us go to the data that our documentary and bibliographical research has exposed,[4] which offer evidence of an only apparent contradiction between the introduction of psychoanalysis in São Paulo and its connivance with conservative—or even reactionary—social policies, as exemplified in the career of the psychiatrist and psychoanalyst Durval Marcondes.

A "Fearless Bandeirante" in Psychoanalysis

In a biography of Durval Marcondes that is part of the *Pioneers of Brazilian Psychology* collection, the author (Sagawa, 2002) says that "exploration by the bandeirantes[5] of unexplored lands was an inspiration of his childhood" (p. 13). And in his speech at the Brazilian Society of Psychoanalysis of São Paulo (SBPSP) on the occasion of his 80th birthday, Marcondes said that his mother, a primary school teacher, had explained to him in early childhood "that *bandeirante* was what one called fearless people, our patricians of old times who were not satisfied with the existing world within their immediate reach, and went into the jungle to discover and conquer spaces and riches in the unknown recess" (Marcondes, 1980, apud Sagawa, 2002).

The image of the *bandeirante* inaugurates his biography to serve as a model, or frame, for the activities that Durval Marcondes developed over

[4] The data presented here are results of the research project "Psychoanalysis and social context in Brazil: transnational flows, cultural impact and authoritarian rule," coordinated by Belinda Mandelbaum and Stephen Frosh, with the financial support of FAPESP [São Paulo Foundation for Research] (Processo 2015/11244-3).

[5] *Bandeirantes* are the Portuguese men who in the colonial Brazil participated in expeditions to explore and conquer the inlands.

six decades of academic and professional life. In this same biography, we read that in 1919 the young Durval, in his first year of college, came into contact with an article by Professor of Psychiatry Dr. Franco da Rocha[6] published in the newspaper *O Estado de São Paulo* under the title "Do delerio em geral" ("Of delirium in general"). In this article, extracted from Franco da Rocha's inaugural lecture in the Medical School that same year, "symptoms and also dreams [were approached] as psychological phenomena" (p. 15). Franco da Rocha in this lecture had spoken publicly about the ideas of psychoanalysis "as a therapeutic and scientific advance of our time" (p. 15). This publication aroused the curiosity of Durval Marcondes, even more so because it integrated knowledge from psychiatry, psychoanalysis and literature to show the sexual component present not only in pathology, but also "in all other people" (p. 16). It seems that the young student foresaw in it the path to follow soon after completing medical training, stimulated by the master himself Franco da Rocha to introduce this new therapy in the field of mental disorders. He opened his private practice in 1924 in the centre of São Paulo and studied psychoanalysis alone. Sagawa says that "Durval Marcondes's private practice was the first psychoanalytic clinic in Brazil and, perhaps, in Latin America" (p. 18). As a new clinical practice offered to the traditional elite and rising bourgeoisie, this would be part of his *bandeirante* trait, a pioneer of new lands in the field of treatment of mental disorders, at the same time when Freud himself developed and published his ideas. "Do they tell you dreams?" Franco da Rocha asked Marcondes, feeling that, although he was a curious enthusiast, it was too late to embark himself on this new professional activity—as he had already built his career, in the early decades of the twentieth century, as the first professor of psychiatry at the São Paulo Medical School, and founder and director of Juquery's Psychiatric Hospital, the main institution for the care of the mentally ill at that time.

sThe support of Dr. Franco da Rocha was fundamental to the young psychoanalyst who, over the following decades, had to face incessantly attitudes of "aggressive repulsion" and "cold omission" (p. 40) by his fellow psychiatrists. It is to his involvement with psychoanalysis

[6] For a detailed account on Franco da Rocha, the first doctor to present Freud in the São Paulo Faculty of Medicine, see Chapter 9 in this volume.

that Marcondes attributed having lost the chair of psychiatry, which until 1923 belonged to Franco da Rocha, in the contest in which, in 1936, he competed with Antônio Carlos Pacheco e Silva, an organicist psychiatrist and a fierce critic of psychoanalytic ideas (Assumpção, 2003; Tarelow & Mota, 2015).[7] This division between the psychoanalyst Durval Marcondes on the one hand and the organicist Antônio Pacheco e Silva on the other, would mark São Paulo psychiatry until the mid-1950s and 1960s, a period of enthusiasm and flourishing of psychoanalysis in several countries of the Western world—and in Brazil, in particular[8]—and of increasing interest on the part of psychiatrists in this new therapy, especially in the case of disorders diagnosed as neurotic.

Psychoanalytic Literary Criticism and the Poetry of Durval Marcondes

Durval also identified himself with Franco da Rocha as a reader of classics in philosophy and literature—in the inaugural lecture mentioned above, the professor cited Nietzsche, Schiller and Goethe, as well as other authors of the psychoanalytic field such as Stekel and Adler. In 1926, the young psychoanalyst wrote the thesis "Aesthetic Symbolism in Literature: Essay on an orientation to literary criticism, based on the knowledge provided by Psychoanalysis," published later in a book with a foreword by Franco da Rocha who, referring to the "prevailing morality, for centuries, dominating the civilised world," says that "Freud jumped the Rubicon; penetrated unabashedly into the forbidden region" (Franco da Rocha, 1926, quoted in Sagawa, 2002). Franco da Rocha also uses here the metaphorical image of the pioneers of new, unfamiliar and

[7] In the following year (1937), the dictatorial government of Getúlio Vargas, which became known as *Estado Novo*, would begin in Brazil. In line with the alliances that this government established with the Axis countries, especially Germany and Italy, Antônio Pacheco e Silva expressed support for the Nazi regime and its psychiatric practices. On the influence of Nazi psychiatry on Brazilian psychiatry in the 1930s, see J. F. Costa (1983).

[8] For an examination of the determinants of the flourishing of Psychoanalysis in Brazil, see J. Russo (2012).

forbidden regions, here Freud and Durval Marcondes himself,[9] since this was probably the first work of literary criticism in Brazil to make use of psychoanalysis as an instrument of interpretation. In it, the symbol is presented "as a kind of occult 'disguise' which allows it to communicate what would not otherwise be accepted by the 'resistance of censorship'" (Marcondes, 1926, quoted in Sagawa, 2002). In other words, inspired by Freud and his master Franco da Rocha, Marcondes expanded from the beginning the application of psychoanalysis beyond the field of treatment of mental disorders, towards the examination of myths and literary texts. He sent his book to Freud and received from him a response in which he recognised Marcondes' commitment to "arouse the interest of your compatriots to our young science" (Sagawa, 2002). An example of his interest in the psychoanalytical analysis of literary texts, with a focus on Brazilian literature, is his study on Aluísio Azevedo's book *Casa de Pensão* [*Pension House*], a work based on a real case, a crime that sensationalised Rio de Janeiro in 1876/1877, involving two students. Marcondes also wrote poems throughout his life though he was not notable for his poetic work. His poem "Symphonia em branco e preto" [Symphonia in black and white] was published in August 1922 in the magazine *Klaxon*, the main publication of the modernists of São Paulo. It is also worth mentioning his participation, with this very poem, in the Week of Modern Art of 1922, a milestone in the debate on the incorporation of foreign ideas, in particular from Europe, in the design of Brazilian cultural identity—in which psychoanalysis, especially Freud's social texts, such as *Civilisation and its Discontents*, *Totem and Taboo*, and *The Future of an Illusion*, have a central place. Although Modernism was mainly an aesthetic movement that did not have as its central objective to face the inequalities in Brazil, several literary and artistic works presented in the Week of Modern Art—from the literature of Mario and Oswald de Andrade to the painting of Tarsila do Amaral—make evident the deep penetration of psychoanalysis as an instrument to question the current patriarchal and sexual morality, in favour of rescuing a native

[9] It's noticeable that, in a period of rapid transformations that characterised the first decades of twentieth century Brazilian society, the designation of the pioneer movements takes its references from the colonial period, when the 'bandeirantes,' all of them Portuguese colonisers, came to explore the new land.

Brazilian Society of Psychoanalysis of São Paulo, created as a Psychoanalytic Group in 1944 and recognised by the International Psychoanalytic Association (IPA) in 1951.

In this specialisation in Clinical Psychology, Marcondes taught theoretical classes in psychoanalysis—mainly Freud's clinical texts—and the students underwent their training at the Mental Hygiene Service under the supervision of Judith Andreucci, Virginia Bicudo and Lygia Amaral. Teaching it at the university, Marcondes contributed to giving Brazilian psychoanalysis scientific and academic status.

Durval Marcondes' ex-students in the 1960s remember him as a teacher of authoritarian and conservative personality. This is what Ester Zita Botelho registers in her doctoral thesis *Os fios da História: reconstrução da história da Psicologia Clínica na Universidade de São Paulo* (*The threads of History: Reconstruction of the history of Clinical Psychology at the University of São Paulo*), presented in 1989 to the Institute of Psychology of USP. Botelho interviewed several alumni of the course of Clinical Psychology to reconstruct this history, and much of her report focuses on the year 1968, a landmark of the student movement that gained a unique specificity in the relationships between students and teachers of the course of Clinical Psychology. One of her interviewees says:

> I think at that time the staff at the Clinic did not accept any reform. They did not have a real academic involvement, they had no idea what was going on. I think they were against any possibility of change. The impression I had at the time was that the Clinic was a thing completely out of the university, separate ...

This alienation of the "Clinic staff" in relation to what happened in the university in years of dictatorial regime, persecution, arrest, torture and death of several students and teachers, seems to be confirmed in the report to Sagawa (2002) of a close disciple of Durval Marcondes, the psychoanalyst Ryad Simon, who also came to be invited by the master to be a professor of Clinical Psychology at the University of São Paulo. Simon says:

> For one of these always unexplained coincidences, on the day of the student occupation of the Faculty of Philosophy, on Maria Antonia Street, Durval was giving a theoretical class to psychology students. It was in the afternoon. The mutinous students invaded the classrooms, interrupted them, and expelled students and teachers. One group entered the room where Durval was teaching. The representative spoke to the master: "We have come to tell you that we are occupying the University." And Durval, unfazed: "I tell you that I am occupying this room." Faced with Durval's firmness, the invaders retreated and waited while he ministered his class to the end, though livid and indignant. Durval was the last teacher to leave the occupied building of the former Faculty of Philosophy. (Simon, 1982, quoted in Sagawa, 2002)

The episode reported occurred within a context that also became a landmark of students' resistance to the dictatorship. In July 1968, the students of the University of São Paulo occupied the Faculty of Philosophy building, staying there until October, when a toll on the street to raise funds for a students' congress eventually triggered a real campus war with students of the conservative Presbyterian University Mackenzie, which was across the street. In this confrontation, a student died. The episode reported by Marcondes' disciple makes clear his resistance to the occupation and his opposition to the students who at the time were spokesmen for the struggle for democracy.

As part of our research on psychoanalysis in Brazil during the dictatorial period, we also interviewed former students of Durval Marcondes at the University of São Paulo. We reproduce the following from what we heard from one of them, who in 1968 participated actively in the student movement:

> *The professors of clinic and psychoanalysis, they were considered of extreme right. At the beginning we did not occupy the clinic but then we faced many complaints about how psychoanalysis was taught at the university and I would say very unpleasant situations and very unpleasant information about those people.*
>
> [Would you say something about that?]

I can say, yes I can. At that time what the students were saying was that those teachers - Durval, Virginia and others - they were also practicing psychoanalysis privately, but the contract they used to have with the university was for full education, and the students... then these students brought official sheets of paper in which those teachers were filling those sheets as if there were some seminars and courses that actually were not taking place and all the signatures were falsified ones in order to justify the existence of the disciplines that in reality were not taught. So, it was a big problem.

[...]

They were Right Wing, so I would say that they were trying to provoke army intervention at the university. They became very nasty to us, some people who went to negotiate with Durval Marcondes, he asked them to leave his house in a very nasty way and then he did something that I feel very sad for, I don't like to talk about that although part of this is in the archives of the Society [of Psychoanalysis]. Durval wrote a letter to my father asking him to contain me and making some threats about bringing my name to the security people and to the army and so on, and my father answered Durval and this letter is in the archives of the Society... I think that when Durval Marcondes died it was part of his files[13]*. My father answered it saying I was independent, he would not, I was an adult, I was independent and he regretted that Durval was taking such a stance, taking this role, and he criticized very much Durval for doing so. It might be difficult for you to follow some aspects of what I am telling. Durval was very much connected to what we used to consider the Right Wing at that time.*

[...]

Then there was a moment when the Dean of the university- he was a very decent man, a very honest man, he was appointed by the dictatorship but, at that time, I would not say that he was a Leftist, he was a Liberal, he tried to reconciliate the students and the professors of the clinic, so Durval, Virginia and two others that I do not remember who, me and someone who was a director of the student union as well, so we went to the Dean... and then they presented all their complaints, horrible complaints about us and then we showed them the lists of the disciplines with the falsified data, it was very easy to see that it was falsified because they were identical, and then the Dean addressed them saying either you resign or I will have to dismiss you

13 We found the original letter in Durval Marcondes' archives in the Memory Center of the Brazilian Society of Psychoanalysis of São Paulo, in February 2019. The letter confirms the testimony.

> *and they decided to resign as a group. Of course what they tell people about this is something completely different from that, they were saying very nasty things happened, some of them became mad at me and the people associated with me, they were very nasty, especially this one who is from the Society as well, who used to teach clinical psychology, Ryad Simon, he said horrible things about me in writing, horrible, horrible things.*
>
> [Writing where?]
>
> *In some thesis, PhD thesis, because the occupation of the clinic and the history of clinical psychology at the university was the subject of many theses… he says that I was a son of a bitch and things of this sort about me.*
>
> [What you've said like confirms something that we've heard, rumours in the corridors of the Institute [of Psychology] saying that Durval Marcondes denounced some people to the security and to the army, do you know something about that?]
>
> *He was very, very close to army officers, but I think that he did not do that, this is a belief, it's not something that I know, not directly. I don't think he gave names to them, probably at the moment when he was angry about the Left and about people, he would give all the coordinates for them [to the army] to identify and locate the person, but I don't believe that he would, like others, give them names. You have the Livro Negro [Black Book] of the university,*[14] *Durval is not there as someone who denounced people. So, it's my personal belief, I don't think he denounced directly, that he gave names.*

Other episodes like this, reported by his former students, seem to confirm Marcondes' reactionary stance, explicitly averse to the students' struggle. Here we have a meeting organised between students and teachers of the Institute of Psychology to deal with curricular issues, but which was interrupted by the news that a student, Iara Iavelberg, a militant in the armed struggle, had been captured by the Army shortly before:

> There was an assembly at the time of the arrest of Iara Iavelberg, where, although our agenda was another, we proposed to make a petition of teachers and students requesting measures to the Dean. The reaction of

[14] *O Livro Negro da USP: o controle ideológico na universidade [The black book of USP: ideological control in the university]* was published by the Teachers' Association of USP in 1979, as a result of a research process regarding the impact of the civil-military dictatorship in the university since 1964.

Durval Marcondes, supported by Clinic staff, was to say that he had come to the assembly to discuss curriculum rather than politics.

The episode is registered in the minutes of the General Assembly of Psychology of 06/29/1968, which includes the record of Durval Marcondes' speech at the occasion[15]: "I did not come here to take part in political movement."

Iara was murdered, possibly inside the Information Operations' Detachment—Internal Defense Operation Center (DOI-CODI) in Salvador, Bahia, shortly thereafter.

Conclusion

We have argued in this paper that Durval Marcondes' position as a founder and huge influence on the development of psychoanalysis in Brazil makes him an important exemplar of the fate of Brazilian psychoanalysis. On the whole, his reputation in the Brazilian scene remains high, with his self-presentation as a "fearless bandeirante" being accepted and largely celebrated in the psychoanalytic movement. There are certainly some grounds for this: Marcondes was clearly an originator of the Brazilian psychoanalytic societies and worked industriously to help establish psychoanalysis as a serious force within Brazilian psychiatry as well as (more tangentially) in the cultural sphere. However, his attitudes and ideas were also characteristic of the orientation of Brazilian psychoanalysis as a social practice, in that they were conservative, normalising and authoritarian. As we have suggested, its modes of importing and incorporating psychoanalysis in the first decades of the twentieth century reproduce patterns that scholars in Brazilian culture have termed *conservative modernisation*, a broad process of rapid cultural change that has left untouched economic, social and political structures in the country. This can be seen in the developmental theory he used (focusing on childhood as a period of adaptation and socialising into cultural norms), his approach to families and specifically to women, and most graphically

[15] A copy of these minutes is included in the doctoral thesis referred to in the text.

his authoritarian modes of teaching and his attitude towards dissident students during the Brazilian dictatorship. Marcondes was of course not the only psychoanalyst who acted in this way or had these attitudes, but his influential position in the Brazilian psychoanalytic movement makes him important in the documentation of the conservative tendencies in that movement, especially in relation to the approach taken towards the dictatorship by the official Brazilian psychoanalytic societies. We need to be careful, it seems, not to assume that those who are "bandeirantes" in one way will necessarily be progressive or even democratic in others.

Acknowledgements The authors are grateful to Renata Conde for her collaboration in the first stages of this research.

References

ADUSP. (1979). *o Livro negro da USP: o controle ideológico na universidade*. USP.

Assumpção, F., Jr. (2003). A ideologia na obra de Antonio Carlos Pacheco e Silva. *Revista Latinoamericana de Psicopatologia Fundamental, 6*(4), 39–53.

Botelho, E. Z. F. (1989). *Os fios da história: reconstrução da história da psicologia clínica na Universidade de São Paulo*. Tese (Doutorado em Psicologia), Universidade de São Paulo, São Paulo.

Coimbra, C. (1995). *Guardiães da ordem. Uma viagem pelas práticas psi no Brasil do "Milagre"*. Oficina do Autor.

Costa, J. F. (1983). *Ordem médica e norma familiar*. Graal.

Fernandes, F. (1975). *A revolução burguesa no Brasil: ensaio de interpretação sociológica*. Zahar Editores.

Frosh, S., & Mandelbaum, B. (2017). 'Like kings in their kingdoms': Conservatism in Brazilian Psychoanalysis during the dictatorship. *Political Psychology, 38*(4), 591–604.

Lima, L. A. G. (2012). Ascensão e queda da infância: um estudo sobre a concepção de criança na psicanálise de Durval Marcondes e seus impactos na Psicologia brasileira. In M. H. S. Patto (Org.), *Formação de psicólogos e relações de poder: sobre a miséria da Psicologia*. Casa do Psicólogo.

Marcondes, D. (1952). *A Medicina e a Psicologia*. Livraria Martins Fontes.

Oliveira, C. L. V. (2005). *História da psicanálise – São Paulo (1920–1969).* Escuta.

Oliveira, C. L. V. (2014). Trajetórias da psicanálise paulista. *Analytica: revista de Psicanálise, 3*(4), 59–97.

Roudinesco, E. (2017). O principal fator para o desenvolvimento da Psicanálise. *Fronteiras do pensamento.* https://www.fronteiras.com/videos/o-principal-fator-para-o-desenvolvimento-da-psicanalise.

Russo, J. (2012). Brazilian psychiatrists and psychoanalysis at the beginning of 20th century: A question for national identity. *Psychoanalysis and History, 14,* 297–312.

Sagawa, R. Y. (2002). *Durval Marcondes.* Coleção Pioneiros da Psicologia Brasileira (Vol. 11). Imago, Conselho Federal de Psicologia.

Tarelow, G. Q., & Mota, A. (2015). Eugenia, organicismo e esquizofrenia: diagnósticos psiquiátricos sob a lente de Antônio Carlos Pacheco e Silva, nas décadas de 1920–40. *Dimensões: Revista de História da UFES* (34).

Vianna, H. B. (1994). *Não conte a ninguém: contribuição à história das sociedades psicanalíticas do Rio de Janeiro.* Imago.

Werneck Vianna, L. (1996). Caminhos e descaminhos da revolução passivam à brasileira. *Dados, 39*(3), 377–392.

13

A Psychoanalyst Between Fame and Oblivion: Karl Weissmann and the Spread of Psychoanalysis in Brazil

Rodrigo Afonso Nogueira Santos

In this chapter, I will present elements of the life and work of Karl Weissmann. He was a man of many faces—a psychoanalyst, disseminator of psychoanalysis, author of several books, bearer of one of Freud's last letters, a magician of hypnotism and a biographer of German philosophers. Despite having occupied important positions during his career as a renowned psychoanalyst and intellectual, he remains unknown among some Brazilian psychoanalysts. I shall be investigating how he has remained in the margins of historiographical investigations, yet is consistently present as an author in the Brazilian history of psychoanalysis. My goal is to shed light on the erasure of certain characters[1] within the official history of psychoanalysis[2] in Brazil.

[1] This issue was raised by Lima (2019).

[2] According to Oliveira (2006), this is the history narrated by the training institutions, especially those linked to the International Psychoanalytical Association (IPA).

R. A. N. Santos (✉)
Universidade de São Paulo, São Paulo, Brazil

B. Mandelbaum et al. (eds.), *Brazilian Psychosocial Histories of Psychoanalysis*, Studies in the Psychosocial,
https://doi.org/10.1007/978-3-030-78509-3_13

The perspective of microhistory serves as an inspiration for this analysis, by recognising the importance of looking at the dimension of the singular. In this sense, I believe that the research on a sole psychoanalyst may throw light on broader debates about the history of psychoanalysis in the country.

Regarding the foundations of microhistory, Revel (2010) states that focusing on the individual does not contradict the social understanding of an issue and that it is possible to think about small units—whether that of a person or a group of people—in the context of multiple spaces and social timing, therefore adding social signification to them.

Taking this perspective into account, I present the biographical elements of Karl Weissmann, an immigrant who developed survival strategies in Brazil. Weissmann experienced several difficulties during his time in Brazil, from financial problems to issues with the police. I inscribe him in a specific tradition within the field of the history of psychoanalysis in Brazil, focusing on his publication of texts in newspapers and magazines to disseminate its ideas.

This chapter has two main aims. The first is to present Karl Weissmann, giving this relatively unknown psychoanalyst a face, with emphasis on his work of spreading psychoanalysis to the lay public. The second one is to contribute to the debate about the erasure of certain psychoanalysts from the official history of psychoanalysis. This introduces new elements to the debate about who should be recognised as a psychoanalyst and who should not.

Karl Weissmann's Early Days and His Work with Psychoanalysis: From Vigorous Psychoanalyst to Magician of Hypnotism

Karl Weissmann was born on 31st August 1910 into a Jewish family in Vienna, Austria. His parents were Karl and Hedwig Weissmann. They moved to Brazil in 1921, with Karl and his three brothers.[3] The family had migrated due to the political tensions in Europe. The growing anti-Semitism was taking shape in diverse parts of the continent (Salzstein, 2001).

When they arrived in Brazil, the Weissmann family started working on cotton farms. Due to the challenging economic conditions, the young Karl and Franz supplemented their income by teaching language classes to foreigners. After the family moved to Rio de Janeiro in 1929, Karl took an interest in psychoanalysis and hypnosis.

In the Brazilian capital, Karl Weissmann learned about the work of the physician Gastão Pereira da Silva (1898–1987), who had dedicated himself to studying psychoanalysis. Pereira da Silva considered himself to be a disciple of Medeiros e Albuquerque[4] (1867–1934) and wanted to present psychoanalysis to the general public.

According to a text written by da Silva in the early 1930s, psychoanalysis should not be an exclusively medical practice[5] (Pereira da Silva, 1932). He asserted that its 'formidable revelations of the *unconscious*' (Pereira da Silva, 1932, p. 72—original emphasis) had become a 'universal philosophy. Freud presents the *spirit*, the *psyche* of man, in an *objective* way' (Pereira da Silva, 1932, p. 73—original emphasis).

Karl Weissmann moved to Belo Horizonte the capital of Minas Gerais, in 1931. Upon arriving there, he began mixing with young intellectuals with diverse interests, like architecture, poetry and journalism. According to the architect Sylvio de Vasconcellos[6] (1916–1979), the group had some core members:

---

3 Karl's brothers were Fritz, Franz, and Stephan Weissmann. Fritz became an important industrialist in Brazil; Franz dedicated himself to sculpting and came to be one of the most prominent artists in the country. Stephan's path is unknown.

4 Medeiros e Albuquerque was an important Brazilian intellectual. He got close to psychoanalysis due to his practice of hypnosis and taught elements of the Freudian doctrine in Rio de Janeiro in the 1910s.

5 Something that Freud himself believed in.

6 Sylvio de Vasconcellos was a prominent architect from Minas Gerais. He became a Professor at the School of Architecture at the Federal University of Minas Gerais. After charges of involvement with communists, he was compulsorily retired during the Brazilian civil-military dictatorship in 1969.

> The fixed members of the group were René de Guimarães, Fritz's cousin, convinced of his resemblance to John Barrymore regarding the profile of his face and poet in his spare time; José Bartolota, of Italian beauty, who only left home after sunset and was also keen on poetry; Juracy, making a living from magazine and newspaper advertising limited to advertisers; Diogo Costa, a journalist with political ideas and Karl Weissmann, whom Henrique had successfully advised to become an English teacher to take advantage of his foreign name. (Vasconcellos as cited in Brasileiro, 2008, p. 257)

Weissmann published the book *Our English Teacher: 50 Lições de Inglez*, in 1934. The dissemination of pedagogical material earned him praise from Minas Gerais intellectuals. Lucio José dos Santos,[7] the former Dean of the University of Minas Gerais, wrote to him on 2nd December 1934: 'I therefore consider your work highly recommendable and am certain that it will have the deserved success. Felicitating you on this, I remain at your service' (Weissmann, 1936, p. 7). The publication of the book made Weissmann a recognised language teacher, and enabled him to teach English and German in important schools in the state.

A year after the publication of his book, Weissmann was investigated by the political police of Minas Gerais. The bulletin of the Security Corps of the Investigations Service of the State of Minas Gerais contains information about his origin, his address in Belo Horizonte and the observation that he was a communist: 'I have to inform you that the following communists currently reside in this capital: Karl Weissmann, professor of English and German, with a room at Ed. Brasil, 814' (Siemg, 1935).[8]

During the Vargas Era[9] in Brazil, foreigners were not favourably regarded. The government believed that immigration should not be

[7] Lucio José dos Santos was an enthusiast of the Integralist movement—an ultranationalist movement inspired by Italian fascism, which operated between 1933 and 1937—as well as president of the Dom Vital Center of Minas Gerais, an important Catholic institution in the country at the time.

[8] Original citation in Portuguese: '*Tenho a comunicar-lhe que residem actualmente nesta capital os comunistas abaixo: Karl Weissmann, professor de inglês e alemão, com sala no Ed. Brasil, 814*' (Siemg, 1935).

[9] President Getúlio Vargas ruled Brazil from 1930 to 1945.

compromised by 'the idea of social corrosion and with the *exotic doctrines*, traits pertinent to the stereotyped image of the *Jews*, evaluated as unassimilable, *communist*, parasitic' (Carneiro, 2018—emphasis added). Catholicism in Belo Horizonte represented the primary opposition to psychoanalysis at the time, considering it to be an 'exotic' doctrine (Santos, 2016). As a Jewish immigrant,[10] a friend of poets and intellectuals[11] and someone who talked openly about psychoanalysis, Weissmann was indeed suspect in the eyes of police during the 1930s.

After Belo Horizonte, Weissmann risked his first venture in psychoanalysis in 1937, when publishing the book *O dinheiro na vida erotica.*[12] He stated that psychoanalysis 'means, above all, the exploration of the unconscious' (Weissmann, 1937, p. 39). Its usefulness would be to shed light on 'human misery,' constituting 'a means of social sanitation' (Weissmann, 1937, p. 45).

The preface to this work, by Gastão Pereira da Silva, defines the author as a *vigorous psychoanalyst.*[13] The book reviewed financial themes in relation to morality in the Vargas Era (Santos & Mandelbaum, 2019) and attempted to explain psychoanalysis to the general public. According to Weissmann, psychoanalysis 'must be disseminated so that it can fulfil its high societal purpose in the present era' (1937, p. 40). Weissmann believed that psychoanalysis would lose its utility and value if it remained limited to being a prerogative of leading scientists or a luxury for superficial amateurs (Weissmann, 1937).

Weissmann forwarded a copy of his book to Freud, who replied with a kind letter in 1938; this was one of the last missives written by the creator of psychoanalysis. In it, Freud praised him for the publication and indicated that Weissmann should pursue his studies, but stated he could not read in Portuguese. The recipient received the letter with joy (Weissmann, 1984) and several newspapers reported the

---

[10] Psychoanalysis was presented as a 'Jewish science in countries dominated by Nazism' (Frosh, 2005).

[11] At the time, other members of the group were also submitted to an investigation (Brasilerio, 2008).

[12] The title can be translated to English as '*Money in erotic life.*'

[13] Pereira da Silva did not consider psychoanalysis to be an exclusively medical practice. This paved the way for Weissmann to work with the theme, even though he was a language teacher.

correspondence. According to Leão Cabernite, another psychoanalyst, Weissmann 'triumphantly displayed it to everyone' (Cabernite cited in Salim, 2010, p. 257). Weissmann referred to the letter in several of his works, including those published in the 1980s.

Weissmann continued to publish, which earned him recognition as an intellectual in Brazil. One of his notable works published in 1945 is a series about thinkers and writers from Germanic countries, like the book *Vida e pensamento de Schopenhauer*,[14] the papers '*Goethe e o gênio paterno*'[15] (1949) and '*Nietzsche e o Radicalismo Psicológico*'[16] (1952). However, his works related to psychoanalysis are the ones that stand out—he published several texts in newspapers from Minas Gerais and Rio de Janeiro. In the text '*Freud e a Civilização*[17] 'which appeared in the newspaper *Folha de Minas*, he presents psychoanalysis as a truly civilising tool. In the author's words, the aims of psychoanalysis are:

> To harmonize psychic life with the social environment; direct energies for useful purposes; free us from the dark fears that enslave us; establish the power we need most after the domination of the outside world: *the power over ourselves*. In its ends, psychoanalysis is strictly within the program of civilization. (Weissmann, 1944, p. 4—emphasis added)

Between the 1940s and 1950s, three different positions illustrate Weissmann's importance as a disseminator of psychoanalysis in Brazil. The illustrated magazine *Cruzeiro*, was one of the major Brazilian publications from the last century and beginning in 1948, he produced a series of texts inspired by psychoanalysis in which he debated family problems. In '*Édipo no drama conjugal*'[18] for example, he asserted that 'a whole series of conjugal blunders that are combated psychoanalytically has its origin in the affective bonds between mother and son, father and daughter, which, unfortunately for many couples, are excessively prolonged' (Weissmann, 1949, p. 86).

---

[14] 'Schopenhauer's life and thought.'

[15] 'Goethe and the paternal temper.'

[16] 'Nietzsche and Psychological Radicalism.'

[17] 'Freud and the Civilisation.'

[18] 'Oedipus in marital drama.'

Weissmann was hired as a psychoanalyst for a penitentiary in the metropolitan area of Belo Horizonte, where he worked from 1953 to 1959. This was remarkable because Weissmann was not a physician and he had received no formal university education whatsoever (the main approaches of psychoanalysis to criminology had taken place in the field of Legal Medicine). Apparently, his hiring is connected to a series of works published by him on psychoanalysis and criminology. The text '*A base anal da criminalidade*'[19] refers to possible psychoanalytic origins of criminality. In it, Weissmann affirms:

> The father of psychoanalysis, contrary to Lombroso's theories about congenital delinquency, established the principle according to which all men, without exception, undergo an anal phase, that is, a delinquent phase, in the course of their development and that they typically remain in it for a worthy part of their lives. The criminals would be solely the individuals who prolong this pre-genital (anal) stage or regress to it due to some difficulty encountered in the further evolution to genitality. (Weissmann, 1952, p. 28)

The third position was that of a star in Brazilian popular culture during the 1950s, presenting hypnosis shows in major theatres in the country. Popular newspapers covered such shows effusively. This earned Weissmann the nicknames of *Magician of Hypnotism* and the *Greatest Hypnotist in the Hemisphere*—cited in his book, *O hipnotismo*[20] (1958), which remains an important reference work in hypnosis until today. In this work, Weissmann highlighted the psychoanalytic foundation of hypnosis: 'The triumphant return of hypnotism on modern psychological grounds is largely due to psychoanalysis. As for their modern techniques, they are a direct consequence of psychoanalytic guidance and penetration' (Weissmann, 1958, p. 26).

Weissmann moved to Rio de Janeiro in 1959, but he did not perform as frequently as before. He had to interrupt his shows in 1961, due to a

[19] 'The anal basis of criminality.'

[20] 'Hypnotism.'

ban imposed by the president Jânio Quadros.[21] The interruption, along with the distance from the stage, marked a new moment in his life. He then turned to publishing and more stable psychoanalytic work in private practice.

Maturity: From the Ghost of Communism to Medical Publications

The publication of the book *A conquista da maturidade*[22] (1961) marked the beginning of this new phase. In it, Weissmann presented his conception of a *mature* subject using his interpretation of psychoanalysis. He defined 'happiness and maturity as a problem of libido and unconscious psyche' (Weissmann, 1961, p. 5). He introduced the concept of maturity into what he calls *psychoanalytic characterology* and defined it as '*fullness without adventurism*' (Weissmann, 1961, p. 6). One might take advantage of 'the prospect of fertile boredom and a profitable monotony' (Weissmann, 1961, p. 6).

Weissmann believed that people become more socially acceptable with psychological maturity and 'at the same time more resistant to the growing demands of civilised life. The path to maturation is undeniably the path to happiness' (Weissmann, 1961, p. 7). In contrast, the path to regression and adult unhappiness would be those of neuroses and psychoses. He then concluded that: 'psychological maturity is not only a matter of fullness and efficiency in life, but also of mental hygiene' (Weissmann, 1961, p. 7). Weissmann highlighted the opposition between the developmental path to maturity and neuroses and psychoses. Maturity is reached after going through the 'three-phase sequence of psychoanalytic characterology that presides over the emotional maturation processes of our personality' (Weissmann, 1961: 109). Weissman then turned his attention to characteristics and elements

---

[21] The Decree number 51.009, from July 22, 1961, forbade 'isolated shows or numbers of hypnotism, and lethargy, of any kind or form, in clubs, auditoriums, stages or radio and television studios' (Brasil, 1961).

[22] 'The conquest of maturity.'

of a mature subject, in topics as diverse as *religion, love of animals* and *sports*.

In 1963 Weissmann published the paper 'Nietzsche and the Anti-Maturism' in the prominent magazine *American Imago*. In it, he debated Nietzsche's work in the light of psychological maturity.

After the publication of the best-seller *A conquista da maturidade* in 1961, Weissmann wrote *Masoquismo e Comunismo: Contribuição a uma patologia do pensamento politico* (1964).[23] In this book, Weissmann articulated his position in the political debate in Brazil[24]: according to him, there was a fundamental rupture between psychoanalysis and communism, leading to an impossibility of integration of the fields, despite all the efforts to achieve it. Weissmann (1964) stated that Freud's anti-masochistic nature would be anti-communist, a characteristic evident in his life and work.

> The experience of the last half-century has unmistakably demonstrated that Freud and Marx mutually exclude each other. The former represents *liberation*, the latter, *liberticide*. *The aim of Marxism* (albeit pretending to be temporary) *is power over others, whereas the goal of psychoanalysis is power over yourself*. (Weissmann, 1964, pp. 20–21)

Weissmann's hypothesis was that leftist movements in politics are linked to pathology: he expressed the goals of his book in its introductory pages, stating that concessions like social relationships and even friendships with communists are acceptable for civil citizens, but therapists and educators have 'the indeclinable duty to fight them, that is, to cure them' (Weissmann, 1964, p. 9).

It is intriguing to observe that, albeit employing a pointed tone in this specific book, Weissmann had never expressed intense anti-communism in his previous works. He also did not return to this theme in the following years, on the contrary, this book appeared isolated in the whole of Weissmann's work—there was only one mention that communism

---

23 'Masochism and Communism: Contribution to a pathology of political thought.'

24 The country was experiencing political tensions involving the spectre of the communist threat in Latin American countries. These tensions culminated in the 1964 civil-military coup, which led Brazil to a 21-year dictatorship.

and fascism represent characteristics of immature subjects in *A conquista da maturidade* (1961). His activity was aimed more at spreading psychoanalysis than at fighting political enemies. What then led Weissmann to produce such a forceful text, precisely in 1964, if this theme was not present throughout his life and work?

The answer might be the police investigation of 1935, mentioned above. Having been targetted for talking about psychoanalysis at a time of political tension involving communism, it is possible that the book was meant to announce his position within the debate, functioning more like a defence strategy than a treatise on psychopathology or an anti-communist manifesto. In fact, Weissmann was mainly interested in other debates and this issue did not gain prominence in his later works, when the anti-communist struggle intensified in Brazil after 1968.[25]

In 1967, Weissmann published *Psicanálise: Ensaios e experiências*[26]: which contained a collection of texts on various subjects, like '*Racionalização e fantasia*,'[27] '*Crime e sexualidade*,'[28] or 'Profissão e pré-genitalidade'[29] (Weissmann, 1967). He also returned to *Cruzeiro* magazine, this time with several psychological tests, inspired by psychoanalysis. These consisted of questions that, according to him, aimed to measure the level of maturity of the magazine's readers.

In the 1970s, another unexpected feat was the publication of a book entitled *Psychoanalysis* in the collection of a publisher specialising in medicine books called *Cultura Médica*,[30] even though Weissmann was not a physician. This collection contained works on anatomy, cardiology, pediatrics and psychiatry. In the Foreword for Weissmann's book, Ismar da Silveira[31] introduced him as an 'internationally renowned psychoanalyst with deep knowledge of his field' (In: Weissmann, 1976, p. 1) and

[25] This was the year of publication of the Institutional Act 5 (AI-5). It marked the beginning of the harshest years of the Brazilian dictatorship, with the increase in persecutions, exiles, tortures, and murders of opponents of the regime.

[26] 'Psychoanalysis: Essays and experiences.'

[27] 'Rationalisation and fantasy.'

[28] 'Crime and sexuality.'

[29] 'Profession and pre-genitality.'

[30] 'Medical Culture.'

[31] At the time, Silveira was the Vice-Director of the Faculty of Medical Sciences at the State University of Rio de Janeiro (UERJ).

reaffirmed the honour of having him among the invited authors. At a time when groups linked to the International Psychoanalytical Association (IPA) in Brazil were working to maintain the hegemony of psychoanalytic practice (Coimbra, 1995) this was a remarkable invitation, since Weissmann did not have an institutional background.

Between 1967 and 1975 Weissmann published numerous papers in the *Revista Brasileira de Medicina*,[32] in a section that alternated its titles between '*Temas em Psiquiatria*'[33] and '*Temas em Psicanálise*.'[34] His reading of psychoanalysis inspired all of his texts,[35] as in '*A sequência trifásica da caracteriologia psicanalítica*.'[36]

In 1985, his book *A conquista da maturidade* was translated into English under the title *Vistas into Maturity*, and published by Vantage Press. He also wrote an obituary for Anna Freud, which was published in the most prestigious newspaper in Rio de Janeiro, *Jornal do Brasil*. In the text, he commented on his exchange of correspondence with Freud's daughter. Karl Weissmann passed away in 1989, at the age of 78.

A Psychoanalyst, but Not so Much: On Censorship and Erasure in the History of Psychoanalysis

This brief overview of Karl Weissmann's life and work raises the question: how did a psychoanalyst who circulated through so many spaces simply disappear from the official history of psychoanalysis in Brazil?

The outline for this answer begins with a significant text by Marialzira Perestrello from 1988, entitled '*Primeiros encontros com a Psicanálise: Os precursores no Brasil (1899–1937)*.'[37] Perestrello was one of the founders

---

[32] 'Brazilian Magazine of Medicine.'

[33] 'Themes in Psychiatry.'

[34] 'Themes in Psychoanalysis.'

[35] Some of them were taken from the book *Psicanálise:Ensaios e experiências* (1967).

[36] 'The three-phase sequence of psychoanalytic characterology.'

[37] 'First encounters with Psychoanalysis: The precursors in Brazil (1899–1937).'

of the Brazilian Society of Psychoanalysis in Rio de Janeiro[38] (SBPRJ). In this text, she affirmed:

> The conference will not be dedicated to the three foreign doctors who came to train analysts in our country, nor to the Brazilian psychoanalysts, *pioneers*, in São Paulo, Rio or Porto Alegre. Nor to the *founders* of the four psychoanalytic societies – recognized by the IPA. Nor to contemporary analysts who have worked hard to *develop* our specialty. It will be about the *precursors*. Those who came *before* us, who met with psychoanalysis many years ago. (Perestrello, 1988, p. 151)

Perestrello distinguished three categories of psychoanalysts within the history of psychoanalysis: the pioneers, the founders and the precursors. She dedicated her paper to those who were self-taught, 'who *really* deepened themselves into psychoanalytic theories, who disseminated them, who tried—as they could—to employ analytical technique in times when there were no trained psychoanalysts nor trainers in Brazil' (Perestrello, 1988, p. 151).

Based on this distinction, the author characterised as precursors those who investigated and practiced psychoanalytic technique before the institutionalisation of the IPA in Brazil and she presented names like Juliano Moreira, Genserico Pinto, Franco da Rocha, Medeiros e Albuquerque, Durval Marcondes,[39] Julio Pires Porto-Carrero, Maurício de Medeiros, Arthur Ramos and Neves Manta.[40]

Perestrello (1988) also mentioned intellectuals from the modernist movement who read Freud and published texts about psychoanalysis in magazines like *Klaxon* (São Paulo), *Revista* (Minas Gerais) and *Verde* (Minas Gerais). She also tried to justify some flaws and criticism previously directed to those without formal training:

[38] This institution attained recognition from IPA in 1959.

[39] She refers to Marcondes as the only precursor-pioneer, for having devoted himself to analytical training with Adelheid Koch.

[40] Except for Medeiros e Albuquerque, all those *precursors* were members of important scientific groups, such as the National Academy of Medicine or the Brazilian League of Mental Hygiene.

> When here in this Society I referred to those who, without training, called themselves psychoanalysts, there was a certain criticism on my part of the precursors. I rephrase what I said earlier. If *censorship* exists, I address those who, in Rio, from the 1940s onwards, were not interested in applying for personal analysis and *formal training*. (Perestrello, 1988, p. 151—emphasis added)

Perestrello's mention of *censorship* apparently did not happen by chance: as a term that circulates through such diverse fields—like journalism, politics and policing—it points to an operation of erasure of certain marks or imprints. Within a text, censorship means deletion, and it 'reveals itself through "blank spaces" or alterations of passages considered unacceptable' (Laplanche & Pontalis, 2001, p. 61).

Who would Perestrello be referring to in that last quote? In fact, there were two noisy absences in her text—those of Gastão Pereira da Silva and Karl Weissmann: they did not appear in the paper as precursors, nor as pioneers. Were they censored in this history?

Pereira da Silva was a doctor and psychoanalyst from Rio de Janeiro, and Karl Weissmann's mentor. Some elements in his trajectory deserve further investigation, as his initial experiences with psychoanalysis happened through the writing of a psychoanalytic-inspired novel. Medeiros e Albuquerque considered the book of good quality, and it became a starting point for the doctor's formation. From then on, his training occurred in an unconventional way.

Pereira da Silva followed Freudian tips he found in *The Interpretation of Dreams* to embark on a process he considered self-analysis, analysing his own dreams. According to him, this self-analysis was a recommendation by Freud:

> Freud said the psychoanalyst needed the analysis of his own unconscious to be a good analyst and advised *self-analysis*, or to allow himself to be analysed, whenever possible, by a colleague. But life had already taught me to analyse myself. I had practiced *self-analysis* intuitively many, many times! I just lacked a method, a technique, and this I learned, later, from Freud himself! (Pereira da Silva, 1978, p. 195)

Parallel to his self-analysis, Pereira da Silva wrote his first books on psychoanalysis, sending one of them to Freud himself: *Para compreender Freud*[41] (1931). The answering letter came in 1934, whereby Freud thanked him for the material and encouraged Pereira da Silva to spread psychoanalysis in Brazil.

Believing there was a direct connection between him and Freud via correspondence, Pereira da Silva dispensed with institutional training. He also rejected didactic analysis because his accreditation as a psychoanalyst came from the letter, which led him to be '*sure* that he *was right*' (Pereira da Silva, 1978, p. 195). From that moment on, feeling encouraged by Freud, Pereira da Silva dedicated himself even more to the dissemination of psychoanalysis in Brazil. He wrote other psychoanalytically inspired novels, in addition to maintaining columns in widely circulated newspapers and radio programs where he discussed Freudian theories. In his book *25 anos de Psicanálise*,[42] he presented himself as 'Gastão Pereira da Silva–Accredited by Sigmund Freud' (Pereira da Silva, 1978, p. 1).[43]

Pereira da Silva marked Weissmann's path in at least four decisive ways: (1) he opened up the possibility of studying and practicing psychoanalysis without requiring medical training; (2) he dispensed with any institutional affiliations, prioritising self-education and self-validation; (3) he paved the way for talking about psychoanalysis to the general public through unconventional means; and (4) he traced a peculiar path of accreditation, for his connection to Freud was due to the receipt of a letter of encouragement, written by the creator of psychoanalysis.

Thus, Pereira da Silva and Weissmann were psychoanalysts who remained outside the scientific institutions where Freudian knowledge circulated. They both maintained this position long after the institutions linked to the IPA were established in Brazil, remaining distant from these institutional spaces throughout their life and work. Therefore, the censorship of their names in the history of psychoanalysis probably happened because they refused to dedicate themselves to the formal training required by the institutions. For these reasons, they did not fit

[41] 'To understand Freud.'

[42] '25 years of Psychoanalysis.'

[43] Original citation in Portuguese: '*Gastão Pereira da Silva—Credenciado por Sigmund Freud*' (Pereira da Silva, 1978, p. 1).

among the precursors, pioneers or founders—for them, there would be no place in the official list.

Another form of censorship in the psychoanalytic environment was the questioning of Weissmann's texts and techniques. In a letter commenting on the situation of psychoanalysis in Minas Gerais in the 1950s, Leão Cabernite wrote: 'I returned to Belo Horizonte, I continued to practice psychoanalysis. On this occasion, Dr. Paulo Dias Correia, Weissmann's brother-in-law, also practiced it. This happened until 1954. [...] At the time, Weissmann was already a "psychoanalyst" at the Neves Penitentiary' (Cabernite cited in Salim, 2010, p. 258). Leão Cabernite and Paulo Dias Correia, both physicians, at the time were training at an institution recognised by the IPA. Therefore, they were practicing 'official' psychoanalysis, while Weissmann was a 'psychoanalyst' in quotes or a psychoanalyst... but not so much.

In fact, Cabernite questioned Karl Weissmann's written work as well: he referred to the book *O dinheiro na vida erótica* (1937) as 'a heap of the author's fantasies, added to Freud's theoretical statements' (Cabernite cited in Salim, 2010, p. 258).

It is important to take into account that the arrival of psychoanalysis in Brazil happened in three diverse fields: 'among modernist avant-garde intellectuals, among representatives of the medical-psychiatric establishment and among the lay public' (Russo, 2002, p. 51). In her text, Perestello (1988) presented only the two former fields, both being groups of intellectuals regarded as precursors of Freudian ideas in Brazil. The latter one—the lay public—is the least investigated (Russo, 2002). This is not surprising, as I have shown throughout this paper, as it reaffirms how there was a real erasure of these psychoanalysts from the official history of psychoanalysis in Brazil.

Lima (2019) states that the history told from official institutions defines relationships between those who are on and off the field, or who can participate in a community of peers. The history additionally holds a timestamp with its particular criteria: 'at bottom, it is a position of organisation of otherness: there is a before and after which, in the now, unfolds in a heterogeneity finally thinkable in the key of "we" and "they"' (Lima, 2019, p. 48). Therefore, the division between precursors and pioneers, psychoanalysts and 'psychoanalysts,' operate a real exclusion of those who are unallocated in these categories.

Intense debates about the *true* psychoanalysis marked Brazil during the dictatorship. Institutions linked to the IPA proclaimed their legitimacy (Coimbra, 1995). Starting in 1967, publications on the history of psychoanalysis in Brazil gained momentum (Oliveira, 2006), precisely written by psychoanalysts associated with these institutions—like Luiz de Almeida Prado Galvão, Darcy de Mendonça Uchôa and Marialzira Perestrello herself. The characterisation of legitimate psychoanalysts as those with institutional training, was presented to the country. Opposed to them remain the censored 'psychoanalysts.' Those, like Karl Weissmann and his teacher, Gastão Pereira da Silva, apparently had no place in the history of psychoanalysis.

Final Considerations

As this research shows, Karl Weissmann is a relevant name in the history of psychoanalysis in Brazil. As an immigrant who went through financial difficulties and trouble with the police in his youth, he then made psychoanalysis a survival tool. He achieved some fame and even stardom due to his hypnotism shows. Indeed, such difficulties seem to have defined Weissmann's place on the fringe of the official IPA institutions. According to Weissman in an interview with the psychoanalyst Marco Antônio Coutinho Jorge, when he started to study and practice psychoanalysis, there were no recognised institutions in Brazil:

> When Kemper came, I was a psychoanalyst at the Penitentiary, with a paycheck for a civil servant, who could barely provide for the family. [...] When, years later, my economic and financial situation improved substantially, I no longer considered making such a financial sacrifice. I already felt like hors-concours. I did not miss the mentioned diploma. (Weissmann, 1984, pp. 171–172)

Weissmann set out on unusual path for other psychoanalysts and occupied several spaces: he published books aimed to disseminate psychoanalysis to the lay public, in addition to his constant participation in high circulation magazines. From *Cruzeiro* magazine to medical journals, his work in promoting psychoanalysis was committed and constant.

With this paper and research, I seek to place Karl Weissmann in the history of psychoanalysis in Brazil alongside Gastão Pereira da Silva. The fact that they are considered illegitimate—or even censored—based on a certain version of history does not erase their deeds. As Russo (2002) stated, the project of spreading the theme to a lay audience included a basic pedagogical objective. Gastão Pereira da Silva did not only spread the content of psychoanalysis, but above all aimed at disseminating a certain way of self-problematising (Russo, 2002), and Weissmann learned from him. Once achieved, this self-problematisation would be dedicated 'to the 'correct' way of naming, circumscribing and interpreting the conflicts themselves. And of course, to the need to talk about yourself, unveil your most intimate feelings, to a specialist' (Russo, 2002, p. 59).

Weissmann publicised a psychoanalysis marked by a developmental perspective, presenting it as a tool for self-control and increasing maturity. He spoke to the general public about everyday issues such as family problems, money, crime, or even sports (Weissmann, 1961). His best-seller *A conquista da maturidade* constituted the high point of his theorisation, as it presented a psychological model to be desired by the reader, who could come close to this ideal by reading the book itself. Weissmann contributed to making psychoanalysis a type of daily language in the 1930s. This had been his objective since his first book.

According to Russo (2002), the spread of psychoanalysis was certainly capable of reaching those sectors of the middle classes. Those people were the most affected by the eternal process of modernisation and transformation of values that Brazilian society was—and still is—going through. In this sense, this type of work gradually prepared the way for the so-called 'psychoanalysis boom' in the 1970s. It was not just a matter of disseminating elements of the doctrine to the public, but of penetrating ordinary life, marking new ways of naming the impasses experienced by the intermediate classes of the population (Russo, 2002).

At the moment when institutions linked to the IPA began to train psychoanalysts on Brazilian soil, the demand was intense. This intense demand was due, at least in part, to the work of dissemination carried out beforehand in the country. Disregarding—or censoring—this horizon of efforts prevents progress in the debate about the spread of psychoanalytic notions among the Brazilian population, as well as its vast effects.

References

Brasileiro, V. B. (2008). *Sylvio de Vasconcellos: Um arquiteto para além da forma* (PhD thesis). Federal University of Minas Gerais, Belo Horizonte.

Carneiro, M. L. T. (2018). Imigrantes indesejáveis: a ideologia do etiquetamento durante a Era Vargas. *Revista USP* (119), 115–130.

Coimbra, C. M. B. (1995). *Guardiães da Ordem: Uma viagem pelas práticas psi no Brasil do 'Milagre.'* Oficina do Autor.

Decreto nº 51.009 de 22 de julho de 1961 (Brasil).

Freud, S. (2014). A questão da análise leiga. In *Obras completas em 20 volumes* (Vol. XVII). Companhia das Letras.

Frosh, S. (2005). *Hate and Jewish science: Anti-semitism, Nazism and psychoanalysis*. Palgrave Macmillan.

Laplanche, J., & Pontalis, J. B. (2001). *Vocabulário de Psicanálise*. Martins Fontes.

Lima, R. A. (2019). Itineraries of the relationship between psychoanalysis and politics in Brazil: A historical overview from the early period to the military dictatorship. *IMAGÓ Budapest, 8*(2), 45–65.

Oliveira, C. L. M. V. (2006). *História da Psicanálise – São Paulo (1920–1969)*. Escuta.

Pereira da Silva, G. (1932). *Para compreender Freud*. Renascença.

Pereira da Silva, G. (1978). *25 anos de Psicanálise*. APPERJ.

Perestrello, M. (1988). Primeiros encontros com a Psicanálise: Os precursores no Brasil (1899–1937). In S. A. Figueira (Ed.), *Efeitos Psi: a influência da Psicanálise*. Campus.

Revel, J. (2010). Micro-história, macro-história: o que as variações de escala ajudam a pensar em um mundo globalizado. *Revista Brasileira de Educação, 15*(45).

Russo, J. A. (2002). A difusão da psicanálise no Brasil na primeira metade do século XX – Da vanguarda modernista à radio-novela. *Estudos e Pesquisas Em Psicologia, 2*(1), 53–64.

Salim, S. A. (2010). As origens da Psicanálise em Belo Horizonte e do Grupo de Estudos Psicanalíticos de Belo Horizonte filiado à Associação Internacional de Psicanálise: A saga de um ideal. *Mental, 8*(15), 255–272.

Salzstein, S. (2001). *Franz Weissmann.* Cosac Naify.

Santos, R. A. N. (2016). *A história da Psicanálise em Minas Gerais: dos primeiros tempos à institucionalização (1925–1963)* (Master thesis). Federal University of São João del Rei, São João del Rei.

Santos, R. A. N., & Mandelbaum, B. P. H. (2019). Karl Weissmann e a psicanálise na Era Vargas: um psicanalista entre a política, a educação e a criminologia. *Memorandum: Memória e História em Psicologia* (36), 1–27.

SIEMG - Serviço de Investigações do Estado de Minas Gerais. (1935). *Comunicação de Diligência efetuada, Prontuário 052.* Belo Horizonte.

Weissmann, K. (1936). *Our English teacher – 50 lições de inglez.* Companhia Editora Nacional.

Weissmann, K. (1937). *O dinheiro na vida erótica.* Brasília Editora.

Weissmann, K. (1944). Freud e a civilização. *Folha de Minas,* 27 de fevereiro, pp. 3–4.

Weissmann, K. (1949). Édipo no drama conjugal. *O Cruzeiro,* 23 de julho, pp. 81–86.

Weissmann, K. (1952). A base anal da criminalidade. *Acaiaca* (36), 28–33.

Weissmann, K. (1958). *O hipnotismo: psicologia, técnica e aplicação.* Livraria Padro.

Weissmann, K. (1961). *A conquista da maturidade.* Editora Civilização Brasileira.

Weissmann, K. (1964). *Masoquismo e Comunismo: Contribuições para a patologia do pensamento político.* Martins.

Weissmann, K. (1967). *Psicanálise: ensaios e experiências.* Livraria Freitas Bastos.

Weissmann, K. (1976). *Psicanálise.* Cultura Médica.

Weissmann, K. (1984). Interview by Jorge, MAC. *Revista da Prática Freudiana* (1), 160–176.

Weissmann, K. (1985). *Vistas into maturity.* Vantage Press.

14

A Psychoanalysis for Subversion: Psychoanalytic Discourse on the 'new Youth' in Dictatorial Brazil (1964–1985)

Aline Librelotto Rubin

The end of Brazil's civil-military dictatorship (1964–1985) was decreed more than three decades ago, but present-day debates alert us to the continuity of certain authoritarian structures and practices, the not-so-subtle vestiges of those times (Teles & Safatle, 2010). An important aspect of this continuity relates to the sovereignty of Brazil's armed forces after the transition to democracy.[1] After twenty-one years of the dictatorial regime, army officials not only negotiated the terms of their exit but they were also given amnesty for their past actions. The 1988 Federal Constitution, still in force today, ended up by 'democratically'

[1] For more information on the dictatorship period and its stages and presidencies, including the so-called abertura, see Skidmore (1989), *The Politics of Military Rule in Brazil, 1964–85*. More specifically on transitional justice, see Edson Teles and Renan Quinalha (2015), *The Scopes and Limits to the Transitional Justice Discourse in Brazil*.

A. L. Rubin (✉)
Universidade de São Paulo, São Paulo, Brazil

B. Mandelbaum et al. (eds.), *Brazilian Psychosocial Histories of Psychoanalysis*, Studies in the Psychosocial,
https://doi.org/10.1007/978-3-030-78509-3_14

regulating military authority, conferring power—potentially incompatible with the rights envisioned by that very constitution—on those who had previously violated those rights (Zaverucha, 2010). The effects of the authoritarian regime are still felt, profoundly marking relations of power and violence in the country.

With the dictatorship ending officially in 1985, the Polícia Militar (PM—Military Police)[2] stopped persecuting political dissidents and refocused their attention on those identified as 'delinquents' and 'traffickers,' who became the 'threat' to the social order. In recent decades, we have witnessed a significant rise in murders (the most common cause of death) among youth, mainly black and marginalised youth.[3] In a country where the current President of the Republic defends the use of guns and excuses police violence, it is evident that not everyone is granted the same right to life, as enshrined in the constitution. Rather, the abuses and cruelty practiced by the PM reveal a very different situation. Towards the end of 2019, for instance, nine youths died following a crackdown by the PM near the 'Baile da 17,' the biggest funk party in São Paulo, in the *favela* of Paraisópolis. Videos circulated across a variety of social networks depicting grave physical abuse, such as police corralling young people in dead-end streets, leading to people being crushed to death. There is an ongoing political dispute over the legitimacy of funk 'bailes,' which is understood as a space of expression for marginalised youth, and the criminalisation of 'fluxos,'[4] which are seen as 'a threat to the social order.' In this sense, some media narratives today criminalise and stigmatise such spaces, automatically associating them with criminal organisations and drug trafficking.

---

[2] This is the name of the corporation that exercises the policy function within the armed forces. For more on the role of the military institution in Brazilian politics and its relation to the civil governments, see: Alfred Stepan (1971), *The Military in Politics—Changing Patterns in Brazil*.

[3] The section 'youth lost' in the 2020 'Atlas of Violence' emphasizes that 'in Brazil, homicide is the principal cause of death among youth,' in particular in the male segment of the population. 30,873 youths were victims of homicide in 2018, which indicates a rate of 60.4 murders per 100 thousand youths, and 53.3% of homicides in the country (2020, p. 20). The literature has used the term 'juvenicídio' ('juvicide') to refer to the mass murder of segments or specific groups within the youth population.

[4] Funk and its spontaneous parties inside the *favelas*, called 'fluxos,' are part of marginalised youth culture and have become spaces as well for political resistance. See Pedro (2017).

The history shows that is not the first time the state has labelled youth culture as a social threat and sought to repress it. During the years of the dictatorial regime, young people, in various forms of political militancy (partisan, student, feminist, racial, cultural) were seen as subversive threats and became special targets of national security policies. In particular, during 1968, a variety of artistic and cultural resistance movements were subject to political repression, such as the well-known 'Tropicalismo,' which saw the persecution, imprisonment, and exile of many of its members. In 1974, as part of the struggle of the Black movement[5] which opposed the widespread notion of a 'racial democracy,' the first Black *carnaval* group was created, calling itself 'Ilê Aiyê.' While seeking to confront racism in Bahia, the group suffered political repression: Antônico Carlos, one of its founders, remarked in an interview that 'any kind of activity and you were right away painted as a communist.'[6] Discouraged by the authorities from calling themselves 'Black Power,' the group marched in the *carnaval* for three years under police guard. Another *carnaval* group that was founded at the same time as 'Ilê Aiyê' in the late 1960s and subjected to similar levels of repression was 'Os Apaches do Tororó': 'the largest in the city, made up of Blacks who chanted songs from *candomblé* and characteristic rituals' (Figueiredo, 2016, p.73). Responding to media defamation and calls from the elites, the authorities blamed the members of these groups for the violence and

[5] The political and cultural resistance movements in the first decade of the dictatorial regime, such as the 'Movimento Estudantil' ('Student Movement') and 'Tropicalismo,' were formed mostly by young people from the urban middle class. However, according to the Relatório da Comissão da Verdade (Truth Commission Report, 2015, p. 1), 'opposition to the military coup in Brazil was not limited to segments of the urban middle class with a white ethnic majority; the Black presence in the movement to combat the regime was also significant. Among the dead and missing are the names of militants of Black origin. Moreover, being largely among the poorest citizens, Blacks were the most affected by the authoritarian policies of the period. According to Kossling (2008, p. 30), 'the rise of Black movements in the late 1970s occurred in the period known as 'abertura política' ('political opening'). The public archives for the period reveal that in the late 1970s and early 1980s there was intense surveillance of Black movements, grounded in the notion of preserving Brazil's 'racial democracy,' in order to avoid 'social antagonisms' (pp. 30–31). It is important to note that, with regard to psychoanalysis, debates including racism, for example, began majorly after the 1980s. As such, the psychoanalytical theorisations we present here do not include a wider discussion of race or social class.

[6] Publicly available at https://www.geledes.org.br/vovo-do-ile-aiye-fala-sobre-a-resistencia-a-ditadura/.

disorder of the Bahia *carnaval*, arresting 120 members for 'disorder' in 1977 (Figueiredo, 2016, p. 74).[7]

The social construction of youth as a subversive threat in Brazil was part of a larger context of transformations that took place around the world at that time. Since the explosion of student-led political mobilisation throughout the world in 1968, and the flood of countercultural movements within the European, American, and Southeast Asian urban middle classes, youths have occupied a central role in social, political, and cultural changes. Barthes noted that after May 1968, the language of students overflowed so completely that, according to him, one might refer to 'the university revolt as a *Storming of the Word* (as in *Storming of the Bastille*)' (Barthes, 2012, p. 194). Therefore, by taking up words and action in opposition to the *status quo*, to authoritarianism, and to a variety of social injustices, youths occupied a strategic position in the political context of social resistance.

The influence of May 1968 arrived in Brazil, bringing with it the interrogation of religious and family values, patriarchy, and an array of other authoritarian traits. The intensification of protests organised by the Movimento Estudantil (Student Movement) that fought against university reform and the authoritarianism of the regime, ended up supplying the additional political instability needed to spur the introduction of the Ato Institucional nº 5 (AI-5, Institutional Act nº 5),[8] which sent the country's social and political framework in the direction of *greater* authoritarianism. Youths and their protests were consolidated as a representation of 'a communist-inspired "subversive reach" and portrayed as a "threat to internal security," from the point of view of the Doutrina de Segurança Nacional (DSN, Doctrine of National Security),' a narrative that was legitimised by the mass-media (do Valle, 2016, p. 34).

---

[7] Repression of the cultural and artistic movements of the Black population had been going on since long before the dictatorial period. At the end of the nineteenth century, Black people were accused of threatening 'civilised' European standards through the 'Africanisation' of Bahia, and were repressed and considered 'savage' and inappropriate for the 'refined' and 'elegant' carnival, in the style of the carnivals of Paris and Venice (Pinho 2004 *quoted in* Figueiredo 2016, p. 75).

[8] This act, issued by President Costa e Silva in December 1968, authorised the president to close the National Congress and Legislative Assemblies and suspended constitutional guarantees such as habeas corpus, which resulted in the 'institutionalisation' of torture.

The idea of subversive youth as a direct risk to social order led to an increase in the attention given to adolescents and young adults during the first half of the 1970s, in the disciplines of the human and social sciences. English historian John Gillis (1981)[9] claimed that some social science theories attributed to youth certain immutable characteristics and a status of passive subjects rather than active agents of change, placing them outside history. According to Gillis: 'Science lent its prestige to the sanctioning of certain selected forms of social behaviour, thereby underlining the boundaries between acceptable and unacceptable behaviour' (Gillis, 1981, p. 212), such as the sexual attitudes of girls, ghetto youth, school dropouts, and youth protest. Such behaviours were classified as dysfunctional and referred to institutions whose objective was to reform those who deviated from the established norm. In this sense, Patto (1995, p. i) claims that the range of 'psy practices'[10] established in Brazil during the 1970s sought to readjust youth bodies seen as deviant, rounding 'the edges of just and healthy resistance responses, pathologizing them in the name of *ordem e progresso*.'[11]

As part of these 'psy practices,' psychoanalysis developed a discourse about adolescence, which had an important role in explaining some of the social and cultural changes involving youth, and also in preventing deviations from a desired normal adolescence. However, psychoanalytic theory had been used to formulate knowledge about the social reality in Brazil before. Psychoanalysis was introduced to Brazil in the early twentieth century as an important scientific instrument for a particular understanding of some social phenomena, such as the race mixture and so-called backwardness of the Brazilians (Facchinetti & Ponte, 2003; Russo, 2012b). Through the application of some psychoanalytic concepts, mainly by psychiatrists, it contributed to a national project of a more developed, modern, civilised country, aiming at the improvement

[9] Gillis wrote the book *Youth and History—Tradition and Change in European Age Relations 1770—Present* in 1981. In Chapter 5 of this book, 'End of Adolescence: Youth in the 1950s and 1960s,' he brings a historical review on the changes that occurred in youth and adolescence during these decades, taking into consideration social class differences.

[10] This same period represented the 'boom' of psychoanalysis in Brazil, when there was a major expansion of the psychoanalytic field, side by side with the consolidation of societies affiliated to the International Psychoanalytic Association in the country (Russo, 2012a; Coimbra, 1995).

[11] 'Order and Progress' i.e. the national flag's motto.

of hygiene standards and the proper development of maladjusted children.[12] Nearly half a century later, the psychoanalyst Durval Marcondes lamented the closing down of the 'Secção da Higiene Mental Escolar' (Department of Mental Health for Schools) and emphasised the importance that the 'Serviço de Orientação Infantil' (Childhood Orientation Service) had in the 'correction' of 'street urchins.' In pointing out the integration of prophylactic measures in mental health in the home and the school in prior decades, Marcondes emphasised the potential application this service might have 'precisely in the era of the *trombadinha* (pickpocket)' (Bicudo, 1980, p. 102). To conclude, he described a moment of 'anguish before the disaster in the education of our youth' and launched his plea to the then-Secretary of State for Education for the 'resuscitation or reanimation' of the service (Bicudo, 1980, p. 103).

Under the rule of an oppressive state apparatus and its strong propaganda, youth opposition had no space in the social arena. In this context, some psychoanalysts[13] associated the dismantlement of society and the social order with youth, in accordance with the disseminated state ideology. Drawing from the psychoanalytic theories emerging from Britain and America, youth protest was conceived predominantly as an individual problem, an unconscious expression of primitive forces leaking into the social bond. This view may be demonstrated with some examples of psychoanalytic production concerning the theme of adolescence and the so-called new youth, taking into consideration the political implications of psychoanalytic discourse that arose from the intersection of psychoanalysis with its social context. On the frontier between normal and pathological, the rebellious and subversive behaviour of youths was theorized in Brazil by a psychoanalysis apparently more normalizing than subversive.

---

[12] See the Chapters 8, 9, and 11 in this volume.

[13] Especially, the first and second generations of the 'official' psychoanalytic movement, who had a medical and psychiatric background.

A Psychoanalytic Take on Youth Protest and the Counterculture

Although adolescents were not a mainstay of psychoanalysts' consulting rooms, there was a growing concern about adolescence and youth in psychoanalysis, both theoretical and clinical. Following the psychoanalyst Freitas (1989), the 1970s was seen as being an 'unfavourable' decade for Brazilian youth, yet decisive for work about adolescence in Brazil. Freitas documented the relationship among youth behaviours, specifically with regard to the counterculture, political repression, and parental demands for their children to be analysed:

> With the student guilds closed, the university silenced, any type of protest suppressed by violence, all that remains are dreams, alienation, and the pleasure of 'the trip'. The consulting rooms fill themselves with drugged-up youth, people without prospects who receive, along with poor education, the influence of a media that has taken on the role of corrupting via consumerism and the exaltation of the 'Brazilian miracle'. The framework was favourable to the putting in practice of theories about adolescence that were still being developed, specific techniques applied to a growing clientele, brought in by parents bewildered by the use of weed or the sexuality of their daughters. (Freitas, 1989, p. 11)

'Bewildered' parents, taken aback by the behaviour of their children, believed that psychoanalysis, with a high reputation amongst the urban middle class, would have something to say about all this. The psychoanalyst Deocleciano Alves (1974) described the 'symptoms' of this new youth that disquieted their families: intense conflict with authorities, anti-social conduct, idiosyncratic manner of dress, a new relationship with sexuality, drug use, involvement in protests and illegal activities, and political activism and the diffusion of socio-political ideas. According to Alves, the radical shift in attitude among adolescents observed in his own clinical practice (youth primarily from the middle and upper classes of the population) was influenced by 'movements and ideas hailing from the most diverse areas of the world' and challenged the 'socio-familial and cultural patterns in place until that point'[14] (Alves, 1974, p. 53).

Among psychoanalytical explanations for the new behaviour of youth, that of Darcy Uchôa (1973)[15] was representative of a prominent psychoanalytical group that held hegemonic sway until the middle of the 1970s. Uchôa proposed that attitudes such as rebellion, ideological and philosophical engagement 'with the need for social and political reform,' were an intellectual defence mechanism resulting from the adolescent's inability to control the biological and psychic changes they were undergoing (Uchôa, 1973, p. 143). He also emphasised that these manifestations of the defence mechanism of the psyche could be seen in the emergence of rebellious university movements and 'powerful violence against the establishment' visible around the world, citing Berkeley in 1964, Columbia in 1968, Paris in 1968, and, in Brazil, the student agitation that had occurred at the University of São Paulo (USP) and Mackenzie University in October 1968.[16]

Uchôa referred to these youth, who were involved in political, social, economic, racial, and cultural conflict, by 'adopted terminology' as 'subversives,' 'communists,' 'anarchists,' 'marginals,' in precise agreement with the narrative of the state. Adding to these 'types,' Uchôa also highlighted, 'an entire category of youth on the frontiers of delinquency, or even already within it,' with strong characteristics of non-conformity,

[14] Alves (1974) points out that his clinical observation does not include youth from rural areas and that different socioeconomic conditions would influence patterns of behaviour.

[15] Darcy Uchôa was a psychiatrist who worked in the 1940s in the major hospices of São Paulo and also in the Hygiene Service of the city. He was one of the six founders of the São Paulo Society of Psychoanalysis and president of it on three occasions, in the 50s, 60s, and 70s.

[16] From June to August 1968, the Faculty of Philosophy, the Clinic of Psychology, and the Residential Complex of the University of São Paulo (CRUSP) were occupied by students. Coimbra (1995) highlights the tension among some of the psychoanalysts from the São Paulo society who were part of the teaching staff at USP in the time of student militancy. The students demanded a position in the institution in view of the political repression that had already been suffered; they received the response that academic space should discuss curricular and not political reforms. Another location occupied by students was the Faculty of Philosophy at USP. During the occupation, the students organized the 30th UNE Congress. On October 2, a toll was paid to collect funds for the congress, which ended in conflict with occupants of Mackenzie University in the building across the street (do Valle, 2016).

non-adaptability, and even extreme violence. After naming diverse movements of 'maladapted youth' around the world,[17] he affirmed that Brazilian youth had adopted the roles of 'playboy' and that 'plebeianism' had become a symbol of the expression, in adolescence and youth, of 'irresponsibility, irrational behaviour, lack of discipline, aggression' (Uchôa, 1973, pp. 143–144).

Despite making reference to the Brazilian reality, both Alves and Uchôa locate those on the edge of delinquency as 'new youths' within a larger global phenomenon. This allows us to compare Uchôa's line of argument with work published by American sociologist Robert Endleman (1970) in the *Psychoanalytic Review*. Endleman set out to investigate the psychodynamic aspects present in participants in North American student protest movements. In his view, despite the possible legitimacy of the questions raised by the students, these rebellions suggested the existence of irrational excesses involving destructiveness with deeply unconscious individual roots (Endleman, 1970). In ways that differ from the familiar Oedipal plot, both Uchôa and Endleman argue that the psychological motive for rebellion would be triggered by unresolved Oedipal conflicts.

For Uchôa, who was working within a Kleinian framework, rebellious behaviour is conceived of as a 'projection' of fantasies related to internal objects that 'emerge' into the social field as a desire to destroy the institutions of authority, such as the government (1973, p. 172). This was a shared view among psychoanalysts who followed the same or similar theoretical framework; however, the explanation of how aggressive impulses related to one's inner world were 'projected' or 'displaced' to real authority in society was not clear, giving it a transcendental tone. This view gave way to the success achieved by one of the most versatile symptoms relative to the 'emergence of psychopathologies of adolescence': 'acting-out' (Baggio, 1983). Seen as a phenomenon necessary to development of adolescence or as a 'form of communication,' 'acting-out' became a regular feature of Brazilian psychoanalytic knowledge

---

[17] Uchôa (1973) cites, among others, 'Pavitos' (Venezuela), 'Hipsters,' 'Teen-agers' (United States), 'Gamberros' (Spain), 'Vitelloni' (Italy), 'Blousons Noirs' (France), 'Teddy Boys' (England), 'Halbstarker' (Germany), 'Zauzou' (Africa), 'Taizo-Zoku' (Japan), and 'Hooligans' (Poland).

production, consistent with the use seen in other psychoanalytic theories from the northern hemisphere during the same period, especially in the English psychoanalytic tradition. For instance, the book *Adolescence and Breakdown* (1975) was published by the members of the Department of Adolescence of the Tavistock Clinic in London and presents 'a unique study of adolescence,' discussing topics such as: 'emotional conflicts, educational drop-outs, social conflict, delinquency, acting-out, rebellion and violence, drugs, depression and suicide, individual treatment and family therapy.' According to Varchevker and Muir in this book, Freud first introduced the concept of 'acting-out' in 1905, in the case of Dora, where 'she acted-out an essential part of her recollections and phantasies instead of reproducing them in treatment.' For Freud, 'acting-out' concerned a re-enactment of a traumatic situation or event, partly disguised and skewed towards the gratification of desire (Varchevker & Muir, 1975, p. 55). It would be with Anna Freud, in 'Problems of psychoanalytic technique and therapy' (1972) that 'acting-out' appears articulated alongside adolescence as being 'age-adequate.' As such, the term was invoked to describe a wide variety of adolescent behaviours, for instance 'burglary, physical attacks or even homicide, but also other situations where there is little or less or no damage involved' (Varchevker & Muir, 1975, p. 55).

For some Brazilian psychoanalysts, 'acting-out' in adolescence explained the mechanism that transformed unconscious, unelaborated conflict into performative acts, and it was used to inform thoughts not only about delinquency, but also youth sexuality. Adolescent behaviours that reached psychoanalysts' divans also reflected the context of social changes won by women during that time, but the sexual liberation offered by countercultural movements of the period was reduced to a 'hedonistic search for sexual satisfaction, facile and too often repeated' (Baggio, 1983, p. 17) that would not lead to real emotional fulfilment. This view surfaces in considerations over the use of the pill, as part of the sexual revolution of young women and of the feminist agenda for independence in the 1960s. From the perspective of psychoanalysts in Rio de Janeiro during this era, the use of the pill was reduced to a form of freedom of expression that could cover up issues and disturbances such as impotence, frigidity, and homosexuality (Schneider et al.,

1973, p. 267). This was reflected during the police raid on the student residence of Universidade de São Paulo in 1968, as the 'subversive materials' recovered by the police included boxes of birth control pills. These were the behaviours lumped together and flattened out as unconscious manifestations, and thus emptied of their singular, emancipatory potential.

If, on the one hand, psychodynamic understandings derived from notions such as 'acting-out' were a psychological explanation (and reduction) of individual, group, social and cultural youth phenomena, then on the other hand, they did not fully explain the uneasiness and disturbance these phenomena provoked in families and in institutions. The concept of 'generational conflict' arose in response to both of these questions.

The (Psychoanalytic) Message of 'Roda-Viva'

'Generational conflict' was another important theoretical articulation within psychoanalysis for thinking about social ills and the cultural and political effervescence of the youth moment. In 1968, a critical year for Brazilian youth resistance movements, the psychoanalyst Virginia Leone Bicudo published the text 'The Message of the Roda-Viva (Whirlwind),' in which she articulates a psychoanalytic[18] analysis of a censored piece by Chico Buarque de Holanda.[19] Bicudo states that the piece 'serves to

[18] To analyse the play, Bicudo says that it is necessary to understand 'human nature and the development of custom and social institutions.' She underscores human activity as the balance between the instincts of life and death, and states that 'the "diffusion" between the two instincts characterizes the infant psyche, a period in which the mind is split.' This operation characterises a 'primitive mental life,' in which the individual is ruled in a narcissistic, omnipotent way. Development and emotional maturity bring about the fusion of these instincts, causing the instincts of destruction to subordinate themselves to the ends of constructive impulses (Bicudo, 1968, p. 235). Here we see that Bicudo's approach to 'human nature' is in accordance with that of practitioners of Ego Psychology.

[19] The show highlighted the dynamics of popular mobilisation, as well as criticising consumer society and the cultural industry. Due to this innovative and in-your-face way of revealing the country's problems, the Teatro Opinião was invaded by the Comando de Caça aos Comunistas (CCC, Commando for the Hunting of Communists) and vandalized, and cast members were assaulted. The CCC's attack overshadowed the aesthetic and revolutionary importance of the work. Source: http://redeglobo.globo.com/globoteatro/bis/noticia/2013/09/roda-viva-peca-de-chico-buarque-e-um-marco-do-teatro-nacional.html.

illustrate conflict between generations and the role of the artist, of youth, and of elders as participants in mental and social conflicts,' representing the 'wheels of society in the present,' which she terms the society of the 'Roda-Viva' (Bicudo, 1968, p. 233). She confirmed that the greater the generational gap, the greater the social antagonism, but also that 'the intensity of the conflict between generations gives an indication of the extent to which different generations maintain unresolved mental and socio-cultural conflicts, such as those referred to in the myth of Oedipus' (Bicudo, 1968, p. 233).

Writing on the eve of the AI-5 being decreed, Bicudo made no explicit reference to the Brazilian reality, although she did state that 'the social reform movement is characterized by its universality and has on its vanguard youth and artists' (Bicudo, 1968, p. 237). In explaining the plot of the play, however, indications of the social and political moment remain: 'the author refers to a people that suffers from hunger and the lack of freedom to express their will' and compensates for their frustration by creating an idol. This 'idol,' an artist who submits himself to the growing culture industry of the 60s, makes protest music. He travels abroad and is accused by the 'capeta' (devil) of betraying the homeland, echoing a national slogan from the period, 'love it or leave it.' Having encouraged students to identify with his cultural politics, this 'social hero' suffers from censorship and is forced to 'commit suicide,' making it appear as an accident. For the widow of the dead man, all that remains is life 'à la hippie' which, emptied of 'all traditional values,' would have the hope of peace, love, and flowers as a universal value (Bicudo, 1968, p. 241).

Following her contextualisation of the piece, Bicudo offers a psychoanalytic interpretation of the characters, affirming that 'the adults in the "roda viva" society are victims of lingering childhood traits in their personalities,' 'which impede mental and social growth' (Bicudo, 1968, pp. 242–243). Thus, in her psychoanalytical reading of a theatre piece with significant political repercussions, Bicudo highlights the role of the characters' primitive mental functioning as part of the conflict established with past generations.

Following Gomes (2018, p. 165), it should be considered that this was 'an article written by the highest-ranking member' of the São Paulo psychoanalytic society at that moment,' and that Bicudo was close to the spheres of political power. The article allowed one to note the journal's position (and, consequently, that of the psychoanalytic society) with regard to an oppressive political regime, and yet do so without tying itself to it. According to Gomes, 'her evaluation was assured by the Kleinian/Bionian conceptual theory of psychoanalysis and the theme could be justified with recourse to "generational conflict," as a psychoanalytical struggle, and not directly to do with political power' (2018, p. 165). In the end, Bicudo appears to offer a kind of censure of the play because its 'gestures and strong language' could 'excite the repressed centres and lead individuals mentally to search for such pleasures, as seems to have occurred, to a degree, with the perverse attacks suffered by artists' (Bicudo, 1968, p. 243). As such, Bicudo affirms that the function of the theatre ought to be otherwise, one of emotional readjustment through the reinforcement of 'positive and constructive aspects' of individuals (Bicudo, 1968, p. 243).

The theme of 'generational conflict' remained part of a central debate among psychoanalysts into the 1970s. Presenting itself as a concept that could explain the dialectic between the individual and the social, it acted as depository and neutraliser of the antagonisms and social unease that hovered around the youth of the period. At the height of political repression in Brazil, 'generational conflict' was the theme of the Fourth Brazilian Psychoanalytical Congress. Similar to Bicudo's proposal, the work of this congress identified generational conflict as a movement begun by youth who had their sights set on renewal, breaks with tradition, and disputes with the establishment—demands resisted by older generations. At the core of generational conflict for Uchôa (1973) were the death instincts of both older and younger generations, insufficiently neutralised by neurotic instinctive life.

According to Gillis (1981), the use of terms such as 'generation gap' and 'generational conflict' to explain some of the youth behaviours demonstrated a particular ideological stance, as some theories drawing on a 'modernization' paradigm in the 1970s saw adolescence as 'the axis on which individual and social progress turned' (Gillis, 1981, p. 215). According to him, 'modern youth was often delinquent – even somewhat rebellious – yet this was acceptable, even desirable, as long as it did not accentuate inherited social cleavages,' therefore 'the generation gap was viewed as a desirable alternative to class, ethnic and sexual conflict' (Gillis, 1981, p. 215). Gillis questioned the difference between 'new' and 'old,' stating that different generations could have different perceptions of the world, but that there still was a continuity within one class, gender, or ethnic culture, across these generations.

> The possibility of approaching social issues starting with the figure of the youth as the representative of what is new, the figure who confronts previous generations – as happened in both psychoanalysis and sociology – defenders of tradition, proved to be a fertile resource for shifting social tensions into a timeless, supposedly universal dimension, as if the conflict of the new versus the old were inevitable. Although it was easy to justify doing so on the basis of the behaviour of the various social actors in question, to take the conflict of generations as the main reason for these different social problems seems to be above all an attempt to naturalise the social tensions of a certain historical moment. (Matheus, 2010, p. 149)

Martins (2004) claims that 'analytical practices' failed to take into account a local reality in which Brazilian youth struggled, informed by their economic and historical enmeshment, to think in universalist psychological formulations (Martins, 2004). Nevertheless, starting in the 1970s, Brazil's psychoanalytic scene began to diversify, as much in its epistemological as in its institutional character, bringing more capacious and politically engaged forms of thinking to the questions around adolescence and the phenomena of youth in Brazilian society. This renewal of the psychoanalytic movement had as much to do with the arrival of the Lacanian movement in Brazil, as with the expansion of projects related to a 'psychoanalytic psychology' (Russo, 2012a). The conservatism that marked 'official' societies (Frosh & Mandelbaum, 2017), faced with these epochal and disciplinary changes, also began to be challenged internally by members of the third and fourth generation. From the end of the 1970s, these challenges led to important institutional reforms and critiques of the psychologising nature of certain psychoanalytic formulations.

Final Considerations

For Gillis (1981, p. 211), historians did not discover youth until it 'forced its way into public consciousness in the 1960s.' After that, new histories and many psychological and sociological studies on youth began to appear, which researchers turned to as a way of accessing a particular historical moment and its way of interpreting social reality. Perhaps the same can be said regarding the psychoanalytic theorisations about adolescence and youth in Brazil, as this work has aimed to demonstrate.

The examples of knowledge production presented here are representations of a style of psychoanalytic thinking that was pre-eminent in Brazil, particularly within psychoanalytic societies linked to the IPA, which held sway over the field until the mid-1970s. Psychoanalysis heard society's demand for a psychological explanation for the new behaviour of its youth—contentious, strange, different—which was worrying families and institutions. If, on the one hand, the psychological response based on development offered an alternative to the violent and eugenic psychiatric practice observed in the growth of psychiatric institutions, this aspect demonstrated an important ideological-political alignment that understood development as an element 'necessary to overcome the diagnosis of an underdeveloped country' (Dunker, 2015, p. 150).

As such, even while bringing in elements of the local social reality, we observed a kind of intellectual 'anthropophagy' (Mandelbaum et al., 2019), which kept Brazilian psychoanalysis in line with northern-hemisphere theorisations—to the detriment of a psychoanalytic articulation that was more than a mere reproduction or perhaps an articulation of social reality. Nonetheless, we would like to draw attention to the important work of Hélio Pellegrino (1987) in his 'Oedipal Pact and Social Pact' and Lélia Gonzales' (1984)[20] 'Racism and Sexism in Brazilian Culture.' These articles, though published in the 1980s during the dictatorship, offered analyses that departed from traditional versions of

[20] Lélia Gonzales was an important Black intellectual and activist, a reference of intersecting thought and an articulator of Marxism and psychoanalysis. See: Flávia Rios (2019) *Améfrica Ladina: The Conceptual Legacy of Lélia Gonzalez* (1935–1994).

psychoanalytic concepts, such as the Oedipus complex, instead articulating these with regard to elements of Brazilian society, Pellegrino through class struggles and the logic of capitalism and Gonzales through an anti-racist agenda.

Lastly, the question of the perpetuation of state violence, for Teles and Safatle (2010), is related to a particular approach to the past taken by Brazilian society, one which passes through negations, silences, repetitions. In this sense, we think that the restitution of the history of psychoanalysis in Brazil and its diverse roles within specific political and social conjunctures may contribute not only to create a space where the bodies that once have been silenced and normalised can reappear but also to inform us about the past in a way that throws some light on today's psychoanalytic theory and practice so that it does not repeat itself.

References

Alves, D. B. (1974). Novos padrões de conduta dos adolescents. *Alter – Jornal de estudos psicodinâmicos, 4*(1–3), 53–59.

Baggio, M. A. (1983). O Perfil psicológico da adolescência. *Boletim Círculo Psicanalítico De Minas Gerais, No, 21*, 13–18.

Barthes, R. (2012/1988). *O rumor da língua*. WMF Marting fontes.

Bicudo, V. L. (1968). A Mensagem de 'Roda-Viva.' *Revista Brasileira De Psicanálise, 2*(2), 232–243.

Bicudo, V. L. (1980). Durval Bellegarde Marcondes – Precursor da Psicanálise na América Latina. *Alter, 12*(3), 101–105.

Castellar, C. (1989). Sociedade, Família e adolescência. In C. Castellar & L. A. Freitas (Eds.), *Crise da adolescência: visão psicanalítica* (pp. 136–140). Rocco.

Comissão da Verdade. (2015). *Relatório - Tomo I - Parte II - Perseguição à População e ao Movimento Negros*. Available at http://comissaodaverdade.al.sp.gov.br/relatorio/tomo-i/parte-ii-cap1.html. Accessed on 2 September 2020.

Coimbra, C. M. B. (1995). *Guardiões da Ordem: Uma viagem pelas práticas psi no Brasil do 'Milagre.'* Oficina do Ator.

do Valle, M. R. (2016/1999). *1968: o diálogo é a violência – movimento estudantil e ditadura militar no Brasil.* Editora Unicamp.

Dunker, C. I. L. (2015). *Mal-estar, sofrimento e sintoma: uma psicopatologia do Brasil entre muros*. Boitempo.

Endleman, R. (1970). Oedipal elements in student rebellions. *Psychoanalytic Review, 57*(3), 442–471.

Facchinetti, C., & Ponte, C. (2003). De barulhos e silêncios: contribuições para a história da psicanálise no Brasil. *Psychê, 7*(11), 59–83.

Figueiredo, A. K. (2016). *Ativismo negro em Salvador no período da Ditadura Militar (1970–1980)* (Master's degree dissertation). Universidade Federal do Recôncavo da Bahia, Bahia, BH.

Freitas, L. A. (1989). Psicanálise de adolescentes, um pouco de história. In C. Castellar & L. A. Freitas (Eds.), *Crise da adolescência: visão psicanalítica* (pp. 9–15). Rocco.

Frosh, S., & Mandelbaum, B. P. H. (2017). 'Like kings in their kingdoms': Conservatism in Brazilian psychoanalysis during the dictatorship. *Political Psychology, 38*(4), 591–604.

Gonzales, L. (1984). Racismo e Sexismo na cultura brasileira. *Ciências Sociais Hoje*, Anpocs, 223–244.

Gomes, R. M. M. (2018). *Revista Brasileira de Psicanálise: representações de ciência, profissão e história no movimento psicanalítico brasileiro (1967 a 1986)* (PhD thesis). UNESP – Universidade Estadual Paulista, Assis, SP.

Gillis, J. H. (1981), *Youth and history. Tradition and change in European age relations, 1770-present*. Academic Press.

Instituto de Pesquisa Econômica Aplicada. (2020). *Atlas da Violência*. Governo Federal. Available at https://www.ipea.gov.br/atlasviolencia/download/24/atlas-da-violencia-2020. Accessed 25 September 2020.

Kossling, K. S. (2008). Movimentos negros no Brasil entre 1964 e 1983. *Perseu: História, Memória e Política, 1*, 31–62.

Mandelbaum, B., Frosh, S., Rubin, A. L., & Theodoro, R. (2019). Antropofagia e Autoritarismo na Psicanálise Brasileira. *Calibán Revista Latino-Americana De Psicanálise, 17*(1), 112–125.

Matheus, T. C. (2010). *Adolescência – História e política do conceito em Psicanálise*. Coleção Clínica Psicanalítica.

Martins, L. (2004/1979). *A 'Geração AI-5' e maio de 1968 – Duas manifestações intransitivas*. Editora Argumento.

Patto, M. H. S. P. (1995). Apresentação. In C. M. B. Coimbra (Ed.), *Guardiões da Ordem: Uma viagem pelas práticas psi no Brasil do 'Milagre'* (pp. i–ii). Oficina do Ator.

Pedro, T. M. G. (2017). É o fluxo: 'baile de favela' e funk em São Paulo. *PROA Revista De Antropologia e Arte, 2*(7), 115–135. Available at https://www.ifch.

unicamp.br/ojs/index.php/proa/article/view/2829. Accessed on 1 September 2020.

Pellegrino, H. (1987). Pacto edípico e pacto social. In L. A. PY et al. (Eds.), *Grupo sobre grupos*. Rocco.

Rios, F. (2019). 'Améfrica Ladina: The Conceptual Legacy of Lélia Gonzalez (1935–1994)', Dossier: El pensamiento de Lélia Gonzales, un legado y un horizonte. *Lasa Forum, 50*(3), 75–79. Available at https://www.google.com/url?sa=t&rct=j&q=&esrc=s&source=web&cd=&ved=2ahUKEwiz09yOu9DuAhV8GbkGHVuDBkIQFjAAegQIBRAC&url=https%3A%2F%2Fforum.lasaweb.org%2Ffiles%2Fvol50-issue3%2FDossier-Lelia-Gonzalez-8.pdf&usg=AOvVaw2mdw1gsSBWiWtosHVEp3s0. Accessed on 15 October 2020.

Russo, J. (2012). The social diffusion of psychoanalysis during the Brazilian military regime: Psychological awareness in an age of political repression. In J. Damousi & M. Plotkin (Eds.), *Psychoanalysis and politics: Histories of Psychoanalysis under conditions of restricted political freedom* (pp. 165–184). Oxford University Press.

Russo, J. (2012). Brazilian psychiatrists and psychoanalysis at the beginning of 20th century: A question for national identity. *Psychoanalysis and History, 14*, 297–312.

Schneider, G., La Porta, E., Cabernite, L., Besouchet, I., & Ribeiro, N. (1973). O Conflito de Gerações. *Revista Brasileira De Psicanálise, 3*(7), 263–320.

Skidmore, T. (1989). *The politics of military rule in Brazil, 1964–85*. Oxford University Press.

Stepan, A. (1971). *The military in politics—Changing patterns in Brazil*. Princeton University Press.

Teles, E., & Safatle, V. (orgs.). (2010). *O que resta da ditadura: a exceção brasileira*. Boitempo.

Teles, E., & Quinalha, R. (2015). The scope and limits of the discourse on 'transitional justice'. In N. Schneider & M. Esparza (org.), *Legacies of state violence and transitional justice in Latin America: A Janus-faced paradigm?* Lexington Books.

Uchôa, D. M. (1973). Conflito de Gerações. *Revista Brasileira De Psicanálise, 7*(3), 141–185.

Varchevker, A., & Muir, B. (1975). Acting-out, rebellion and violence. In S. Meyerson (Ed.), *Adolescence and breakdown. A study of adolescence* by Member of the Tavistock Clinic and other British experts. George Allen & Unwin Ltd.

Zaverucha, J. (2010). Relações civil-militares: o legado autoritário da Constituição brasileira de 1988. In E. Teles & V. Safatle (Ed.), *O que resta da ditadura: a exceção brasileira* (pp. 41–76). Boitempo.

15

Gay Psychoanalytic Candidates in São Paulo, Today: A Recollection of Interviews

Lucas Charafeddine Bulamah and Daniel Kupermann

Shortly after I finished my book *History of an Unwritten Rule: The Proscription of Male Homosexuality in the Psychoanalytic Movement*[1] (Bulamah 2020), I (LB) was faced with many questions regarding the realities of homophobia in psychoanalytic institutions that were closer to me than the ones the book had accounted for. In the original research for the book, I aimed to understand this homophobia, which was represented by the exclusion of gay candidates from psychoanalytic training offered by the International Psychoanalytical Association (IPA), mainly as a by-product of how psychoanalysis had been institutionalised and popularised.

L. C. Bulamah (✉) · D. Kupermann
Universidade de São Paulo, São Paulo, Brazil

[1] An English translation of the book, originally named in Portuguese *História de uma regra não-escrita: a proscrição da homossexualidade masculina no movimento psicanalítico* (São Paulo: Annablume), will hopefully soon be available. The first edition of the book was published in 2016 and a new and slightly extended version was launched in 2020.

B. Mandelbaum et al. (eds.), *Brazilian Psychosocial Histories of Psychoanalysis*, Studies in the Psychosocial,
https://doi.org/10.1007/978-3-030-78509-3_15

In terms of methodology, and due to the restricted availability of the archives, I restricted myself to researching already-published materials regarding gay candidates being rejected by 'official' IPA-recognised psychoanalytic trainings. There were limited sources of people willing to expose such practices in European Psychoanalytical Societies, so the investigation was restricted mainly to recollections of North-American psychoanalysts and Institutes during the latter part of the twentieth century about the vocal denunciations of exclusion and overall prejudice that took place there, and the measures taken by the IPA on the issue. The denouncements were proportional to the loudness and public virulence with which North-American psychoanalysts demonised homosexuality[2] in the last century. The protestors also borrowed their momentum from the Civil Rights Movement and the Stonewall Riots, which had helped sexual minorities to vocally confront the oppression from the State, the Church and the psychiatric/psychoanalytical establishment.

There was a pronounced lack of published materials available regarding homophobia in Latin America, and particularly regarding Brazil, but this does not mean that homosexual candidates were openly accepted to psychoanalytic training in IPA-licensed Institutes in Brazil. Similarly to European Psychoanalytical Societies, it could be speculated that Brazilian and Latin American Societies were equally homophobic when it came to the issue of gay candidates or psychoanalysts, but that the victims of the prejudice were as discreet about the discrimination as the institutions. I was able to collect some interviews with psychoanalysts affiliated (or perhaps rejected by) the local Psychoanalytical Society in São Paulo. The interviewees were interested in the topic of my book on the 'unwritten rule,' which some of them already knew before, and were able to give some opinions or experiences regarding this.

[2] It should be noted that I chose to investigate homophobia against gay men, since female homosexuality, while far from being accepted, was targeted by a very different prejudice which arose from a distinct understanding of female sexuality by the psychoanalytic discourse (and overall sexism). Besides, lesbians were much less accounted for in denunciations of institutional homophobia than gay men.

My main inspiration for this piece of work was the oral research completed by Mary Lynne Ellis (1994) in Great Britain, who gathered accounts of gay candidates who had been rejected from training in the Institute of Psychoanalysis and other British Societies. She interviewed representatives of these institutions to find out why they were not welcoming to these candidates. The responses were elusive, when not outright homophobic, but disguised with a psychoanalytical masquerade that claims that gay analysts are not able to analyse heterosexual issues due to gay men's position in the castration complex. In Brazil, there has been no inquiry into the issue of gay men on the 'official' psychoanalytic training circuits, except for a single investigation on Brazilian psychoanalysts' (of varied institutional and training backgrounds) opinions regarding homosexuality, which touches slightly on the subject (Maya, 2007). Therefore, this can be seen as a first effort to collect the pieces of a still untold history.

Founded in 1927, the *Sociedade Brasileira de Psicanálise—São Paulo* (SBP-SP in the Portuguese acronym) was the first Psychoanalytic Society in Latin America and is currently one of the largest in the continent. According to official numbers published on their website,[3] it currently has 490 associated and effective members, with 361 affiliated members (which includes those who are still undergoing training analysis).[4]

The SBP-SP is quite proud of its genealogy, as can be seen in the *Family Album* (Sociedade Brasileira de Psicanalise, 1994), a collection of memories from the then 50-year-old Society, told from the perspective of its adherents. Among the many personalities that mark the history of the SBP-SP, there is one which holds a quite mysterious place. Theon Spanudis, someone who would appear first as a notable art collector and enthusiast in 1950s São Paulo, was one of the first training analysts 'imported' into Brazil to improve the then fledgling psychoanalytic Society. The Turkish-born, German-raised and Vienna-trained Spanudis was a highly cultured and much respected training analyst who, nonetheless, left the Society seven years after he arrived. Oliveira (2006) tells us

---

[3] https://www.sbpsp.org.br/quem-somos/a-sociedade/.

[4] For the most thorough and rigorous historical account of Psychoanalysis in São Paulo (which includes the SBP-SP), I recommend Lucia Valadares' *História da psicanálise—São Paulo (1920–1969)*, published by Escuta in 2006.

that his departure was traumatising to the group that had formed around him and it remains shrouded in silence and disavowal:

> [it] happened because of two factors: the severe psychic disturbances he suffered and were diagnosed as schizophrenia, and many hospitalisations throughout his life. Also, there was his overt homosexuality, which left him in an even more difficult and fragile position in the IPA-affiliated institution, which not only condemned, but defined homosexuality as a perversion and prohibited the affiliation of homosexual candidates. (p. 247)

Usually, the rejection of gay candidates from psychoanalytic training occurred in the first stage of selection during the admission interviews. The interviews would ordinarily be conducted separately by at least two, and in the case of the SBP-SP often three, psychoanalysts from the Institutes. The only published material that touches the topic of homophobia in the São Paulo Society consists of a passing mention of it in a larger debate about training analysis. In 2008, a roundtable carried out by the *Jornal de Psicanálise* (Journal of Psychoanalysis), published by the SBP-SP can be used to briefly illustrate the issue not only in Brazil, but also in Argentina and Italy. The debate over the changes that occurred in official IPA policies in the professional training of psychoanalysts, culminated in discussion of the issue of homosexuality of the candidates. In his contribution, Abel Fainstein, from the Argentine Psychoanalytic Association (*Asociación Psicoanalítica Argentina*—APA) said that when he began his professional training over 30 years ago: 'homosexuality was clearly within the list of perversions that had to be cured' (p. 39). However, more recently, the Argentinian society raised objections to an analyst in his country who explicitly considered homosexuality to be a perversion, which highlighted a 'change in the imaginary about homosexuality' (Bolognini et al., 2008, p. 38).

Luiz Carlos Menezes,[5] from the SBP-SP, recalled the discomfort that a well-known psychoanalyst, Luiz Meyer, had caused during the 1990s, during a meeting of interviewers that dealt with selection criteria. In that

---

[5] All persons interviewed for this paper agreed to have their testimonies published.

meeting, he represented an openly gay candidate he had interviewed and, in his view, should have been accepted. 'There was a certain attitude of the IPA in regards to that' (p. 39) Menezes stated. When participating in the discussion, Meyer mentioned the saga of North-American homosexual psychoanalysts[6] to illustrate how wrong theories were about male homosexuality at the time of the application process and during the training analysis. Stefano Bolognini, from the Italian Psychoanalytic Society (*Società Psicoanalitica Italiana*—SPI) commented on two gay men who were going through the application process: one of them had had his application denied, since it was concluded that he was deeply disturbed. The second applicant, who had already been rejected at his first application because he was gay, had applied again, and Bolognini accepted his application because he seemed to be 'a reflexive and creative person (…) who had an uncommon ability of internal and interpersonal contact' (p. 42).

> In my interview with Luiz Meyer, the psychoanalyst pointed out something of a characterological division of candidates that took place during admission interviews: 'A candidate aiming to undergo training is seen by three interviewers and submitted to an assessment, with varying criteria, and curiously there was always a conjunction of judgements. There was always a group that said 'this one is great', 'this one we'll reject', and there is the 'debatable' group of applicants.'

The candidate that Meyer had represented had belonged to this group of 'debatable' applicants, as he 'talked openly and said that he was homosexual, and had a partner' and he spoke freely about his conjugal life without any pronounced defence or even hesitation. Moreover, to Meyer, he was 'a stable and mature subject, who was interested in and knowledgeable of psychoanalysis… so, there was no real reason, right?'.

There was no objective reason given for the refusal of the applicant for the SBP-SP training offered. Meyer's defence of the candidate was not taken into account, even though he struggled for his position to

---

[6] Meyer was referring to Richard Isay and especially Ralph Roughton, who were the first psychoanalysts to come out as gay men after years of pretending to be heterosexuals. Cf. Isay (1996) and Roughton (2003).

be considered. This happened in 1993, before the 'international winds'[7] that were instrumental in a change of attitude regarding gay candidates both in the São Paulo Society and in other IPA Institutes. 'Nowadays, in the Society, a person will not be ruled out of training for being homosexual,' says Meyer.

Meyer no longer participates in the conversations and decisions of the faculty in charge of the admission interviews. However, Liana Pinto Chaves, the Secretary of Admission and also a training analyst, was able to provide information on the current state of affairs regarding the consideration of gay candidates in the Society. She completed her psychoanalytic training in the London-based Institute of Psycho-analysis.[8] I enquired if there was currently any kind of debate about homosexuality and psychoanalytic training. Chavez responded that so far, since she left the Institute in 1979, it was not something that had she had heard of, nor was it published in any institutional by-law.

Given her position as the Secretary of Admission of the SBP-SP, I was naturally curious to know how the interviewers approve or reject candidates. She told me that:

> In the interviews, what we try to assess is the possibility of emotional contact, for example. The sensibility, fluency, if we can evaluate the familiarity of the person with his own mental life. That is what we try to assess, roughly.

With those criteria in mind, we would ask why a gay candidate could not satisfy them a priori. Chavez's first answer which was also voiced

---

[7] Ralph Roughton's declaration in the International Congress of the IPA, in Barcelona, 1997, that he was gay and already a seasoned psychoanalyst from Emory, Atlanta, strongly reverberated among the IPA-affiliated Societies. This was especially because Roughton's image and identity had been spread through the institutions through a debate in *International Psychoanalysis*, an official albeit short-lived journal of the IPA. Even if Luiz Meyer was not present when Roughton publicly made his *outing* in Barcelona (unlike Liana Chaves and Oswaldo Netto, who were there), he testifies to Roughton's impact, attributing to him a good part of the changes that happened both in the IPA and the SBP-SP.

[8] According to Ellis (1994), even if it was not as strongly hit by the protests from the gay community as the North-American Psychoanalytical Societies, the London-based Institute of Psychoanalysis was the one who took the biggest hit when protests against homophobia arrived in Great Britain, since many of its members were strongly against the entrance of gay candidates.

in the debate promoted by the *Revista de Psicanálise* (Bolognini et al., 2008), was that there was a tendency then to conflate homosexuality with perversion. However, she stated that the contemporary trend is to consider the sexual orientation of the candidate not as an 'element of exclusion, of alienation' in itself. Nevertheless, 'issues of character,' such as perversion, are still relevant.

As there has never been an explicit rule to refuse openly gay candidates, Liana Chavez says that, in the SBP-SP, she was never confronted with explicit guidance towards the rejection of them. In effect, we could think that the immediate association of perversion and homosexuality served as a judgement regarding the impossibility of a training admission in the psychoanalytic Society. On that topic, Chavez has a very practical example, of an analysand who was afflicted both by the AIDS epidemic at the end of the last century, and from the dangers of the clandestine sexual commerce and massive stigma that struck marginal sexualities:

> I saw a homosexual patient, the first patient I had when I came back to Brazil. He was a psychiatrist and died from AIDS-related complications. I don't think that he was qualified to be an analyst, not because he was a homosexual, but because of his absolutely suicidal behaviour. Since this was before AIDS, this man… after he did those kinds of follies, he swallowed loads of anti-infection pills. Being a doctor, he was self-medicating the next day, with an enormous load of medicines to avoid infectious diseases.

Based on these attitudes, Chavez is careful to note that the patient would not be admitted to psychoanalytic training not on the basis of his sexuality per se, but because of his 'perversity and suicidal behaviour.' Additionally, even if she was directly responsible for the most immediate stage of selection of candidates to training, Chavez did not participate or have any contact with discussions about cases when candidates were refused after their interviews on the basis of their homosexuality.

However, in a very similar account to the one reported by Luiz Meyer, a psychoanalyst—who prefers to remain anonymous—seems to have had his admittance deferred solely on the base of his sexual orientation. The then candidate, now a reputed psychoanalyst with a recognised academic trajectory, recounted that he had been interested in psychoanalysis since childhood, and at a certain point in the 1980s, his own psychoanalyst had become a training analyst in the SBP-SP. 'As my analyst became a training analyst,'[9] says the interviewee,

> The possibility was open for me to think about a training that was interrupted in the interviews. My curriculum was accepted, and I remember being very excited. The first interview was utterly ridiculous, a thing that wasn't an interview, really. It was just a ceremonial welcoming from a totally uninterested person… The following two interviews were different, there wasn't any kind of unease.

I asked him if there was any sort of feedback from the interviews, besides the impression of an interviewer's lack of interest, to which the psychoanalyst responded:

> No, there wasn't any response after I was denied entrance, no justification, but since in one of the interviews I opened that I was already married, you know? And… I was married and, well, that should have been it. Because afterwards, I mean, I'm only speculating, because there wasn't anything specific said or written about that. I said that I was married to a man, I've been with this man ever since. By chance or maybe not that much and… Then I think one thing is linked to the other.

The account of this psychoanalyst is very similar to the report given by Luiz Meyer regarding the candidate he sought not to be denied.[10] Both applicants were in stable, long relationships, talked free and openly about the gender of their partners as if it was not an issue (and again, why should it be?), and presented a vivid and experienced interest in psychoanalysis. The route to become an analyst at that time was still primarily bound to the official training circuits (the Societies affiliated to the IPA) and the prejudice of some members and silent accordance of most of

[9] His own analyst, who knew very well he was gay, had encouraged him to undergo training at the Society.

[10] Even if we would hardly find any utility in speculating about the identity of both candidates, it is worth mentioning that the distance between Meyer's interviewee and the one referred here is of 10 years.

them, could have discouraged the psychoanalyst from following on with his training. It is worthy of note that the 'unofficial,' non-IPA-related circuits of psychoanalytic training (the Lacanian ones, for example), were more critical and also more inclusive, and have been growing in scale and importance for some time now in São Paulo. It would not be an overstatement that here and elsewhere, such circuits should be accounted as one of those 'winds' that have been forcing the official Societies to change their practices.

The degree of openness and lack of scrutiny with which homophobic discourses circulated among psychoanalysts is also noticeable, no matter the theoretical makeup that underpinned the utterances. After a long academic trajectory in psychoanalysis, at the beginning of his private practice, the interviewee said that:

> when I was about to see my patients, I heard from a colleague – who ended up being the first to refer me to patients – 'but you are a homosexual, are you really going to practice psychoanalysis?' And I said 'well, yes?' 'Because your relationship to the Law, whether you want it or not, is another one. You should consider that…' And I was very upset, because it was a psychoanalytical critique, supposedly psychoanalytical, but it was just prejudice disguised as psychoanalysis. A very cultured person, very educated. I suffered a lot from that because, well, it's my project. And then I heard more… that since my relationship to the Law was another one, because I'm a homosexual, maybe I shouldn't see male heterosexual patients, since I couldn't deal with castration.

On one occasion, he was asked by a friend about his being excluded from the SBP-SP psychoanalytic training and was asked: 'why in the world did you have to tell them that?' This is a comment that is not unfamiliar to many gay candidates who prepare themselves for the interviews. As an irony of fate and a comical side note, the psychoanalyst said that his practice is marked by numerous heterosexual patients that end up getting pregnant during the psychoanalytic process.

Even if accounts of gay candidates being rejected from training are known among members of the SBP-SP and to some of its representatives, the Society is regarded as much more inclusive than other IPA-affiliated

Institutes across the globe.[11] Moreover, Meyer states that the Society has never restricted training to medical practitioners, in distinction from the Rio de Janeiro Society, for example. Aside from not allowing lay candidates at its beginnings, the Rio de Janeiro Society historically faced three major splits, which resulted in four distinct Psychoanalytical Societies. Meyer himself summarises a consensus from the members of the SBP-SP:

> The Society has its own way of avoiding conflict. You can see that in Rio there are three Societies, Porto Alegre has three, as well as London… our Society looks forward to, as it were, living with differences.

Among these 'differences,' there is a psychoanalyst who is noted by his presence and activity in the SBP-SP. A medical practitioner, trained psychiatrist and member of the Society, Oswaldo Ferreira Leite Netto was immediately cited by all of the interviewees as someone who has both addressed directly the matter of psychoanalytic homophobia and been used as an example to illustrate that the Society is no longer homophobic. The ubiquity of Netto in the accounts of the interviewees covers the issue of the gay candidate/psychoanalyst in the São Paulo Society with a very distinctive personalistic façade, unlike any account I have seen before. It is as if everybody would say: 'the Society is not homophobic, we have Oswaldo Netto among us.'

With regard to homophobia in the wider São Paulo Society, the trajectory and events narrated by Oswaldo Netto elicit a portrait of the journey of the psychoanalytic candidate during the last decades of IPA dominance, along with the dilemmas faced by an openly gay man who wished to undergo training and practice the Freudian legacy. Netto comes from the most progressive pedagogical circuits of São Paulo, during a time marked both by the escalation of the State's repressive apparatus during the Brazilian civil-military dictatorship, and by the growth of pockets of resistance in the city. Through his youth and medical training, he gave

[11] Cf. Ellis (1994), Cunningham (1991), Roughton (2003), Drescher (2008), Bulamah and Kupermann (2018).

a remarkable account of how psychoanalysis was entangled with psychiatry during those years, similar to the circumstances in the United States until the latter half of the last century:

> Back then, everyone who was cool wasn't looking for a psychiatric training to be a psychiatrist, the way things go nowadays, Clinical Psychiatrist. There was no such thing back then. In general, psychiatrists were the ones who were interested in psychoanalysis.

Besides, according to Netto, even in its official and institutionalised form, psychoanalysis was seen as the path to a subversive technique and knowledge about the subject (and not something out-of-touch or close-minded, which was an impression reinforced by the Lacanian groups). The subversiveness matched both Netto's interest in, and his experiences with, the associations that resisted the Civil-Military Dictatorship. 'As a good Bolshevik—to whom sex and love was a waste of time and revolutionary energy,' Netto joked, 'I didn't have anything to answer when I was asked about my relationship status' in the admission interviews, because he was single when he applied for training.

It should be noted that Netto's personal analysis, which was undertaken years before his admission to the SBP-SP and throughout his training, was marked by a proper psychoanalytical attitude by his training analyst. Even if Netto says that his sexuality was a conflicting matter in itself, it is noticeable that there was never an effort from his analyst to go beyond listening and analysing the conflicts, towards the dangerous (and unfortunately common) goal of 'curing' him of homosexuality. The action of this 'classic Bionian' on him 'was always very liberating... at least my homosexuality was always validated, authorised and de-pathologised in my own analysis.'

However, for the recent history of SBP-SP, Netto's most important actions are twofold. First, his initiatives to bring to light the issues of homosexuality and homophobia in institutionalised psychoanalysis through study groups and papers[12] were widely read by Brazilian psychoanalysts. Secondly, but no less important, was his position as the head of

[12] See, for example, Martins et al. (2014).

a psychoanalytical branch in the powerful Institute of Psychotherapy of the Hospital das Clínicas for more than twenty years. In a time when psychoanalysis seems ever more separate from clinical psychiatry, both in Brazil and elsewhere, it is striking that the Freudian discipline keeps attracting attention among young medical practitioners who end up undergoing psychoanalytical training.

In contrast to the many study groups offered by the SBP-SP Scientific Committee, which were usually joined by only a few people, the homosexuality and homophobia study group organised by Netto began with forty people. In this group, participants not only debated the taboo topic of the homosexual candidate, but some of them openly identified as gay men undergoing psychoanalytic training, were eager to talk about their experiences and understood the importance of being subjects of a history that until very recently had identified them only as objects.

Many members of this study group were not only associated members of the SBP-SP, but were also introduced to psychoanalysis after their psychiatric training in the Institute of Psychiatry of the Hospital das Clínicas, through the psychoanalytical course that Netto taught. The interest of these young practitioners in undergoing psychoanalytic training at the SBP-SP was praised by the older members of the institution, because they not only seemed to bring an air of freshness and renovation, but also to provide a throwback to the days when psychoanalysis used to be of such an interest to psychiatrists.

Rodrigo Lage, psychiatrist and associated member of the SBP-SP, was introduced to psychoanalysis at the aforementioned course at the end of the psychiatric training, during his residency from 2001 until 2003. He recounted that:

> I ended the residence with a very mechanistic training, anchored mainly in biological psychiatry, but at the same time I was very ambivalent… because I was undergoing clinical supervision with Oswaldo, which was very psychoanalytic.

I asked Lage if he considered himself as part of a larger process in the IPA, as it opened up to some matters in a less prejudicious attitude, and his answer concerned both his presence and the impact of his identity (also contingent to the critical mass he takes part in) and also the initiative of de-pathologising homosexuality and problematising homophobia:

> I think I'm a part of this process, meaning that... it was a huge group of psychoanalysts that joined this homosexuality and psychoanalysis study group. Not only analysts identified as gay, but a wide group of analysts in our generation, to whom this is not really a problem. Or even better, it is a problem, meaning that it shouldn't be ignored or denied. Because a great change that I see is that maybe there was before a certain discourse like 'well, this is not a problem, this person can operate analytically', but this is a problem, since many people sometime end up being barred at the admission interviews because of matters clearly riddled with prejudices. I think a change is beginning, even among psychoanalysts who are not gay and say that 'this is an anachronism, this damages psychoanalysis' thinking structure, this denies what is most radical in Freud.'

Even if the candidate passed the interviews in any way and could camouflage himself enough in the training analysis—or put himself in an extraordinarily submissive position to the point of succumbing to the analysts' compulsory heterosexuality during the most conservative periods of the psychoanalytical societies affiliated to the IPA—undergoing clinical supervisions with members of the Society would still be a liability in training, because it was one of the operators for institutional heterosexism (Mitchell, 1981). Similar to his personal analysis, considered by Lage as 'very much free' from heterosexist restraints and attitudes, the supervisions he underwent received the same judgement:

> I never felt this, the 'petulance' of homophobia, in my supervisions and training analysis. But one thing that is very entangled with the surveillance of homosexuality, to those groups that are occupied with it, are the attempts to associate behaviours, modes of existence, marriage, children, long-term relationships as if they were determinant to a certain kind of psychism. A specific subjective life, that is, the vigilance not only rests upon sexual orientation, but is a subjective structuring. I haven't felt oppressed in my personal analysis, nor in supervisions, and I don't think that is a rule at all... I was lucky, somehow.

It is also important to report that Lage also expanded the theme of heterosexism to include not only sexual orientation, but also the reproductive, monogamic family and the role of the State in regulating what should, or should not be, deemed to comprise a family unit. This expansion reaches to the point of contemporary queer theory's critique of the structure and violence of gender norms and the technologies employed to maintain them.

In the end, Rodrigo Lage echoed all interviewed psychoanalysts in promoting the idea that the SBP-SP has been through a period of embracing themes that used to be alien to the institution (such as using psychoanalysis to interrogate political themes, including the gay issue), and also to candidates and members who would be aprioristically framed as problematic and, therefore, excluded. This might lead us to believe that the SBP-SP is engaging in a process of opening up to those figures that used to represent the outer limits of possibility for the official psychoanalytical training in São Paulo, as elsewhere. However, the stories told by the local representatives of the IPA-affiliated Society reproduces the same script that the IPA as a whole enacts, with some exceptional local specificities that do not alter the general picture.

Local specificities are, for example, the tradition in SBP-SP of accommodating conflicts inside a frame, avoiding major splits, dissidences and the founding of other Societies and, also, the original openness to lay candidates. The debate is still alive regarding whether these characteristics could help understanding in part why the SBP-SP is seen as more receptive or liberal to openly gay candidates. Certainly (and very explicitly) it is, again, very open regarding admittance of non-medics and distinct psychoanalytic traditions to its body. Rodrigo Lage, for example, feels that his interest in French and even Lacanian psychoanalysis is not only accepted, but also stimulated among members and groups of the Society.

With regard to the wider picture, why does the local reality not seem to change this historical frame? In the interviews recounted, as in every investigation of homophobia in psychoanalytical institutes, two main figures can be noted as the enunciators of psychoanalytic prejudice: the psychoanalyst who is aware of prejudice, and the candidate or even trained psychoanalyst who denounces the prejudice that he himself has faced. Richard Isay, Ralph Roughton, John Fryer (*Doctor H. Anonymous*)—among many others who did not want their identities to be revealed—for example, are representatives of the latter group, to whom we could add the anonymous psychoanalyst shown here to have been barred in the admission interviews.

Oswaldo Netto and Rodrigo Lage not mentioning homophobia as the wall that set them apart from the possibility of training at the SBP-SP, insulated them in the Institute or had forced them to a late *coming out* after years of hiding under heterosexual masks, is indeed a sign of change. On the other hand, as we have also seen, there have always been psychoanalysts like Liana Chaves and Luiz Meyer, who did not accept and tried to fight psychoanalytic homophobia whenever they had the chance from inside the institution, even if they did not identify themselves as gay. They align themselves with the likes of Robert Stoller and Judd Marmor, allies in the disassembly of a machine that, since the death of Freud, was ingrained in the IPA as a form of gathering social prestige and *status quo* while throwing away the critical and deconstructive power of psychoanalysis.

However, there is a third element that, even in its muteness and invisibility, personifies the history of institutional homophobia—both the homophobia denounced thoroughly (in the United States, for example), and that which did not create the same reaction, such as in São Paulo. This element is the interviewer who denies the entrance of the gay candidate, or the supervisor who states that the direction of treatment given by his student is wrong because the analysand keeps longing for same-sex relationships, or the training analyst who makes explicitly clear that his analysand, or the candidate undergoing training, is about to be 'cured,' and almost made a heterosexual. Even if we imagine that this no longer happens, the candidate and analysand is not going to become an analyst (at least today, not an analyst trained by the SBP), because he is considered to be 'incurable.' Nowadays, when it is almost impossible that an openly discriminatory opinion could be voiced without immediate backlash, those who would voice them have retreated, but almost every interviewee that was present here gave an account about someone who was openly discriminated against solely on the basis of their non-normative sexualities.

Some of these accounts were so traumatic that it is better they remain unpublished, so as to protect the victim from reliving the trauma, and there is still an effort to cover up the more brutal perpetrators of homophobic and heterosexist violence, seemingly to protect the institution that still accommodates them. In the absence of more explicit material, I present this research not only as a hypothesis, but as an experience.

This chapter points to the fact that there is a progressive and significant change happening not only in the North-American or European IPA Societies. If we take São Paulo as a representative of the Southern psychoanalytic institutions, homosexuality does not seem to crash into a presumptuous institutional border like it did before. However, given that there is a traditional way of alleviating conflict to maintain its integrity, the enunciators of the homophobic silence of the institutionalised psychoanalytic movement in São Paulo seem to slowly wither, in a silence not unlike the one that allowed the unwritten rule to act for such a long time.

References

Bolognini, S., Horta, A., Helena, B., & Maria, F. (2008). Debate—A análise didática. *Jornal De Psicanálise, 41*(74), 25–54.

Bulamah, L. (2020). *História de uma regra não escrita: a proscrição da homossexualidade masculina no movimento psicanalítico.* Zagodoni.

Bulamah, L., & Kupermann, D. (2018). The proscription of male homosexuality in the history of the institutionalized psychoanalytic movement. *Ágora, 21*(3), 301–312.

Cunningham, R. (1991). When is a pervert not a pervert? *British Journal of Psychotherapy, 8*(1), 48–70.

Drescher, J. (2008). A history of homosexuality and organized psychoanalysis. *The Journal of the American Academy of Psychoanalysis and Dynamic Psychiatry, 36*(3), 443–460.

Ellis, M. L. (1994). Lesbians, gay men and psychoanalytic training. *Free Associations, 4*(4), 501–517.

Isay, R. (1996). *Becoming gay: The journey to self-acceptance.* Vintage.

Martins, E. S. T., Leite, R. L., Porto, T. S., & Netto, O. F. L. (2014). Psicanálise e homossexualidade—da apropriação à desapropriação médico-moral. *Ide (são Paulo), 36*(57), 163–177.

Maya, A. (2007). O que os analistas pensam sobre a homossexualidade? *Psychê, 11*(21), 85–104.

Mitchell, S. A. (1981). The psychoanalytic treatment of homosexuality: Some technical considerations. *International Review of Psychoanalysis, 8*, 63–80.

Oliveira, C. L. M. V. (2006). *História da psicanálise—São Paulo (1920–1969).* Escuta.

Roughton, R. (2003). The international psychoanalytical association and homosexuality. *Journal of Gay & Lesbian Mental Health, 7*(1), 189–196.

Sociedade Brasileira de Psicanalise. (1994). *Álbum de família: imagens, fontes e idéias da Psicanálise em São Paulo.* Casa do Psicólogo.

16

Pioneers of Lacan's Ideas in Brazil: An Essay on the History of the Psychoanalytic Movement

Francisco Capoulade

In 2019, at the First International Symposium on the History of Psychoanalysis in Latin America, I began to collate information about the events surrounding the initial reception of the ideas of the French psychoanalyst Jacques Lacan in Brazil. My practice as a psychoanalyst in the city of Campinas-SP gave me easy access to such information. I began to gather reports from observers of these events—among them Durval Checchinato and Geraldino Alves Ferreira Netto—and indirect witnesses. Along the way, I was able to find at least two relevant documents. The first was unpublished and refers to the postgraduate course in clinical psychology at the Pontifical Catholic University of Campinas, and the second was a document written by Jacques Laberge about the foundation of the Centre of Freudian Studies (CFS) and the first meetings that were held there during the 1970s.

F. Capoulade (✉)
IPEP—Instituto de Pesquisa e Estudos em Psicanálise nos Espaços Públicos, São Paulo, Brazil

B. Mandelbaum et al. (eds.), *Brazilian Psychosocial Histories of Psychoanalysis*, Studies in the Psychosocial,
https://doi.org/10.1007/978-3-030-78509-3_16

The research is at an initial stage and aims to understand the first proponents of Lacan's ideas in Brazil. It has raised the following questions: What academic background did they have? What were the cultural characteristics demonstrated in their interpretation of Lacan's thought? What social and political context did they occupy? How did they create psychoanalytic clinics? In this, I found useful Finchelstein's (2007) idea of a 'transnational perspective,' which is where the appropriation of psychoanalysis is considered in a broader context of circulation and dissemination, as well as a perspective that goes beyond geographical lines, and that builds transnational networks of intellectual exchanges (Plotkin & Damousi, 2009).

The first part of my research focussed on the history of the PUC-Campinas document and the founding document of the Centre of Freudian Studies (CFS) between 1974 and 1979. The founders were located across Brazil, which, while challenging in terms of travel and communication, enabled the wider distribution of the ideas of psychoanalysis across the country, at a time when travel and dissemination would otherwise be restricted by time or finances.

Transmission of Psychoanalysis at University

At the end of 2017, I was able to interview Geraldino Alves Ferreira Netto, during which, he provided me with the first document. He touched on the subject, almost unwittingly, that he had taken a postgraduate course and that it would have been there that Lacan or rather Lacan's ideas were first presented to him. Ferreira Netto confirmed that he had attended the course during 1974 and 1975 and the document was signed by the course coordinator Prof. Luiz Carlos Nogueira, who also appeared in the foundation document of the CFS.

I then went to PUC-Campinas to make sure that there was indeed some document that would confirm what I had in hand. I contacted Professor Vera Cury,[1] who was the coordinator of the postgraduate

[1] I would like to express my gratitude to Professor Vera Cury for providing the document cited in this essay.

psychology course at the time: she promptly sent an electronic document. The document sent was a copy of the course curriculum, entitled 'Analytical Techniques I,' which was taught by Durval Checchinato and was part of the postgraduate course in clinical psychology. The document contained an outline of the subjects to be covered in the course including Saussurian linguistics, Structuralism, the history of the Freudian School in Paris, and the constitution of the subject, as well as clinical seminars.

The recommended bibliography did not contain any text by Lacan, even in French, since there was still no translation into Brazilian Portuguese.[2] The Saussure General Linguistics Course contained a text on Structuralism: one by Anika Rifflet Lemaire that was entitled *'Jacques Lacan*[3] *- an introduction to Lacan'* and a text with an English title *The physical control of the mind*.

This document was dated 1974 and contains two important pieces of information: firstly, it confirms the secondary and tertiary bibliographic sources that encapsulate the discipline. Secondly, it demonstrates the preference for a reading of Lacan that is guided by a debate with linguistics and structuralism.

On the first aspect, it is important to point out that, according to sources (Ferreira Netto and Laberge), Durval Checchinato attended a number of Lacan's seminars during his time in France and was accepted as a member of the École Freudienne de Paris in 1976. This would have been the same year that Laberge was also accepted.[4] This allows us to infer that having mastered the French language, he was able to enjoy both written and spoken elements of Lacan's teaching. Ferreira Netto stated that: 'Durval had arrived from France, he trained there. So, he was much more aware of things' (interview recorded on 11/15/2017).

---

2 The first Brazilian translation of Lacan's texts appeared in 1978.

3 This text was translated by Checchinato and was widely disseminated during that period. Regina Steffen, a psychoanalyst who works in Campinas, with whom I exchanged a lot of information about the beginning of the diffusion of Lacan's ideas in Brazil, was part of the group formed by Checchinato at the end of the 1970s and attests to the importance of this text for psychoanalysts in formation.

4 This information concerns an informal conversation in which Laberge tells me that both he and Checchinato were received as members of the *École Freudienne de Paris* in 1976. However, Roudinesco and Plon (1998), in the *Dictionary of Psychoanalysis*, in the entry Brazil, state that the year of receipt of Checchinato was 1973.

However, the fact that no text by Lacan appears in the bibliography of this discipline is noticeable. In fact, Ferreira Netto (who attended this course and was part of the study group that was created at that time) said in the same interview that Lacan's texts were used in French by the students; even if they had some difficulty, they all tried to read in French. In his words:

> In 1975, this group in the presence of Durval – it was he who set the tone to put Lacan in evidence, he had a very good basis – began to study, albeit with very few resources. From 1975 to 1979 we had no Lacanian text in Portuguese. What we had was the *Écrits*, seminar 1, seminar 2, seminar 11 and seminar 20. So, it meant the following: to learn Lacan at that time you had to know French. The luck was that this whole group that was here in Campinas, and I entered exactly at that moment as a student, I read in French. Then we would take the *Écrits* and read them in locks and ravines because each one understood in his own way. And the seminars helped us a lot. I had seminars 1 and 2 there from Lacan's beginning, still from the theory of the imaginary. Seminar 11 already puts Lacan in the symbolic and a little of the real. And Seminar 20, then, already went beyond any possibility of understanding at the time. (Interview recorded on 11/15/2017)

The texts indicated by Ferreira Netto had been published between 1974 and 1979, which was confirmed by the work of psychoanalyst and historian Roudinesco.

> After the publication of volume XI in 1973, two other volumes were published in 1975 according to this principle: volume I (1953-4) and volume XX (1972-3). It will then be three years before volume II (1954-5) appears, 1978. (Roudinesco, 2008, p. 55)

In addition to these seminars, Lacan's collection of texts, *Écrits*, was published in 1966 in France.

Checchinato had a religious and erudite background and his psychoanalytical trajectory in France enabled him to correspond with important names from the psychoanalytical scene of the 1960s and 1970s (Roudinesco, 2008). He was pivotal in the reception and dissemination of

Lacan's ideas, having been a pioneer and a true advocate of Lacanian psychoanalysis in Brazil. From his work derived the Campinense Psychoanalysis Society (later renamed as the Campinense Psychoanalysis Association), of which he was for a time one of the presidents. Nevertheless, we need to investigate Checchinato further in order to answer clearly the questions raised at the beginning of this chapter.

Secondly, we will see in the founding document of the CFS the influence of linguistics and anthropology on the movement of these first Lacanians.

The two documents issued by PUC-Campinas comprise a discovery that establishes Lacan's ideas were in circulation during the early 1970s, allowing us to see that this academic undertaking was a fundamental element in the formation of various psychoanalysts, which is reinforced by Ferreira Netto himself, who still works as a psychoanalyst in the city of Campinas.

About the Foundation

In July 2019, I received the following email from Durval Checchinato:

> Dear Francisco,
>
> I received your invitation. I appreciate it. However, although I have lived with Lacan and the great masters of this golden age of psychoanalysis in France, as with Serge Leclaire, Maud Mannoni, Jean Clavreul, Moustapha Safouan, and others, I do not feel comfortable recording anything. In fact, within my limitations, I think this would be of less importance. I prefer to leave my writings as a testimony of my studies and clinical practice. I also let my students witness my clinical work.
>
> A hug for you and good work.
>
> Durval.

At this point, we had already conducted the interview and Checchinato had given me the original founding document of the Centre of Freudian Studies (CFS). The conversation was friendly and fruitful.

The second document is an account of the national meetings of the CFS, which gains importance when considered in the wider context. The document was written by Jacques Laberge and was presented at the 6th National Meeting of the CFS in January 1978. The material that I had access to was the same text, but revised a year later.[5]

In yellow, typewritten pages, Laberge's text is entitled 'The History of a Project, the Centre of Freudian Studies' and briefly narrates the foundation of the CFS through a summary of what happened at each of the six meetings. The text also allows us to observe the spirit through which various characters are connected in order to think and practice psychoanalysis based on Lacan's ideas.

> Talking about institutionalization is an invitation to chart our paths and review the progress made. When, on July 16, 1975, I travelled to São Paulo to meet Durval Checchinato and Luiz Carlos Nogueira, a long series of displacements began, which will always prove necessary for symbolic creativity, and the contestation of constantly renewed dual relationships. The geographical challenge of distance entails sacrifice, in its appearance as an obstacle, [but it] operated, and still operates today, as an occasion for encounter and questioning, as well as permission for a salutary slide. From an informal conversation on 16 July, came the idea of holding the First National Meeting. It was the founding decision. (Laberge, 1985, p. 5)

On 16 July1975, Laberge and Ivan Corrêa travelled to São Paulo to meet Durval Checchinato and Luiz Carlos Nogueira, which was their first personal contact. According to Laberge, Jeanne-Marie Machado de Freitas Interlandi was also present, but she does not appear in the meeting minutes, despite the personal meeting occurring before the formal meeting. Jeanne-Marie Machado de Freitas Interlandi was a teacher at USP and a sociologist, but no other information on her is available.

The first formal Meeting took place on 4 October 1975, in Ilha do Sul, Pinheiros, São Paulo. In attendance were Durval Checchinato, Ivan Corrêa, Jeanne-Marie Machado de Freitas Interlandi, Jacques Laberge

[5] In August 2020 in a Skype conversation with Jacques Laberge, who currently lives in Recife, he added details of this period and soon after our conversation he sent me a copy of the same text that had been published in 1985 on the occasion of the celebration of the 10th anniversary of the CFS.

and Luiz Carlos Nogueira. The first objective was to spread Lacan's thought in the media (newspapers, for example). It was a closed group that expressed a wish to be open to everyone, analysts or not, 'spoken before speaking,' a contradiction pointed out by Laberge.

The group decided not to adopt the word 'school' since such a term would tend to institutionalise even more what is not in principle meant to be institutionalised. Thus, the name Centre for Freudian Studies seemed more appropriate to them, for a centre, they thought, would be a less institutionalised term. However, the issue of identity hung over the group:

> The return to Freud corresponds to a practice. To call oneself a Freudian is to affirm this return. But the question arises: are others Kleinians, or more eclectic; are we more Freudian or more Lacanian? The answer 'more Freudian because more Lacanian', however elegant, leaves the question hanging. (Laberge, 1985, p.6)

The meeting provided actions for each of the attendees: Laberge was responsible for the areas of studies and publications, Checchinato for analytical practice issues and Nogueira for the secretariat.

On the same afternoon of 4 October, Checchinato spoke briefly in an open meeting about Lacan and the *École Freudienne* on the subject of 'How to express our connection to Paris and to experience this inspiration?' Emphasis was placed on the ruptures of 1953 and 1964, to provide a better understanding (an issue that resurfaced at the 4th meeting). The theme of the training analysis and the subversion proposed by Lacan was on the agenda, that is, now it is the patient who becomes his own training analyst.

Checchinato was in charge of presenting clinical work and discussing theoretical aspects for this presentation: his work with psychotics is noteworthy. There was also a debate on the time and duration of the session, it was unanimous that the 50-minute sessions were an obsession that did not respect anyone's singular time.

The following day (second and last), Laberge also presented a 20-page paper on the transference in Lacan. 'It was the first text written for the meeting: a panoramic view of the theme, from Lacan's first allusion to the transference, in 1946, until 1964, after which he did not have the unpublished texts.' The issue was to be of great relevance to the group, which is why it was introduced and discussed at subsequent meetings. It is important to note that Laberge excluded Lacan's reflection on the transference from Plato's Banquet since this text had come into his hands 'at the last minute.' This was one of the main reasons that made him propose to return to the subject in subsequent meetings.[6]

The second Meeting was spread across 6–8 February 1976 in the same place as the first. People from other states were beginning to join the movement, among which included Edilene, Lena and Maria do Carmo from Recife; Maria Isabel and Chantal from Rio de Janeiro; Pérsio and Sebastiana Guimarães from Curitiba.

Checchinato, Pérsio and Sebastiana Guimarães, and Ivan Corrêa all presented clinical cases in the first half of the meeting, while Laberge presented his summary of the seminar on transference in the other half. It can be seen how concerned Checchinato was to work with clinical issues. This is explicit in practically all the meetings reported in this document.

An important decision taken at this meeting was the creation of a CFS collection, with the book *The navel and the voice: psychoanalysis of two children* by Denis Vasse being the inaugural text.

At the third Meeting,[7] Laberge brought the following statement that had been published by Luiz Carlos Nogueira in the 1976 newsletter: 'We have been informed of the existence of the Freudian College in Rio de Janeiro, which has the same objectives as the Centre for Freudian Studies. We are planning a meeting to fuse both' (Laberge, 1985, p. 8). It seems that the term fusion, according to Laberge, did not sound good and put the two groups in a position of mistrust, 'fear of being swallowed up by each other' (Laberge, 1985, p. 9).

Magno Machado Dias (director since 1971) was also present at the third Meeting. He spoke about the Borromean knot and said that the

[6] In conversation with Laberge, I asked about these texts. He told me that they will probably be published in the coming years. But first, in this year 2021, he intends to publish tales and stories about the legends of fishermen in Recife, a subject he commented on with Lacan in the 1970s and which Lacan asked him to send him, something that never happened.

[7] The absence of Alduísio Moreira de Souza, one of the founders, was a striking point in this meeting.

college would assume responsibility for the organisation and payment of expenses of the next meeting. Laberge was quoted as saying: 'There were misunderstandings, disagreements at that meeting. Fight of heirs? Ghost of fusion? The style did not help either. But the history goes round and round' (ibid.).

The subject of transference was still fashionable, with other members allowing themselves to talk about it from other (French) authors of psychoanalysis: Dolto, Maud and Octave Mannoni, Leclaire.

The fourth Meeting took place in Brasilia in February 1977 and focussed on the Lacanian subject. It appears to have been an important moment for the movement. During the meeting, members presented papers articulating the theme of the subject from a range of theoretical perspectives, dialoguing between psychoanalysis and psychology, linguistics and anthropology. Themes, such as 'The movement of return to Freud and the issue of the subject,' 'The subject in linguistics and psychology,' were presented, and the work of authors such as Chomsky, Levi-Strauss, Herder, Humboldt and Saussure was referred to.

The theme of the subject, as proposed by Lacan, begins to gain strength in this meeting, producing a kind of decentralisation. This means the division into groups and subgroups by states across Brazil. According to Laberge, São Paulo's lack of attendance at the third Meeting was especially problematic.

> Significant detail: the link between regional groups and national meetings. Luiz Carlos observed one day that the group from São Paulo broke up because few attended the 3rd Meeting (What good can come out of Recife?) and only started again after the 4th Meeting, that of Brasilia. (…) The national meetings carry out certain displacements that reappear in the regional groups and allow the emergence of new characters in the following meetings. It is interesting to note that the people from Recife who presented work from the 3rd Meeting had gone to São Paulo for the previous meeting. Geographical displacement appears as a condition for new displacements for those who belong to the Centre of Freudian Studies (Laberge, 1985, p.10)

When considering the aspects of psychoanalytic theory, it is important to consider the geographical spread as it reflects the nature of the subject as decentralised, without essence and lacking synthesis. This decentralisation, on the other hand, has contributed to greater articulation between interlocutors in positions of equality, and no longer relies upon relationships between the masters of a particular place and the pupils of other places; 'if it is to perpetuate the position of a chronic student, there is no encounter that will make up for it' (Laberge, 1985, p.10). This appears to form the basis of a claim to authority by the São Paulo group; however, as far as we can see, this was not accepted either by the Recife group or by the others. What does this mean? Would this be an opportunity to think about post-colonial issues within this nascent movement? This seems to be an urgent reflection to be undertaken within the psychoanalytic movement in Brazil.

The fifth Meeting took place in Campinas and dealt again with the Lacanian subject at the same time that the theme of the psychoanalytic institution returned. Checchinato used an expression of Leclaire to start this meeting: 'the subject gives vertigo.' For Laberge, the subject and institution were relatively conflicting, antagonistic themes. It could be a need to find support again or a floor to stand on. However, the group soon asked itself: 'what kind of floor do we want? (…) To speak of the "Institution" at the meeting on the "Subject," is to recognize that the Centre wants to live under risk, "to be scratched" by the subject. The desire to risk the Centre by compromising it as the subject of the unconscious' (Laberge, 1985, p. 11).

Laberge sought to read the history of psychoanalysis to understand the institution. He criticised the training analysis and then extended this criticism to the *pass*, saying that in the same way, one ends up achieving the same result, a hierarchy. He says, 'despite Lacan's attempt to distinguish degrees and hierarchy, it seems that the much-criticised hierarchy of the International Association has found its way back into the School' (Laberge, 1985, p. 12). This impasse is not limited in scope and remains as a current concern; however, Laberge points to a provisional situation where 'being an analyst is not primarily depending on the institution but refers to the subject himself. There we find ourselves more at the level of desire, desire provoked in the couch, in studies, in supervision' (Ibid.). This is what we understand as the tripod of training in psychoanalysis. But Laberge goes further in his questions: Could there be someone who authorises himself as a psychoanalyst forever? This question remains to be answered.

Laberge, in his eagerness to think of the subject and institution, declares that there is no Centre with a single project. The role of the institution, in this case, would be to consider the projects of each one. In other words, the Centre's project should be based on the participants' projects. If this is not the case, the institution swallows them all. It is first and foremost a matter of each one to find their place in the Centre, be it the beginner who elaborates questions from his first readings of psychoanalysis, or the experienced psychoanalyst who does so from his repeated re-readings.

> How to articulate this space, from the primacy of the signifier, from the questioning of the radicality of the unconscious with other discourses? Several differences arise here, because the interests vary: literature, politics, philosophy, mathematics, linguistics, communication, history, mythology, religions, anthropology, poetry, psychology, the *discourse of the oppressed.*[8] And if Lacan operates his return to Freud from Saussure and Jacobson, in reference to Hegel and Plato's dialogues, why couldn't we, returning to these references, characterize our return through works of Machado de Assis, of Guimarães Rosa, of Graciliano Ramos, of Fernando Pessoa, of the indigenous or northeastern legends, of Capistrano de Abreu's historical speech? (Laberge, 1985, p. 13)

Laberge takes a radical approach to psychoanalysis, and even the training of psychoanalysts, from post-colonial issues and issues of national interest, as thought by Machado de Assis in his text *Instinct of Nationality* (1873). Laberge raises the question: What is the difference between being a psychoanalyst in Paris or in Brazil? None? And the particularity of questions of power and domination, of the marginalisation of the people, with regard to societies and governments as institutions, is there anything to challenge us when we come together in an institution? (Laberge, 1985, p. 13).

It is quite likely that Laberge's studies as a Jesuit contributed fundamentally to psychoanalytic thought in the Brazilian context, not only

[8] My emphasis.

that, but the approach to Lacan and his ideas were facilitated by a more pluralistic and, I would say, secularised perspective, proper to Jesuits. His text makes the concern for the dissemination of psychoanalysis clear, for the training of psychoanalysts and, most importantly, for the commitment to a contextualised and problematised experience, based on local discourses from each region of this country with continental dimensions, even with international interlocutors. The social dimension is contemplated in what Laberge calls the discourse of the oppressed, but what did he mean by that? What is the possibility of including this type of discourse in the psychoanalytical context of that time?

It should also be noted that some of the founders and participants in this movement had a background education in religious institutions, such as Checchinato himself, Laberge and Ferreira Netto, to name a few, which raises the question: What were the consequences of this training for the reception and dissemination of Lacan's thought and for clinical practice? Perhaps another essay could begin to answer these questions.

Final Considerations

This essay aims to present at least two important events in the history of the psychoanalytic movement in Brazil: firstly the teaching of Lacan's ideas at PUC-Campinas in 1974, and secondly, the organisation of national meetings of people interested in those ideas, which culminated in the foundation of the Centre for Psychoanalytic Studies. According to the information provided by these documents, these events seem to be connected and have particular relevance for the psychoanalytic movement. It is possible to observe much of their effects to this day, both in the institutions of psychoanalysis that have derived from these events (I could at least mention the CFS based in Recife and the Campinense Psychoanalysis Association (CPA),[9] based in Campinas-SP), and in the

[9] It is important to say that at the end of writing this essay I received the information that the CPA (in Portuguese ACP) is in the process of cataloguing all its documents. Remembering that it is one of the oldest Lacanian institutions in Brazil, this information can be very valuable for future researchers and those interested in the history of the psychoanalytic movement.

testimony of the psychoanalysts who took part in these meetings and continued in their offices for the following decades. I hope that future research can further clarify these events and the characters who received, disseminated and practised Lacanian psychoanalysis in Brazil.

References

Assis, M. (1873). Notícia da atual literatura brasileira: instinto de nacionalidade. In *Obra completa* (3rd ed.) Rio de Janeiro: Aguilar, v. 3, 801–809.

Finchelstein, F. (2007). Introducción. *Estudios Interdisciplinarios De América Latina Y El Caribe, 18*(1). http://www3.tau.ac.il/ojs/index.php/eial/article/view/428.

Laberge, J. (1985). História de um Projeto, o Centro de Estudos Freudianos. *Revista Céfiso* no.4, Tomo 1, Edição comemorativa dos Dez anos de fundação do C.E.F. do Recife.

Plotkin, M., & Damousi, J. (2009). *The transnational unconscious: Essays in the history of psychoanalysis and transnationalism.* Palgrave-Macmillan.

Roudinesco, E. (2008). *Jacques Lacan: esboço de uma vida, história de um sistema de pensamento.* Tradução Paulo neves. Companhia das Letras.

Roudinesco, E., & Plon, E. (1998). *Dicionário de Psicanálise. Tradução Vera Ribeiro eLucy Magalhães.* Zahar.

17

Mythification Demand? The Assimilation of the Black Legend of Jacques Lacan in Brazil

Fuad Kyrillos Neto and Rodrigo Afonso Nogueira Santos

Introduction

In 2016, the book *The Black Legend of Jacques Lacan: Élisabeth Roudinesco and Her Historical Method*, by Nathalie Jaudel, was published in Brazil as a criticism of *Jacques Lacan: An Outline of a Life and History of a System of Thought*, by Élisabeth Roudinesco. The text by Jaudel is not a proposal for another biography, but according to the author, Roudinesco has tried writing a history in which she has been a character herself. Therefore, to Jaudel, Roudinesco's negative transference to Lacan carried her away, resulting in a distancing from the teachings and clinical practices of the psychoanalyst.

F. K. Neto (✉)
Universidade Federal de São João Del Rei, São João del-Rei, Brazil
e-mail: fuadneto@uol.com.br

R. A. N. Santos
Universidade de São Paulo, São Paulo, Brazil

B. Mandelbaum et al. (eds.), *Brazilian Psychosocial Histories of Psychoanalysis*, Studies in the Psychosocial,
https://doi.org/10.1007/978-3-030-78509-3_17

Jaudel's (2016) criticisms were authoritative for some analysts, and, consequently, colleagues started to question the relevance of Roudinesco's work. By way of illustration, for example, consider a meeting that occurred between colleagues about ongoing postgraduate studies in psychoanalysis. In the course of this discussion, the colleague advised us to avoid Roudinesco's books and stated that he had also warned his students about them. He mentioned Jaudel's work as a reason for his actions, claiming a lack of conceptual rigour by Roudinesco as Lacan's biographer. The colleague also questioned the seriousness of her work as a psychoanalyst. What caught our attention was that he started to question the credibility of all work published by Roudinesco based on criticism of a single book.

We then became curious about Jaudel's book: noticing that, in Brazil, the publication is part of a collection maintained by the Brazilian School of Psychoanalysis (EBP). Jaudel graduated in Law at Sciences Po Paris. She is also a member of the *École de la Cause Freudienne,* which was founded by Jacques-Alain Miller, Lacan's son-in-law and first president of the World Association of Psychoanalysis (WAP). Reviewing her affiliations, we started questioning: Are we facing yet another rift between psychoanalytic institutions?

For this paper, we intend to examine the criticisms made by Jaudel of Roudinesco's book through the analysis of its methodology and take into consideration dissension within the Brazilian Lacanian field. We hypothesise that the disagreement among psychoanalysts can refer to institutional arrangements—and to their transferential dynamics—rather than being a merely theoretical debate. The causes of such crises are not always significant theoretical divergences among groups, but the emotionality in these tensions shows that there is a component of irrationality here, including the attempt to stain the whole body of work of a psychoanalyst through the criticism of a single book.

From its arrival in Brazil in the 1910s, psychoanalysis has experienced several institutional splits. These rifts have developed among psychoanalysts and have happened alongside local debates, such as the issues of national identity and hygienist policies. Over the course of more than one hundred years of psychoanalysis' history, crises, ruptures and splits, it is evident that issues repeat themselves. In the Lacanian field in Brazil, in 1998 a schism occurred in the EBP that was part of a wider movement, which overtook the WAP, and these events are the subject of this paper.

Was It a Methodological Mistake?

To Jaudel, the work by Roudinesco contains a series of methodological issues that turned her into a kind of paradigm of the black legend that persists about the psychoanalyst, even among all those who diverge from Lacan's views (Jaudel, 2016).

In her criticism of the historical method used in the work about Lacan, the author considers that Roudinesco is excessively captured 'by the memorial process to do the work of a historian, overly historian to apprehend the irreducible uniqueness of her theme, and abusively psychoanalyst to escape from the temptation of posthumous interpretation [of Lacan's thought and life]' (Jaudel, 2016, p. 12).

In Jaudel's conception, the text by Roudinesco neglects what Lacan used to say about himself and about the practice to which he had dedicated a significant part of his life. Roudinesco disregards the axiom that she should not be the historian of the history in which she is included. To Jaudel, the text about Lacan is symptomatic of our modernity, which craves for the triumph of the imaginary.

To support this thesis, Jaudel organises her book in three parts. The first part is entitled 'Judge and part.' She dedicates it to showing Roudinesco's text is nurtured by 'feelings and resentments' (Jaudel, 2016, pp. 21–22), emphasising the difficulties of separation between memory and history in the proposed historical method. According to Jaudel:

> [...] the work by Elisabeth Roudinesco seems paradigmatic of the way it contaminates the history of our days, especially because it inspires itself in being at the service of a particular memory. (Jaudel, 2016, p. 22)

The author raises the tone of her criticism in the part where she demonstrates the blooming of the negative transference: she states that *An Outline of a Life...* is a 'portrait dictated by the negative transference and mistrust, from a great transient thinker to a perpetually evil man' (Jaudel, 2016, p. 75). One of the passages Jaudel uses as an example is an account of a visit by Lacan to a library during his trip to the United States. After one hour of conversation, he left with a bag of books without paying for them. Roudinesco narrates that she had watched the scene—and Jaudel deduces that this 'I watched it' means that she was already keeping an eye on him. To Jaudel, the sentence chosen by Roudinesco—'the expenses were on him [the bookstore clerk]'—gives an 'unpleasant impression produced by the story' (Jaudel, 2016, p. 86).

In the third part, entitled 'Where the arrow misses its target,' Jaudel states the production of 'a fictional other' (2016, p. 145).

> [...] By sustaining sayings from his contemporaries rather than what he has said about himself, she can only capture an image – a reflex of Jacques Lacan in the mirror, deformed by the self of his interlocutors, a shadow of himself: partner and being. (Jaudel, 2016, p. 145)

In the final section, she argues that her discomfort is due to Roudinesco ignoring that Lacan called himself a psychoanalyst. Almost nothing about his practice arouses interest in Roudinesco, except for the duration of sessions, 'the matter of money, and both the transgressions he had allowed himself and the objections made about his technique by some people' (Jaudel, 2016, p. 239).

Is It a Black Legend? Notes About Method in Roudinesco's Work

In this section, we will present methodological elements of Roudinesco's work as the categorical statement that her work would have been 'contaminated' by a negative transference requires a more thorough examination.

In her book *Généalogies*, Roudinesco expatiates on the references that guide her. She considers her investigation an articulation effort between Lacan—the subject—and the thinking system that he had constructed:

> In general, stating that the development of a thought can reflect the life of an author is as fake as denying all the relation between the singularity of an existence and the invention of a conceptualisation. The historian must take into account all the forms of historical experience: subjective experience, history of ideas, social and intellectual history. (Roudinesco, 1994, p. 104)

Such debates direct us to the matter of biographies within the field of history. According to Dosse (2015), there are multiple ways of writing about a life. The author highlights three grand styles in biographies: heroic, modal, and hermeneutic.

Heroic biographies aim to present a panorama of the great existence of the biographed, extolling their characteristics and suppressing controversies at times. Modal biographies give priority to the collective dynamics, rather than narrating the individual experience and they present institutional debates, for example, to 'decentralise interest in the singularity of the recovered path, to visualise it as representative of a broader perspective' (Dosse, 2015, p. 195). Hermeneutic biographies are an effort to place the investigated subject in the context of his time and the character is portrayed as someone traversed by several stories that are simultaneously constituted by him:

> The modern regime of historicity deconstructs the tutelary figures who lend themselves to identification. This deconstruction offers possibilities to plural figures. The biographer can then make the best out of the most common indexes according to lines of multiple intensities. The linearity postulated by classical biography will no longer be considered untouchable. The fact that the man is considered fundamentally plural, maintainer of various bonds, alters the approach of the biographical genre. (Dosse, 2015, p. 297)

We classify the text by Roudinesco as hermeneutic biography as she indicates her efforts to inscribe Lacanian thought in multiple debates that have crossed his life. It is equally remarkable how she seeks to situate the effects of Lacanian thought in several records of French intellectual life, especially those connected to psychoanalysis.

Roudinesco also recognises two impasses that have crossed her work. The first one refers to a question from Jacques Derrida: 'How are you going to tell about the happenings you were part of? Are you going to narrate in the first person?' (Roudinesco, 1994, p. 85).

Roudinesco was aware of the problems associated with writing a history that she was involved in, so she dedicated part of *Généalogies* to presenting her personal relation with Lacan and provided a background of the generation of intellectuals who comprised the trajectory of *A History of Psychoanalysis in France*, including herself. She did not set out to write a story presumably noted from outside, so instead decided to present her own relations with these happenings and recognised her place within this universe.

The second impasse is the absence of written archives. There has been a decimation of the archive, which was supported in part by Lacan himself, who had kept his work essentially oral:

> To retrace the intellectual and private itinerary, in the absence of a 'true' correspondence – 250 letters, only – and without any work notes, I only had fragments of sources scattered in the homes of everyone who knew Lacan in the past, during his childhood, the pre-Lacan Lacan, and whose archives were available. (Roudinesco, 2011, p. 58)

In fact, Lacan's childhood was virtually unknown and the work with sources, something necessary to write about Lacan's life, brought a series of predicaments:

> We do not indeed know almost anything about Lacan's childhood, about this childhood from which I have managed to collect the only possible traces through oral testimonies – from his brother Marc-François, with whom I had a long and unprecedented correspondence to this date; from his sister, whom I had interviewed several times. (Roudinesco, 2011, p. 58)

Thus, Roudinesco does not refuse to present the dilemmas and limits of her endeavour. Furthermore, writing a biography should not assume the exhaustion of the debate. The aim is the presentation of a subject compatible with the sources to which one has access. In these terms, her work configures a possible biography, but never a definitive one.

Where the Arrow Misses the Target... What Does It Strike?

There is an apparent mismatch between what Jaudel expects of a biography and the book by Roudinesco. Jaudel highlights likely inaccuracies in Roudinesco's work, regarding them as effects of a supposed negative transference. In contrast, we consider Lacan's biography as a near impossible one, given the difficulties of working on the life of the psychoanalyst. The inevitable inaccuracies of every biographical work do not point to the presentation of a virtuous nor wicked subject, but instead to the limits of the biographical endeavour.

Regarding this alleged demotion of Lacan, which Jaudel denounces, we cite the words by Catherine Millot in *Life With Lacan*:

> In the private domain, Lacan was a man of absolute simplicity. Not in the sense that we would say of a simple person as a great one of this world who indulged himself in relating to inferior people. He was only strange, in his relationships with others, the complications arising from this dimension of intersubjectivity that we call psychology. [...] His simplicity resided equally in not hesitating to ask what he wanted as directly as possible. (Millot, 2017, p. 36)

Millot writes as someone who got to know Lacan beyond his couch. According to her, the French psychoanalyst presented himself as someone who did not display exuberant personal characteristics—neither excessively good nor astonishingly bad, just alien. However, the tension between Roudinesco's work and Jaudel's reading is real. This may be due to issues arising outside of the strictly theoretical debate.

We ask what target might Roudinesco have struck to receive such harsh criticisms, especially when they fall outside the traditional theoretical or historiographic debates. In an interview, Roudinesco presents one of the reasons for writing a history of Lacan's life and work:

> Lacan's heirs, even if they differ within Lacanianism, misread it. They mythicise it. [...] The Lacan of the Lacanians shows up transfigured. He fits a soap opera: a good father and someone who loves his grandchildren. It is grave. I believe in renewal, but I fear the erudite Lacan is a victim of the Manichaeism of his followers. [...] *The worship of Lacan is characteristic of all religious organisations.* (Roudinesco, 1998, pp. 24–25, emphasis added)

To historicise Lacanian thought, one of the features Roudinesco targets is the mythology of the figure of Lacan. She places him as a subject who is crossed by impasses and passions, ascensions and declines. Myths are images capable of invoking all the feelings that, through the idealism provided by them, bring people together for a cause (Shore, 1996). Hence, by targeting the myth of Lacan, Roudinesco's text would also have a direct impact on those who cluster around this figure as a cause.

According to Roudinesco, Jacques-Alain Miller—Lacan's son-in-law—stands out among those who support such mythification. She referred to him several times as a 'party chief,' because of how he conducts the WAP (Roudinesco, 1998). In fact, the disagreements between Miller and Roudinesco are recurrent and have incurred litigation more than once. Would she have struck that target?

We believe there is a clue to resolve this question in Jaudel's institutional connection because she is also linked to the WAP, and Miller is her primary reference. Jaudel even announces Roudinesco's work as a failure because of the 'aporias of the biographical enterprise by itself when it lacks the *compass* that allows one to orient oneself in the labyrinth of an existence' (Jaudel, 2016, p. 10, emphasis added). The significant '*compass*' is present in several parts of Jaudel's text where she ultimately offers us the key, which would be the north, for the *Orientation* of her reading: 'Without the compass provided by Jacques-Alain Miller's Lacanian Orientation Course, this book would not have been born' (Jaudel, 2016, p. 269). When assuming Miller as her compass, Jaudel identifies the beacons that guide her hypothesis. This is a well-explored dynamic by Lacanian psychoanalysis regarding transference as a love directed to knowledge. The analysand places the analyst as the subject supposed to know, who knows a consistent knowledge, a knowledge that knows; but at this point, a paradox develops: from the point of view of the analyst, the knowledge does not know. The analyst must conduct the analysis keeping in mind that not knowing as truth, recognising the inconsistency of his knowledge (Lacan, 1951/1988). Thus, the game of transference should not remain on the Imaginary. The analyst might adopt a tactic that allows him to act more freely and not to risk running into the game with his own being. This strategy is the use of the word, that is, the Symbolic, because 'he would be better advised to take his bearings from his lack of being (manque à etre) rather than from his being' (Lacan 1958/1998, p. 596).

It is worth noticing, 'transference is not a phenomenon that exists only in analytical situations, it exists everywhere where there is power and identification' (Safatle, 2017, p. 213). Roustang (1987) points to the impasses that can derive from the relationship between transference and institution, especially when what is at stake is the figure of the leader. According to him, this can produce effects of infatuation and servitude, depending on the uses of transference in the groupings of psychoanalysts. When Jaudel defines Miller as a *compass*, she attunes herself not to the foundations of a teaching—that of Lacan's—but to the figure of a subject who guides and, above all, knows.

As follows, the institutional and transferential dimensions of the debate do not seem innocuous. It looks like Roudinesco, from the point of view of her detractors, might have threatened the myth of Lacan—which is necessary for those who consider themselves as direct heirs. More than a conceptual debate, there is a transference issue with the master and it reveals itself within the significant oscillations between a myth and a renovating intellectual. Jaudel's reading of Roudinesco's book allows us to question the modalities of transference between peers in psychoanalytic institutions.

Next, we reflect on the peculiarities of the transference with the master in Brazilian institutional settings to map some of the conditions of the reception of the *Black Legend*.

A Brazilian Target? On the 1998 Schism

During the Brazilian military dictatorship, psychoanalysis was disapproved of by sections of society. The defence of the psychoanalyst's neutrality towards the patient, the formal primacy of the contract and the moral and political asepsis of treatment represent sensitive points to many critics, who also claim that the psychoanalyst is a professional who adapts the subject to the current rules (Coimbra, 1995).

The first association of Lacanian psychoanalysts in Brazil dates back to 1975 and coincides with the beginning of efforts to reframe the years of lead and the novel Brazilian institutional arrangements by part of the society, which intensified after the promulgation of the Federal Constitution in 1988.

The affiliation among Lacanians is contemporary to the New Cinema and the *Tropicalia* movements, wherein the alliance is a proposal of an association to establish new social bonds. According to the Lacanian maxim: 'the analyst authorises himself' (Lacan, 1967/2003).[1]

Several institutional efforts marked the first twenty years of the Lacanian movement in Brazil, which was inspired by varied readings of Lacan's work. After years of considerable fragmentation, there was a concerted attempt to articulate different Brazilian Lacanian strands in the 1990s. In March 1995, Miller signed a letter of congratulation on the creation of the Brazilian School of Psychoanalysis. Recalling the route to it, he stated that 'a lot of time was spent in subordinated dissensions. An appeal to the French was made while fearing imperialism' (Miller, 1995). In another passage, he makes an appeal for the acceptance of the 'One of the School in Brazil': 'The One of the School is fragile, and anything that reinforces it will be welcome with one condition – that the Multiple will accept it willingly' (Miller, 1995). This is an attempt to unite Brazilian Lacanians in a School directed by Miller, however, the functioning of the School quickly illustrated many of the issues that would form an institutional crisis.

[1] 'Here, in a proposal to mitigate phallicisation within psychoanalytic institutions, the School would not carry out the function of authorising an analyst. It would rather recognise and ensure those who graduate in it, stating one's practice as an analyst' (Lacan, 1967/2003).

In 1998, the EBP split. Observations made are taken from the compilation of documents about this movement entitled *A Cisão de 1998* ('The 1998 Split'). This was not an isolated occurrence and led to the parting of about a third of EBP members and adherents and was part of a broader movement that infected the WAP—under Miller's direction—which brought together schools in Spain, France, Belgium, Venezuela, Colombia, Chile, Peru and Argentina. This crisis happened because of the tension between the peculiarities of the functioning of the Schools and the organisation of the WAP that encompassed them (Ribeiro, 1998).

The concentration of power in the leadership was responsible for triggering the statutory crisis in the Rio de Janeiro section, which involved the whole EBP. The general delegate of the WAP performed an external intervention in this section by appointing a secretary to take part in a reunion, convened by the WAP, with members of the Rio section. This secretary would work as mediator and moderator, as well as someone who was able to intervene in the meeting (Quinet, 1998).

This generated a series of events, leading to a crisis in the Rio section, which triggered the split. A seminar by Antônio Quinet in Belo Horizonte was cited as competition against the activities of the Minas Gerais section. Even though Quinet had stated that the EBP board approved his lecture, rumours spread that his activity happened regardless of the will of the Minas Gerais section.

A 'mistake' on the folders printed for the Colette Soler visit to Rio de Janeiro was responsible for another nuisance in the WAP. Instead of 'EBP-Rio,' the folders announced it as a (national) EBP event: Miller subsequently accused the Rio section of wanting to compete against the national meeting that would take part in Salvador. The section board, then, wrote a note to acknowledge the misunderstanding.

Miller also disagreed with the publication of Soler's book, which was composed as a result of the seminars she taught in Rio. Miller claimed that the book was a repetition of his own work, *Lacan elucidado* ('Elucidated Lacan'), and that Soler had inserted a few texts to make her book look longer than his (Quinet, 1998).

It is also worth noticing that Miller's leadership faced resistance in the hub formed by Rio, Toulouse and Madrid. The proposition of *Jumelage*—in English, the word means 'twinning,' referring to the creation of twin cities to exchange experiences in psychoanalysis—created more tensions. Quinet went to Toulouse as Rio's twin and taught in conferences there. Judith Miller—Lacan's daughter, who was married to Jacques-Alain Miller—intervened in the arrangement and called it inappropriate. She claimed the idea was to do as in Cuba, taking medicines to and helping people from the Third World (Ribeiro, 2018).

During the International WAP Congress in Barcelona, a series of letters from EBP members and correspondents seeking to leave the organisation arrived. Those letters put the WAP general delegate (Miller) at the centre of divergences as they indicated issues with Miller's authoritarianism, his predilection for conflicts—many of them without basis, such as the accusation of plagiarism against Colette Soler, disrespect towards the Statutes, and his pretension to reduce the reading of Lacan's work to his own interpretation.

The 1998 schism produced several effects, one of which was the foundation of the Lacanian Field Forums that were 'born from an opposition to the misuse of the One in psychoanalysis, after the 1998 crisis, aiming at an institutional alternative guided by the teachings of Sigmund Freud and Jacques Lacan' (EPFCL, 2018). This was a significant rupture in the already fragmented Lacanian psychoanalysis.

In the following section, we intend to present elements of the history of psychoanalysis in Minas Gerais by contextualising the rejection of Roudinesco's work by certain analysts in the Brazilian state.

A Case from Minas Gerais: The Imaginary Dimension of Transference as Authoritarianism

The psychoanalytic movement in Minas Gerais retains a unique organisation. A priest and psychoanalyst named Malomar Lund Edelweiss founded the first institution of psychoanalysis in the state in 1963. This institution, under the name of the Brazilian Circle of Depth Psychology-Minas Gerais Section, was initially linked to the thought of Igor Caruso and changed its name to the Psychoanalytic Circle of Minas Gerais (CPMG) in the 1960s.

By the end of the 1970s, a group of dissidents from the CPMG formed the Mineiro College of Psychoanalysis. This was the first institution to open itself up to the ideas of Lacan through the psychoanalyst Célio Garcia. As a place for studying and training psychoanalysts, this was the seeding for the latter EBP. According to Arlindo Pimenta (2013), the Mineiro College provided a path for Lacan's ideas to take shape through the formation of the Group of Studies Freud-Lacan (GEFLA). The GEFLA evolved into 'the Symposium, Matheme and later to the Brazilian School of Jacques-Alain Miller' (Pimenta, 2013, p. 37).

The International Psychoanalytical Association (IPA) only acknowledged the Psychoanalytic Society of Minas Gerais in 2015. The delayed implementation of an institution linked to the IPA made it possible for Lacanian groups to gain strength without proper opposition from another strand of psychoanalysis. We acknowledge that until the 1970s, the institutions linked to the IPA were centres of graduation for a self-proclaimed legitimate/true psychoanalysis (Coimbra, 1995). Hence, the absence of such a centre in Minas Gerais led to a consolidation of Lacanian studies in the state without many obstacles. Therefore, the EBP-Minas Gerais Section was able to establish itself without challenge since its foundation in 1995, as a peerless force. Even consolidated institutions were not capable of sustaining a counterpoint to the EBP but according to Arlindo Pimenta,[2] regarding the CPMG, Lacan's teachings were only accessible to those who agreed to submit to 'Mr. Miller's epistemic tyranny' (Pimenta, 2013, p. 37), whose policy led members of his School to occupy university and public service seats. In this sense, students would necessarily have to go through Miller's ideals to become formal psychoanalysts. Within this policy of unilateralism, CPMG was considered 'a place of criticism and devaluation [...]. Our concern, then,

[2] Arlindo Pimenta is an important psychoanalyst from Minas Gerais and one of the leading characters in the history of CPMG.

was how to gain access to Lacan's teaching without having to pay taxes to Mr. Miller' (Pimenta, 2013, p. 37).

In this context, it seems that the 1998 spin-off did not have as many marked effects as it did in other Brazilian states, like Rio de Janeiro and São Paulo. On the contrary, EBP-MG grew considerably in the following years. This can be attested to by the inauguration of the Institute of Psychoanalysis and Mental Health of Minas Gerais, linked to EBP-MG, in 1998. The Institute of Psychoanalysis became an important place for studies and diffusion of psychoanalysis in the state.

However, twenty-one years after the schism, important ruptures and complaints of authoritarianism were still felt in the institution. According to Francisco Paes Barreto,[3] one of the pioneers of Lacanian psychoanalysis in Minas Gerais, the EBP has a 'vertical, totalitarian, conformist, discriminatory policy, in which the imaginary effects prevail, with a fierce power struggle, not without marked obscenity' (Barreto, 2019). Barreto states that the behaviour of EBP's membership is similar to that of 'a battalion or a *cult*, and not an open and diverse set. The dissenting point of view is not accepted, it is never handled as a contribution, but as a deviation from the proper *orientation*, or even as a sign of enmity' (Barreto, 2019, emphasis added).

There seems to be a reason for the vertical policy in the EBP-MG, which borders on authoritarianism, in the interpretation of what should be Jacques-Alain Miller's role. This, according to Barreto (2019), led to a totalitarian approach:

> In the early days, there was an inevitable junction between Lacanian orientation and the character Jacques-Alain Miller. There was no way to separate them. These were the heroic times of a movement. It also happened with Freud and Lacan. However, for a long time, the disjunction became not only possible but also necessary. Yes: it is necessary to make the separation between the figure of the leader and the Lacanian orientation, as a step to neglect group policy and privilege the policy of

[3] Barreto is the founder and president of the Mineiro College of Psychoanalysis, analyst and member of the Brazilian School of Psychoanalysis (EBP) and of the World Association of Psychoanalysis (WAP), and General Director of the Institute of Psychoanalysis and Mental Health of Minas Gerais from 1998 to 2001. He was preceptor of the Psychiatry Residency at the Galba Velloso Hospital and at the Raul Soares Institute for twenty years.

> the non-whole. This operation has another obvious reason to happen: the character Jacques-Alain Miller is not eternal. In the policy of the Brazilian School of Psychoanalysis, however, it seems that the imaginary link with Miller prevailed over the epistemic link. (Barreto, 2019)

There are similarities between Barreto's critics and the ones that marked the 1998 spin-off. These resemblances exist both in relation to the dynamics of the institution's functioning and to the role played by Miller in the effort to sustain the place of One in the School. The effect of this position of claiming the One is unequivocal:

> To claim the One of the exception to sustain the School is trying to make the institutional power function exclusively to guarantee the monopoly of psychoanalysis on the part of One. Thus, it does not seem difficult to conclude that reducing Lacan's statement to the reading of One is irrevocably the second death of Jacques Lacan. (Teixeira, 1998, p. 187)

Therefore, it looks like that the reference to Miller as the supposed holder of the accurate reading of Lacan continues having extensive effects of transference and institutional consequences.

Despite all his criticism, Barreto considers himself a Millerian, stating he is situated, 'according to a formula I heard in Paris, in the "field opened by Freud, radicalised by Lacan and elucidated by Miller." I do not see myself, however, as Lacanian. I see myself as Millerian' (Barreto, 2019). He directs his critiques to the place that Miller occupies as the alleged One of the School, instead of directing it to the orientation of Lacan's teaching. However, he still calls attention to the signifier 'Millerian': of the various readers and commentators on Lacan's work, Miller seems to be the only one who owns such a characterisation by name. What does it suggest? Are we talking about an imaginary link to Lacan's heir as a guarantee of the purity of psychoanalysis?

At this point, we refer to the debate about the relation between transference and institution. As Barreto suggests, being a Millerian requires agreement with the reading of Lacan as interpreted by Miller. Recalling Jaudel's words, admitting to being a Millerian means to turn Miller into a *compass* or as *north*. Transforming an author into the only authorised reader of Lacan, of course, bears its consequences. It appears to be an act of faith rather than an epistemic link. According to a statement attributed to Laurent during a WAP council seminar, there was a 'crisis of trust' in the institution. 'I'm from a generation that has believed in Jacques-Alain Miller since 1966' (Izcovich, 1998).

To rely on Lacan's teaching is not the same as to admit the status of belief in an heir of Lacan. As Roudinesco and Barreto point out, such belief places psychoanalysis closer to religious organisations. This paves a way for the exclusion of difference, of the unmatched, of the odd: 'the heirs of Lacan, the analytical community that wants to continue with its School, want to constitute a community of peers' (Ribeiro, 2000, p. 88).

Accordingly, if Colette Soler was expelled from the group of authors appointed by EBP at the time of the schism, Roudinesco might also have become another *persona non grata*. This situation was consolidated with the publication of *The Black Legend of Lacan*. Her text, aiming to strike at the myth of Lacan, seems to have equally struck those who pose themselves as direct and authorised heirs of his teachings.

Thus, we support the hypothesis that the reception of the *Black Legend* among certain psychoanalysts from Minas Gerais—especially the Millerians—reignites an old debate about which authors must be authorised and which ones should be banned from the Lacanian circle. According to Ribeiro (2018), who disconnected himself from the EBP in the 1998 spin-off, the schism represented a relief. In a new democratic climate, psychoanalysts could finally write a paper 'without having to quote Jacques-Alain Miller' (Ribeiro, 2018, p. 148). From these deductions, we are able to consider some motivations for the swoop among psychoanalysts. This happens in the context of emergence of the mastery discourse of several Lacanian analysts.

Final Considerations

In this paper, we have discussed the exclusion of Élisabeth Roudinesco from the list of supported authors by certain analysts in Minas Gerais: but her case is not an isolated one, as this also happened to Colette Soler. During the schism in 1998, Soler's name was excluded from the list of authors authorised by the EBP.

We should also take into account that psychoanalysis in Minas Gerais faced several problems regarding the training of analysts and the formal acknowledgement of an official institution. Because of the lag in obtaining support from the IPA, the psychoanalysts from Minas Gerais got official status from WAP that had already existed in other places of Brazil, coming from Lacan's heir. However, the assumption of an official—or true—psychoanalysis does not necessarily provide good results, as Coimbra (1995) shows.

In the Statute of the EBP, the institution asserts its aim to promote the development of psychoanalysis in Brazil and, by following the path started by Jacques Lacan, 'to contribute to restore *the truth of psychoanalysis*, to transmit his knowledge, to offer it to scientific control and debate, and to found, consequently, the qualification of the psychoanalyst' (EBP, 2019, emphasis added).

In that manner, the effects of the publication of *The Black Legend* in Minas Gerais seem to mark rather an episode of transference with the figure of Jacques-Alain Miller and not a strictly conceptual debate. These networks of transference oriented towards the leader of the institution, end up slipping into the phantom of purity or legitimate psychoanalysis. This phantom has accompanied psychoanalysis in Brazil since its first institutional steps. The assumption of a true or legitimate psychoanalysis is precisely from where the outcasts emerge—those who do not seek their north with the correct *compass*.

As in the 1998 spin-off, the proscription of Roudinesco in the mid-2010s, the management of transference from the alleged One in psychoanalysis happened through imposition. This stance, however, disregards the basic principles of the clinical activity itself and the effects can be the most harmful ones. According to Lacan himself, 'the inability to sustain a praxis in an authentic manner, falls back, as is usually the case in man's history, on the exercise of power' (Lacan, 1958/1998, p. 592).

Among all the effects, we must note there is a place for a certain belief in Miller, which is present in the discourse of some analysts. This points to another problem in relation to the fundamentals of psychoanalysis: 'Spiritual direction, in the sense of the moral guidance that a Catholic might find in it, is radically excluded here' (Lacan, 1958/1998, p. 592). In this sense, it is curious that both Roudinesco and Barreto compare the functioning of WAP—and EBP—to religious groups, regarding the belief in an unquestionable leader.

We agree with Safatle (2017) that there is a double movement in which the transference allows an instability of power relations to circulate. The transference is equally made and unmade of this instability:

> To comprehend the transference is to understand how it is done and undone, it is to comprehend how its liquidation is the opening of the subject to what we could call power relations without domination. This is a central political issue for Lacan, namely, *politics requires institutions in which the settlement of the transference can be recognised*. (Safatle, 2017, pp. 212–213)

To us, it genuinely seems that Roudinesco hit the target of the myth of Lacan. This has had an effect on those who arrange themselves around Lacan's rightful heir and the School of Psychoanalysis he runs. The signifier *Millerian* is an evidence of this stability of transference. This comes from the search for an orientation, for a psychoanalysis that could be recognised as legitimate.

The proscription of Roudinesco among psychoanalysts from Minas Gerais points to critical elements of the history of psychoanalysis in the Brazilian state. Therefore, we conclude this is only an episode in a complex debate and not its end.

References

Barreto, F.P. (2019). *A política da Escola Brasileira de Psicanálise em questão*, viewed 26 April 2020. http://www.franciscopaesbarreto.com/a-politica-da-escola-brasileira-de-psicanalise-em-questao/.

Coimbra, C. (1995). *Guardiães da ordem: Uma viagem pelas práticas psi no Brasil do 'milagre.'* Oficina do Autor.

Dosse, F (2015) *O Desafio Biográfico: Escrever uma Vida.* São Paulo: Edusp,.

EBP—Escola Brasileira de Psicanálise. (2019). *Quarta alteração do Estatuto da Escola Brasileira de Psicanálise – Escola do Campo Freudiano*, viewed 19

September 2020. https://www.ebp.org.br/wp-content/uploads/2020/05/Estatuto_da_EBP-.pdf.
EPFCL—Escola de Psicanálise dos Fóruns do Campo Lacaniano. (2018). *Carta de Princípios*, viewed 10 October 2020. https://www.campolacaniano.com.br/apresentao-c1rj3.
Izcovich, L. (1998). Carta a Eric Laurent. In M. A. C. Ribeiro (org.), *A cisão de 1998* (pp.143–146). Marca d'Água.
Jaudel, N. (2016). *A lenda negra de Jacques Lacan: Élisabeth Roudinesco e o seu método histórico*. Contracapa.
Kehl, M. R. (2010). Tortura e sintoma social. In E. Teles & V. Safatle (Eds.), *O que resta da ditadura: a exceção brasileira*. (pp.123–132). Boitempo.
Kupermann, D. (1996). *Transferências cruzadas: Uma história da psicanálise e suas instituições*. Editora Revan.
Lacan, J. (1967/2003). Sobre o psicanalista da Escola. In *Outros escritos* (pp. 249–264). Jorge Zahar.
Lacan, J. (1951/1998). Intervenção sobre a transferência. In *Escritos* (pp. 214–225). Jorge Zahar.
Lacan, J. (1958/1998). A direção do tratamento e os princípios de seu poder. In *Escritos* (pp. 591–652). Jorge Zahar.
Miller, J. A. (1995). *Carta de Jacques-Alain Miller à Escola Brasileira de Psicanálise*, viewed 4 October 2020. https://www.ebp.org.br/wp-content/uploads/2020/02/22Carta-de-Jacques-Alain-Miller-a%CC%80-Escola-Brasileira-de-Psicana%CC%81lise22-Jacques-Alain-Miller.pdf.
Millot, C. (2017). *A vida com Lacan*. Zahar.
Pimenta, A. C. (2013). Da dilemática à dialética. *Reverso, 35*(66), 33–40.
Quinet, A. (1998). Pacto, que pacto? In M. A. C. Ribeiro (org.), *A cisão de 1998* (pp 123–133). Marca d'Água.
Ribeiro, M. A. C. (2018). 20 anos de Escola. *Revista De Psicanálise Stylus, N., 36*, 139–146.
Ribeiro, M. A. C. (2000). A cisão de 1998. *Pulsional, Revista de Psicanálise*, 137, 83–89.
Ribeiro, M. A. C. (Ed.). (1998). *A cisão de 1998*. Marca d'Água Livraria e Editora.
Roudinesco, E. (1994). *Jacques Lacan: Esboço de uma vida, história de um sistema de pensamento*, Companhia das Letras.
Roudinesco, E. (1998). Lacan anjo e demônio. In J. M. Silva, *Visões de uma certa Europa*. EDIPUCRS.
Roudinesco, E. (2006). *A análise e o arquivo*. Jorge Zahar.
Roudinesco, E. (2011). *Lacan, a despeito de tudo e todos*. Jorge Zahar.

Roustang, F. (1987). *Um destino tão funesto*. Livraria Timbre Taurus.

Safatle, V. (2017). Lacan, revolução e liquidação da transferência: A destituição subjetiva como protocolo de emancipação política. *Estudos Avançados, 31*(91), 211–227.

Shore, C. (1996). Mito. *Dicionário do pensamento social do Século XX* (pp. 469–470). Jorge Zahar Editores.

Teixeira, M. A. (1998). Carta a Jacques-Alain Miller. In M. A. C. Ribeiro (org.), *A cisão de 1998.* (pp. 185–187). Marca d'Água.

Index

B. Mandelbaum et al. (eds.), *Brazilian Psychosocial Histories of Psychoanalysis*, Studies in the Psychosocial,
https://doi.org/10.1007/978-3-030-78509-3

The manufacturer's authorised representative in the EU is Springer Nature Customer Service Centre GmbH, Europaplatz 3, 69115 Heidelberg, Germany. If you have any concerns regarding our products, please contact ProductSafety@springernature.com

Printed and bound by CPI Group (UK) Ltd, Croydon, CR0 4YY
22/09/2026
02221066-0015